Ophthalmic Optics and Visual Function

Ophthalmic Optics and Visual Function

Editor

Kazuno Negishi

MDPI • Basel • Beijing • Wuhan • Barcelona • Belgrade • Manchester • Tokyo • Cluj • Tianjin

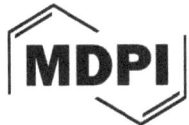

Editor
Kazuno Negishi
Keio University School of Medicine
Japan

Editorial Office
MDPI
St. Alban-Anlage 66
4052 Basel, Switzerland

This is a reprint of articles from the Special Issue published online in the open access journal *Journal of Clinical Medicine* (ISSN 2077-0383) (available at: https://www.mdpi.com/journal/jcm/special_issues/visual_function).

For citation purposes, cite each article independently as indicated on the article page online and as indicated below:

LastName, A.A.; LastName, B.B.; LastName, C.C. Article Title. *Journal Name* **Year**, *Volume Number*, Page Range.

ISBN 978-3-0365-4475-5 (Hbk)
ISBN 978-3-0365-4476-2 (PDF)

© 2022 by the authors. Articles in this book are Open Access and distributed under the Creative Commons Attribution (CC BY) license, which allows users to download, copy and build upon published articles, as long as the author and publisher are properly credited, which ensures maximum dissemination and a wider impact of our publications.

The book as a whole is distributed by MDPI under the terms and conditions of the Creative Commons license CC BY-NC-ND.

Contents

About the Editor vii

Kazuno Negishi
Special Issue on Ophthalmic Optics and Visual Function
Reprinted from: *J. Clin. Med.* **2022**, *11*, 2966, doi:10.3390/jcm 11112966 1

Kiwako Mori, Hidemasa Torii, Yutaka Hara, Michiko Hara, Erisa Yotsukura, Akiko Hanyuda, Kazuno Negishi, Toshihide Kurihara and Kazuo Tsubota
Effect of Violet Light-Transmitting Eyeglasses on Axial Elongation in Myopic Children: A Randomized Controlled Trial
Reprinted from: *J. Clin. Med.* **2021**, *10*, 5462, doi:10.3390/jcm10225462 5

Tadahiro Mitsukawa, Yumi Suzuki, Yosuke Momota, Shun Suzuki and Masakazu Yamada
Effects of 0.01% Atropine Instillation Assessed Using Swept-Source Anterior Segment Optical Coherence Tomography
Reprinted from: *J. Clin. Med.* **2021**, *10*, 4384, doi:10.3390/jcm10194384 21

Satoshi Ishiko, Hiroyuki Kagokawa, Noriko Nishikawa, Youngseok Song, Kazuhiro Sugawara, Hiroaki Nakagawa, Yuichiro Kawamura and Akitoshi Yoshida
Impact of the Pressure-Free Yutori Education Program on Myopia in Japan
Reprinted from: *J. Clin. Med.* **2021**, *10*, 4229, doi:10.3390/jcm10184229 31

Yukari Tsuneyoshi, Sachiko Masui, Hiroyuki Arai, Ikuko Toda, Miyuki Kubota, Shunsuke Kubota, Kazuo Tsubota, Masahiko Ayaki and Kazuno Negishi
Determination of the Standard Visual Criterion for Diagnosing and Treating Presbyopia According to Subjective Patient Symptoms
Reprinted from: *J. Clin. Med.* **2021**, *10*, 3942, doi:10.3390/jcm10173942 41

Miki Kamikawatoko Omoto, Hidemasa Torii, Sachiko Masui, Masahiko Ayaki, Ikuko Toda, Hiroyuki Arai, Tomoaki Nakamura, Kazuo Tsubota and Kazuno Negishi
Short-Term Efficacy and Safety of Cataract Surgery Combined with Iris-Fixated Phakic Intraocular Lens Explantation: A Multicentre Study
Reprinted from: *J. Clin. Med.* **2021**, *10*, 3672, doi:10.3390/jcm10163672 51

Eun Young Choi, Raymond C. S. Wong, Thuzar Thein, Louis R. Pasquale, Lucy Q. Shen, Mengyu Wang, Dian Li, Qingying Jin, Hui Wang, Neda Baniasadi, Michael V. Boland, Siamak Yousefi, Sarah R. Wellik, Carlos G. De Moraes, Jonathan S. Myers, Peter J. Bex and Tobias Elze
The Effect of Ametropia on Glaucomatous Visual Field Loss
Reprinted from: *J. Clin. Med.* **2021**, *10*, 2796, doi:10.3390/jcm10132796 61

Bojan Pajic, Horace Massa, Philipp B. Baenninger, Erika Eskina, Brigitte Pajic-Eggspuehler, Mirko Resan and Zeljka Cvejic
Multifocal Femto-PresbyLASIK in Pseudophakic Eyes
Reprinted from: *J. Clin. Med.* **2021**, *10*, 2282, doi:10.3390/jcm10112282 77

Adeline Yang, Si Ying Lim, Yee Ling Wong, Anna Yeo, Narayanan Rajeev and Björn Drobe
Quality of Life in Presbyopes with Low and High Myopia Using Single-Vision and Progressive-Lens Correction
Reprinted from: *J. Clin. Med.* **2021**, *10*, 1589, doi:10.3390/jcm10081589 91

Kazutaka Kamiya, Fusako Fujimura, Takushi Kawamorita, Wakako Ando, Yoshihiko Iida and Nobuyuki Shoji
Factors Influencing Contrast Sensitivity Function in Eyes with Mild Cataract
Reprinted from: *J. Clin. Med.* **2021**, *10*, 1506, doi:10.3390/jcm10071506 . . . . **101**

Erisa Yotsukura, Hidemasa Torii, Hiroko Ozawa, Richard Yudi Hida, Tetsuro Shiraishi, Ivan Corso Teixeira, Yessa Vervloet Bertollo Lamego Rautha, Caio Felipe Moraes do Nascimento, Kiwako Mori, Miki Uchino, Toshihide Kurihara, Kazuno Negishi and Kazuo Tsubota
Axial Length and Prevalence of Myopia among Schoolchildren in the Equatorial Region of Brazil
Reprinted from: *J. Clin. Med.* **2021**, *10*, 115, doi:10.3390/jcm10010115 . . . . **109**

Kazuno Negishi, Ikuko Toda, Masahiko Ayaki, Hidemasa Torii and Kazuo Tsubota
Subjective Happiness and Satisfaction in Postoperative Anisometropic Patients after Refractive Surgery for Myopia
Reprinted from: *J. Clin. Med.* **2020**, *9*, 3473, doi:10.3390/jcm9113473 . . . . **121**

Alberto Domínguez-Vicent, Loujain Al-Soboh, Rune Brautaset and Abinaya Priya Venkataraman
Effect of Instrument Design and Technique on the Precision and Accuracy of Objective Refraction Measurement
Reprinted from: *J. Clin. Med.* **2020**, *9*, 3061, doi:10.3390/jcm9103061 . . . . **133**

Sujin Hoshi, Kuniharu Tasaki, Takahiro Hiraoka and Tetsuro Oshika
Improvement in Contrast Sensitivity Function after Lacrimal Passage Intubation in Eyes with Epiphora
Reprinted from: *J. Clin. Med.* **2020**, *9*, 2761, doi:10.3390/jcm9092761 . . . . **143**

Miyuki Kubota, Shunsuke Kubota, Hidenaga Kobashi, Masahiko Ayaki, Kazuno Negishi and Kazuo Tsubota
Difference in Pupillary Diameter as an Important Factor for Evaluating Amplitude of Accommodation: A Prospective Observational Study
Reprinted from: *J. Clin. Med.* **2020**, *9*, 2678, doi:10.3390/jcm9082678 . . . . **151**

Arne Ohlendorf, Alexander Leube and Siegfried Wahl
Advancing Digital Workflows for Refractive Error Measurements
Reprinted from: *J. Clin. Med.* **2020**, *9*, 2205, doi:10.3390/jcm9072205 . . . . **161**

Hou-Ren Tsai, Tai-Li Chen, Jen-Hung Wang, Huei-Kai Huang and Cheng-Jen Chiu
Is 0.01% Atropine an Effective and Safe Treatment for Myopic Children? A Systemic Review and Meta-Analysis
Reprinted from: *J. Clin. Med.* **2021**, *10*, 3766, doi:10.3390/jcm10173766 . . . . **173**

About the Editor

Kazuno Negishi

Kazuno Negishi is a professor and chair of the Department of Ophthalmology, Keio University School of Medicine, Tokyo, Japan. She specializes in cataract and refractive surgery, and her research interests include ophthalmic optics, visual function, myopia control, and presbyopia. Dr. Negishi serves as the president of the Japanese presbyopia society, executive vice president of the Japanese Society of Ophthalmic Optics, and chief editor of the anterior segment section in the Japanese Journal of Ophthalmology.

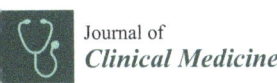

Editorial

Special Issue on Ophthalmic Optics and Visual Function

Kazuno Negishi

Department of Ophthalmology, Keio University School of Medicine, 35, Shinanomachi, Shinjuku-ku, Tokyo 160-8582, Japan; kazunonegishi@keio.jp

Exploring quality of vision is one of the most important issues in modern ophthalmology, and research into ophthalmic optics and visual function is essential for making progress in this field. Several factors affect quality of vision, and among them, refractive error/aberrations [1,2], accommodation [3], and tear film [4] are major.

People's lifestyles have changed dramatically in recent decades, and a variety of digital devices, including personal computers and gadgets, are used extensively in daily life for social and professional purposes across all age groups. These changes have resulted in a range of ocular and visual symptoms [5].

Uncorrected/under-corrected refractive errors, aberrations, and presbyopia accelerate the multifaceted symptoms of the so-called digital computer syndrome, including eye strain, asthenopia, and other symptoms [5,6]. Dry eye may also accelerate the symptoms, because the tear film plays an important role as the first refractive ocular component, and the alterations in the tear film dynamics may cause vision-related and ocular surface-related symptoms [4].

The recent lifestyle change may also contribute to the increased prevalence of myopia because environmental factors are considered to be important for myopia progression [7–9].

This Special Issue of *JCM* on "Ophthalmic Optics and Visual Function" is a collection of articles that highlight innovative findings with the potential of enhancing diagnosis and monitoring ophthalmic conditions and treatments, especially of the anterior segment.

The issue includes 16 manuscripts: two original papers on refraction measurement, four on presbyopia diagnosis and treatment, two on myopia treatment, four on other topics, and one review paper and three original papers on myopia control.

Regarding presbyopia, Yang et al. evaluated the impact of myopia severity and the type of visual correction in presbyopia on vision-related quality of life (QOL) and reported that highly myopic presbyopes had a worse overall QOL and functionality, both with and without glasses, compared to presbyopes with low myopia, although progressive addition lens users had a better perception outcome than single-vision distance lens users in both groups [10]. Kubota et al. investigated the factors that cause presbyopia other than advanced age and reported that age and the difference between the maximal and minimal pupillary diameters were both significantly and independently related to accommodation amplitude and age under 44 years but not age 45 years and older [11]. Tsuneyoshi et al. reported that patients became aware of presbyopia in their late forties, although some had difficulty with near-vision-related tasks before becoming aware of presbyopia [12]. These studies suggest that proper intervention for presbyopia may improve the quality of vision and vision-related QOL.

Yotsukura et al. reported the prevalence of myopia in equatorial Brazil and suggested that the light environment, in addition to other confounding factors, affects the axial length and refractive errors [13]. Ishiko et al. reported the effect of educational pressure on myopia progression and reported that the progression rates and increased prevalence of high myopia were observed only during high-pressure education [14]. Tsai et al., who conducted a systematic review and meta-analysis with the latest evidence on the efficacy and safety of 0.01% atropine in myopic children, concluded that the drug had favorable

Citation: Negishi, K. Special Issue on Ophthalmic Optics and Visual Function. *J. Clin. Med.* **2022**, *11*, 2966. https://doi.org/10.3390/jcm11112966

Received: 23 May 2022
Accepted: 23 May 2022
Published: 24 May 2022

Publisher's Note: MDPI stays neutral with regard to jurisdictional claims in published maps and institutional affiliations.

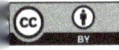

Copyright: © 2022 by the author. Licensee MDPI, Basel, Switzerland. This article is an open access article distributed under the terms and conditions of the Creative Commons Attribution (CC BY) license (https://creativecommons.org/licenses/by/4.0/).

efficacy and adequate safety for childhood myopia over a 1-year period [15]. Mori et al. conducted a randomized controlled trial on the effect of violet light-transmitting eyeglasses on axial elongation in myopic children and reported that the mean change in axial length in the violet light glasses group was significantly smaller than in the placebo glasses group when the time spent performing near work was less than 180 min and when the subjects were limited to those who had never used eyeglasses before this trial [16].

These reports support the relationship between environmental factors and myopia progression as previously reported and added new findings.

Other studies in this Special Issue are on the visual function related to cataract [17] and lacrimal passage intubation [18], clinical results and QOL related to surgeries [19–21], refractive measurement [22,23], and others [24,25].

As Guest Editor, I thank the reviewers for their professional comments and the JCM Editorial Office for their robust support. I believe the readers of this Special Issue will find the articles very useful.

Funding: This research received no external funding.

Conflicts of Interest: The author declares no conflict of interest.

References

1. Wen, D.; McAlinden, C.; Flitcroft, I.; Tu, R.; Wang, Q.; Alió, J.; Marshall, J.; Huang, Y.; Song, B.; Hu, L.; et al. Postoperative efficacy, predictability, safety, and visual quality of laser corneal refractive surgery: A network meta-analysis. *Am. J. Ophthalmol.* **2017**, *178*, 65–78. [CrossRef] [PubMed]
2. Yamaguchi, T.; Satake, Y.; Dogru, M.; Ohnuma, K.; Negishi, K.; Shimazaki, J. Visual function and higher-order aberrations in eyes after corneal transplantation: How to improve postoperative quality of vision. *Cornea* **2015**, *34* (Suppl. 11), S128–S135. [CrossRef] [PubMed]
3. del Águila-Carrasco, A.J.; Kruger, P.B.; Lara, F.; López-Gil, N. Aberrations and accommodation. *Clin. Exp. Optom.* **2020**, *103*, 95–103. [CrossRef] [PubMed]
4. Koh, S.; Tung, C.I.; Inoue, Y.; Jhanji, V. Effects of tear film dynamics on quality of vision. *Br. J. Ophthalmol.* **2018**, *102*, 1615–1620. [CrossRef]
5. Sheppard, A.L.; Wolffsohn, J.S. Digital eye strain: Prevalence, measurement and amelioration. *BMJ Open Ophthalmol.* **2018**, *3*, e000146. [CrossRef]
6. Jaiswal, S.; Asper, L.; Long, J.; Lee, A.; Harrison, K.; Golebiowski, B. Ocular and visual discomfort associated with smartphones, tablets and computers: What we do and do not know. *Clin. Exp. Optom.* **2019**, *102*, 463–477. [CrossRef]
7. Jones, L.A.; Sinnott, L.T.; Mutti, D.O.; Mitchell, G.L.; Moeschberger, M.L.; Zadnik, K. Parental history of myopia, sports and outdoor activities, and future myopia. *Investig. Ophthalmol. Vis. Sci.* **2007**, *48*, 3524–3532. [CrossRef]
8. Rose, K.A.; Morgan, I.G.; Smith, W.; Burlutsky, G.; Mitchell, P.; Saw, S.M. Myopia, lifestyle, and schooling in students of Chinese ethnicity in Singapore and Sydney. *Arch. Ophthalmol.* **2008**, *126*, 527–530. [CrossRef]
9. Cooper, J.; Tkatchenko, A.V. A review of current concepts of the etiology and treatment of myopia. *Eye Contact Lens* **2018**, *44*, 231–247. [CrossRef]
10. Yang, A.; Lim, S.Y.; Wong, Y.L.; Yeo, A.; Rajeev, N.; Drobe, B. Quality of life in presbyopes with low and high myopia using single-vision and progressive-lens correction. *J. Clin. Med.* **2021**, *10*, 1589. [CrossRef]
11. Kubota, M.; Kubota, S.; Kobashi, H.; Ayaki, M.; Negishi, K.; Tsubota, K. Difference in pupillary diameter as an important factor for evaluating amplitude of accommodation: A prospective observational study. *J. Clin. Med.* **2020**, *9*, 2678. [CrossRef] [PubMed]
12. Tsuneyoshi, Y.; Masui, S.; Arai, H.; Toda, I.; Kubota, M.; Kubota, S.; Tsubota, K.; Ayaki, M.; Negishi, K. Determination of the standard visual criterion for diagnosing and treating presbyopia according to subjective patient symptoms. *J. Clin. Med.* **2021**, *10*, 3942. [CrossRef] [PubMed]
13. Yotsukura, E.; Torii, H.; Ozawa, H.; Hida, R.Y.; Shiraishi, T.; Teixeira, I.C.; Rautha, Y.V.B.L.; Nascimento, C.F.M.d.; Mori, K.; Uchino, M.; et al. Axial length and prevalence of myopia among schoolchildren in the equatorial region of Brazil. *J. Clin. Med.* **2020**, *10*, 115. [CrossRef] [PubMed]
14. Ishiko, S.; Kagokawa, H.; Nishikawa, N.; Song, Y.; Sugawara, K.; Nakagawa, H.; Kawamura, Y.; Yoshida, A. Impact of the pressure-free Yutori Education Program on myopia in Japan. *J. Clin. Med.* **2021**, *10*, 4229. [CrossRef]
15. Tsai, H.R.; Chen, T.L.; Wang, J.H.; Huang, H.K.; Chiu, C.J. Is 0.01% atropine an effective and safe treatment for myopic children? A systemic review and meta-analysis. *J. Clin. Med.* **2021**, *10*, 3766. [CrossRef]
16. Mori, K.; Torii, H.; Hara, Y.; Hara, M.; Yotsukura, E.; Hanyuda, A.; Negishi, K.; Kurihara, T.; Tsubota, K. Effect of violet light-transmitting eyeglasses on axial elongation in myopic children: A randomized controlled trial. *J. Clin. Med.* **2021**, *10*, 5462. [CrossRef]

17. Kamiya, K.; Fujimura, F.; Kawamorita, T.; Ando, W.; Iida, Y.; Shoji, N. factors influencing contrast sensitivity function in eyes with mild cataract. *J. Clin. Med.* **2021**, *10*, 1506. [CrossRef]
18. Hoshi, S.; Tasaki, K.; Hiraoka, T.; Oshika, T. Improvement in contrast sensitivity function after lacrimal passage intubation in eyes with epiphora. *J. Clin. Med.* **2020**, *9*, 2761. [CrossRef]
19. Omoto, M.K.; Torii, H.; Masui, S.; Ayaki, M.; Toda, I.; Arai, H.; Nakamura, T.; Tsubota, K.; Negishi, K. Short-term efficacy and safety of cataract surgery combined with iris-fixated phakic intraocular lens explantation: A multicentre study. *J. Clin. Med.* **2021**, *10*, 3672. [CrossRef]
20. Pajic, B.; Massa, H.; Baenninger, P.B.; Eskina, E.; Pajic-Eggspuehler, B.; Resan, M.; Cvejic, Z. Multifocal femto-presbyLASIK in pseudophakic eyes. *J. Clin. Med.* **2021**, *10*, 2282. [CrossRef]
21. Negishi, K.; Toda, I.; Ayaki, M.; Torii, H.; Tsubota, K. Subjective happiness and satisfaction in postoperative anisometropic patients after refractive surgery for myopia. *J. Clin. Med.* **2020**, *9*, 3473. [CrossRef] [PubMed]
22. Ohlendorf, A.; Leube, A.; Wahl, S. Advancing digital workflows for refractive error measurements. *J. Clin. Med.* **2020**, *9*, 2205. [CrossRef] [PubMed]
23. Domínguez-Vicent, A.; Al-Soboh, L.; Brautaset, R.; Venkataraman, A.P. Effect of instrument design and technique on the precision and accuracy of objective refraction measurement. *J. Clin. Med.* **2020**, *9*, 3061. [CrossRef] [PubMed]
24. Choi, E.Y.; Wong, R.C.S.; Thein, T.; Pasquale, L.R.; Shen, L.Q.; Wang, M.; Li, D.; Jin, Q.; Wang, H.; Baniasadi, N.; et al. The effect of ametropia on glaucomatous visual field loss. *J. Clin. Med.* **2021**, *10*, 2796. [CrossRef] [PubMed]
25. Mitsukawa, T.; Suzuki, Y.; Momota, Y.; Suzuki, S.; Yamada, M. Effects of 0.01% atropine instillation assessed using swept-source anterior segment optical coherence tomography. *J. Clin. Med.* **2021**, *10*, 4384. [CrossRef]

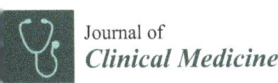

Article

Effect of Violet Light-Transmitting Eyeglasses on Axial Elongation in Myopic Children: A Randomized Controlled Trial

Kiwako Mori [1,2,†], Hidemasa Torii [1,2,†], Yutaka Hara [3], Michiko Hara [3], Erisa Yotsukura [1,2], Akiko Hanyuda [1,2], Kazuno Negishi [1], Toshihide Kurihara [1,2,*] and Kazuo Tsubota [1,4,*]

1. Department of Ophthalmology, Keio University School of Medicine, 35 Shinanomachi, Shinjuku-ku, Tokyo 160-8582, Japan; morikiwako@gmail.com (K.M.); htorii@keio.jp (H.T.); erisa.yotsuku@icloud.com (E.Y.); akiko-hanyuda@hotmail.co.jp (A.H.); kazunonegishi@keio.jp (K.N.)
2. Laboratory of Photobiology, Keio University School of Medicine, 35 Shinanomachi, Shinjuku-ku, Tokyo 160-8582, Japan
3. Hara Eye Clinic, 1-5-27 Suehiro, Ohtawara City 324-1142, Japan; yharaohtawara@gmail.com (Y.H.); michiko.h.mama55@icloud.com (M.H.)
4. Tsubota Laboratory, Inc., 304 Toshin Shinanomachi-ekimae Bldg., 34 Shinanomachi, Shinjuku-ku, Tokyo 160-0016, Japan
* Correspondence: kurihara@z8.keio.jp (T.K.); tsubota@tsubota-lab.com (K.T.); Tel.: +81-3-5315-4132 (T.K.); +81-3-6384-2866 (K.T.)
† These authors are contributed equally to the work and request the double first authorship.

Abstract: The fact that outdoor light environment is an important suppressive factor against myopia led us to invent violet light-transmitting eyeglasses (VL glasses) which can transmit violet light (VL), 360–400 nm in wavelength, for the suppression of myopia, and can meanwhile block harmful ultraviolet waves from sunlight. The current study is a double-blinded randomized clinical trial to investigate the myopia-suppressive effect of VL glasses compared to conventional eyeglasses (placebo glasses) that do not transmit VL. The subjects were children aged from 6 to 12 years old, the population in which myopia progression is generally accelerated, and the myopia suppressive effect was followed up for two years in a city in Japan. Periodical ophthalmic examinations, interviews, and measurements of reflection and axial length under mydriasis were performed at the initial visit (the baseline) and at 1, 6, 12, 18, and 24 months. The mean change in axial length in the VL glasses group was significantly smaller than in the placebo glasses group when time for near-work was less than 180 min and when the subjects were limited to those who had never used eyeglasses before this trial ($p < 0.01$); however, this change was not significant without subgrouping. The suppressive rate for axial elongation in the VL glasses group was 21.4% for two years.

Keywords: violet light; eyeglasses; myopia; axial length; refraction; myopia control; double blinded randomized controlled trial

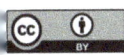

1. Introduction

Myopia is reported to progress due to both genetic and environmental factors [1], but its precise mechanism remains unclear. Only a few safe and secure preventive measures against myopia progression have been established; in addition, the population suffering from myopia has expanded, exceeding one billion people [2].

When myopia progresses and turns into high myopia, the axial length grows and the shape of the eye changes, which may lead to blindness because of sequelae such as myopic maculopathy, glaucoma, and retinal detachment [3,4]. In a domestic epidemiological study, the Tajimi study, it was shown that high myopia accounted for 20% of all myopia cases and ranked first as the cause of WHO-defined blindness [5]. Additionally, it is reported that one diopter suppression of myopia reduces 20% of the possibility of blindness caused by high myopia [6,7]. In order to avoid blindness, prevention of axial elongation and eye deformation is critically important [8]. Therefore, early intervention to prevent myopia progression is highly significant, as it can considerably reduce the risk of sequelae of high myopia, which may lead to blindness.

It is crucial to control environmental factors to suppress the progression of myopia. There are some studies regarding environmental factors in relation to myopia progression, such as the Orinda Study [9], the Singapore Cohort Study of the Risk Factors for Myopia [10], and the Sydney Myopia Study [11,12]. These studies revealed that myopia could be accelerated by urban habitation, long-term near work, higher education, and high intelligence quotient (IQ), while outdoor activities suppressed its development. Two hours or more of daily outdoor activity can reduce the onset rate of myopia, irrespective of whether parents are myopic or not, which is one of its genetic factors [13,14]. There were a couple of major RCTs regarding the correlation of outdoor time with myopia. Cao et al. reported the significance of outdoor time for myopia prevention in their systematic review and meta-analysis, based on randomized controlled trials [15]. According to their report, an additional 20 min of recess outside the classroom could help to slow down the change speed of the refractive error [16]. RCTs conducted in China revealed that 40 min of school outdoor activity was added to the outdoor group, and the changes in both refractive error and axial length were slower than those of the control group [17]. A similar finding in another RCT conducted in Taiwan showed similar results [14]. Though it has been considered that the light that is critical for myopia prevention in an outdoor environment is very high intensity of illumination, even low illumination intensity could have myopia suppressive effects on myopia [18].

Although many researchers have performed investigations to reveal the reason for the effectiveness of outdoor activities on myopia prevention, there are studies focused on a light wavelength that exists in the outdoor environment. The current environment regarding myopia is characterized by ultraviolet-blocking materials such as windows and eyeglasses [19]. Previous studies have revealed that red, green, blue, and violet have the potential to suppress myopia [20–25]; among these wavelengths, violet light (VL: 360–400 nm) is the most potent [26]. Conventional eyeglasses do not penetrate the ultraviolet wavelength, but they also cut off VL [19]. VL eyeglasses were invented to solve these issues and this study was performed to verify their effect.

There have been some previous studies concerning VL. Torii et al. demonstrated that VL suppressed axial elongation and myopic shift of the refractive error in a lens-induced myopia model using chicks [19]. The same results were demonstrated in other reports using mouse models [24,26]. The mechanism of VL in suppressing myopia progression was revealed to maintain choroidal thickness through OPN5 in the retina [26,27]. OPN5 is an opsin, one of the photoreceptors in the retina, which is sensitive to VL [26]. OPN5 is reported to be associated with the circadian rhythm, vasculogenesis, and thermogenesis [26,28,29]. Another study revealed that EGR1, a myopia-suppressive gene, is associated with VL. EGR1 expression was dominant in the myopia-suppressed enucleated eyes illuminated by VL in chicks [19]. Torii et al. also conducted a retrospective study comparing axial elongation for one year between a partially VL-blocking contact lenses (CL) group, comprising 31 eyes of 31 patients (age range, 13–18 years; mean age, 14.7 ± 1.3 years), and a VL-transmitting CL group comprising 116 eyes of 116 patients (age range, 13–18 years; mean age, 15.1 ± 1.4 years). This study revealed 0.19 mm of mean axial elongation in the partially VL-blocking CL group and 0.14 mm of mean axial elongation in the VL-transmitting CL group ($p < 0.05$) [19]. Another retrospective study revealed that axial elongation in 10 subjects with −6 D or less refractive errors implanted with non-VL-transmitting phakic intraocular lenses (pIOL) was 0.38 mm, and axial elongation in 13 subjects with −6 D or less refractive errors implanted with VL-transmitting pIOL was 0.09 mm for 5 years ($p < 0.05$) [30].

VL exist in the outdoor environments; however, they hardly exist in indoor environments because most of them are blocked by windows [19]. Likewise, VL do not reach our eyes since they are blocked by ordinary eyeglasses [19].

Thus, we invented eyeglasses that transmit VL and block harmful short ultraviolet (UV) light from sunlight. We designed the study to investigate the myopia-suppressive effect of our eyeglasses, violet light-transmitting eyeglasses (VL glasses), for two years, comparing with conventional eyeglasses (placebo glasses) that do not transmit VL.

2. Materials and Methods

2.1. Study Design

This was a prospective randomized double-blind placebo-controlled trial conducted for 2 years. The study was performed in compliance with the Declaration of Helsinki, Ethical Guidelines for Medical and Health Research Involving Human Subjects, and local regulatory requirements, and was also conducted under the approval of all study institutional review boards (IRB) and ethics committees. This trial was approved by the Certified Review Board of Keio (Approval No. N20188004). This trial was also registered by Japan Registry of Clinical Trials with the registration number jRCTs032180418. This randomized control trial followed CONSORT guidelines.

2.2. Study Organization

The participants were recruited at Hara Eye Clinic, Tochigi, Japan. The analysis of statistics was outsourced to an independent company (Satista, Inc., Kyoto, Japan), without any relationship with JINS HOLDINGS, Inc., Gunma, Japan, the sponsor of this clinical study, and interpretation after the results of the analysis was performed by the department of ophthalmology and laboratory of photobiology, Keio University School of Medicine, Tokyo, Japan.

2.3. Participants and Sample Size

The participants were enrolled from July 2016 to August 2018 and followed-up for 24 months. As for the sample size, previous research results of MyoVision (Zeiss International) showed values of 0.78 ± 0.29 mm for axial elongation and -1.65 ± 0.80 D for refractive change for two years while wearing conventional eyeglasses [31]. When considering that the suppressive effect of an outdoor environment is 30%, it can be estimated that axial elongation is 0.55 mm and refractive change is -1.16 D for two years. Upon establishing the sample size, along with axial length and refractive change, each group required 34 cases, under the condition that the effect size was 0.23, the standard deviation was 0.29, $\alpha = 0.05$ (both sides), and $1-\beta = 0.90$ when axial length was the primary outcome. When it was assumed that the dropout rate was 15%, each group required 40 participants, meaning the total sample size would be 80 participants. When refractive change was the secondary outcome, each group required 57 participants, under the condition that the effect size was 0.49, the standard deviation was 0.80, $\alpha = 0.05$ (both sides), and $1-\beta = 0.90$. Since the refractive change was the secondary outcome in this study, the total sample size was 140 participants when the drop rate was assumed to be 15%. The first participant was enrolled on 17 August 2016. Though the pace of the enrollment was initially steady, it gradually dropped and could not reach the target number by the end of the scheduled recruitment period. Therefore, the recruitment period was extended twice, and the total number of participants was finally 113 (Figure 1).

Children who met all the criteria were included in the study; (1) those who were aged 6–12 of both gender at the moment of consent; (2) those who spent at least 1 h per a day outdoors; (3) those whose cycloplegic refraction in each eye was between -1.50 D and -4.50 D, (4) those who had one or two parent/s with myopia; (5) those who were able to wear eyeglasses habitually and who could fulfill clinical visits in accordance with the study protocol; (6) those who had no ocular diseases besides ametropia; and (7) those who could provide written informed assent from the study subjects (hereinafter referred to as "subject(s)") themselves and informed consent from their legal guardian(s).

Children who met at least one of the following criteria were excluded from the study; (1) those who had worn bifocals or progressive power lenses; (2) those who had worn orthokeratology lenses; (3) those with anisometropia exceeding 1.50 D; (4) those with astigmatism exceeding 1.50 D, (5) those with manifest strabismus; (6) those with a history of refractive surgery; (7) those with a history of keratoconus, herpetic keratitis, or papillary hyperplasia, etc.; (8) those participating in an ongoing similar study; or (9) those who had been judged to be ineligible to participate in the study by the investigators.

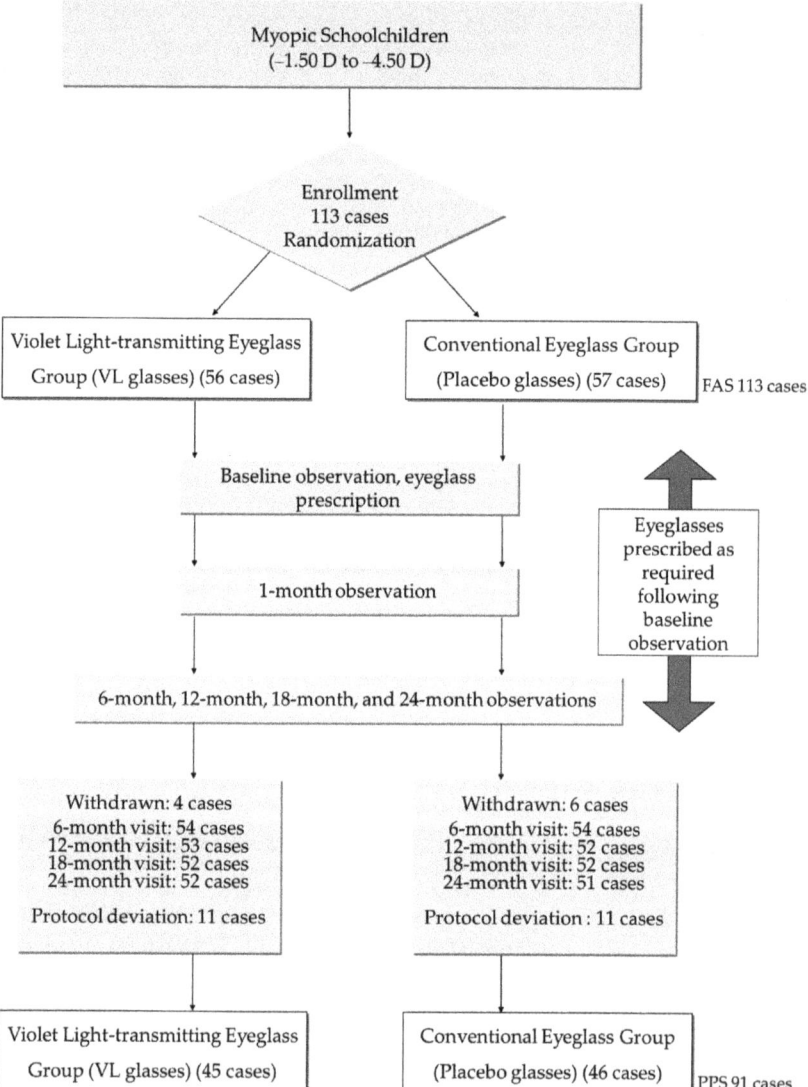

Figure 1. Flowchart of the double-blind randomized clinical trial time points and number of participants. Details of the reasons for withdrawal and protocol deviation are described in Table S1. FAS: full analysis set; PPS: per protocol set.

2.4. Randomization and Masking

Randomization followed the EDC system. Static allocation of stratification by (1) age and (2) gender, i.e., random substitution block method, was performed, and schoolchildren were assigned to either a VL glasses group or a placebo glasses group. The principal investigator and the co-investigator/s were not informed about the details of the allocation steps.

2.5. Intervention

The intervention group was obliged to wear VL glasses for 24 months, whereas the control group was instructed to wear conventional eyeglasses (placebo glasses) that did not transmit VL (Figure 2).

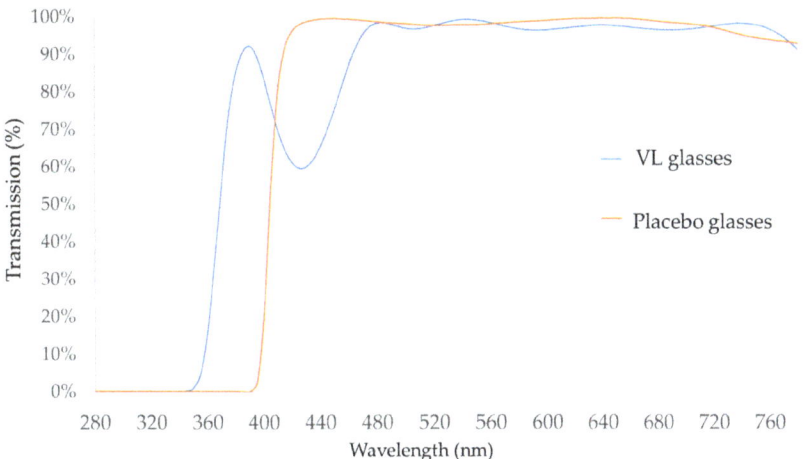

Figure 2. Characteristics of the eyeglasses used in this study: the transmission rate (%) at each wavelength of the light with VL glasses (blue) and with placebo glasses (orange) is shown. VL glasses transmit light 360–400 nm in wavelength, whereas placebo glasses block the light of the wavelengths less than 400 nm.

2.6. Procedure for Follow-Up Examinations

The primary investigator or co-investigator prescribed refraction correcting eyeglasses based on the result of a visual acuity examination under cycloplegia which was conducted at the baseline. Whether the glasses were VL glasses or placebo glasses was not disclosed to the primary or co-investigator at prescription. At the point of regular eye examination, 1, 6, 12, 18, and 24 months after the baseline, over the 24-month research period, new correcting glasses of each type were prescribed to gain 20/20 or more of visual acuity. Barring these points, the same correcting glasses of each type were prescribed only in case of accidental damage or loss of eyeglasses, and the prescriptions were not allowed to be changed.

At the first encounter, details of the study design and the rights of the participants were explained. An eye examination was performed to measure subjective/objective cycloplegic refraction and axial length following written informed consent. The best corrected visual acuity of subjective refraction was measured under cycloplegia to prescribe the eyeglasses. Objective refraction was measured with a closed-field type auto ref/kerato/tono/pachymeter (TONOREF®III, NIDEK, Tokyo, Japan) with 0.01 D increments. The measurement of objective refraction under cycloplegia was performed one hour after the application of 1% cyclopentolate hydrochloride eyedrops (Cyplegin® 1% ophthalmic solution, Santen, Osaka, Japan). Axial length was measured with an IOLMaster 500 (Carl Zeiss Meditec, Jena, Germany). Interviews of the participants were performed at every visit. Participants' age, gender, number of parents with myopia, living environment, and lifestyles such as time for sunlight exposure, near work, sleep, and physical activities were asked. The time for sunlight exposure and near work was calculated with weighted means of 5 weekdays and 2 weekends. Regular eye examination was performed at 1, 6, 12, 18, and 24 months from the baseline to measure the visual acuity of the prescribed eyeglasses, best corrected visual acuity, subjective refraction, objective refraction under cycloplegia, and axial length. Regarding adverse events, surveillance of each participant during the whole period of this study was performed to report in the form of case reports.

2.7. Outcomes

The primary and the secondary outcomes were the change in axial length and objective refraction, i.e., spherical equivalent refraction (SER), under cycloplegia for 24 months, respectively.

2.8. Statistical Analysis

All data were analyzed based on the intention-to-treatment principle. The primary analysis was performed in the per-protocol set (PPS), and robustness of the results was explored through sensitivity analysis in the full analysis set (FAS).

The repeated-measure outcomes were analyzed with a linear mixed-effects model for repeated measures (MMRM) that included intervention, dummy variables for time, intervention-by-time interactions as covariates, and the subjects as a random effect. Furthermore, in this model, all measurements obtained from both eyes were used and entered as repeated effects. The covariance structure was a completely general (i.e., unstructured) covariance matrix. The results were reported as the least squares means with 95% confidence interval (CI) at each time-point.

The odds ratios (OR) and 95% confidence intervals (CI) were calculated by univariate logistic regression analysis for independent risk factors associated with rapidly progressed myopia, i.e., increase in axial length by 1.2 mm or more, and deterioration of SER by −2.5 D or less at 24 months. Multivariate analysis was performed with adjustment by gender, "already wearing glasses at first visit", and parental myopia. There are some papers regarding the definition of rapid progression of myopia. Rapid progression of myopia is mostly defined as −1 D or less of decrease in refractive errors per year [32,33]. In the meantime, it is reported that 1.25 D of deterioration of myopia categorized in fast progression of myopia tends to progress more in the following year [34]. In this study, because of the preceding reasons, the degree of −2.5 D or less of progression of myopia for two years was defined as fast/rapid progression of myopia and its exacerbating factor was investigated.

Subgroup analysis according to factors considered to be related to the outcome (i.e., baseline age, already wearing glasses at first visit and baseline time of near-work) was conducted with the MMRM. The time of near-work was calculated by weighted means of 5 weekdays and 2 weekend days.

A p-value of <0.05 was considered statistically significant, and all p-values were two-sided without multiplicity adjustment. All statistical analyses were performed using SAS 9.4 Foundation for Microsoft Windows for x64 (SAS Institute Inc., Cary, NC, USA).

3. Results

3.1. Flow of Participants

A total of 113 children were enrolled in this trial. Of these, 57 participants were assigned to the placebo glasses group (placebo group) and 56 participants to the VL glasses group (VL group) (Figure 1). During the follow-up period, 32 participants dropped out; 22 participants deviated from the protocol and 10 withdrew their consent to participate. As a result, a total of 91 participants—46 in the placebo group and 45 in the VL group—completed this trial. The investigators, including orthoptists and ophthalmologists, were masked with regard to the allocation of the groups.

3.2. Participant Profiles

The profiles of the participants are shown in Table 1. No significant differences were found between the two groups with respect to age or gender. In addition, SER and axial length at the first visit showed no significant differences. The mean ages of the participants in the placebo and the VL groups were 9.5 ± 1.5 years (mean ± SD) and 9.3 ± 1.5 years; the mean SERs of right eyes were −2.66 ± 0.85 and −2.82 ± 0.87 D; the mean SERs of left eyes were −2.66 ± 0.87 and −2.90 ± 0.92 D; the mean axial lengths of right eyes were 24.53 ± 0.67 and 24.45 ± 0.93 mm, and the mean axial lengths of left eyes were 24.54 ± 0.67 and 24.45 ± 0.97 mm, respectively. No significant differences were found between the two groups except time for near work.

Table 1. Characteristics of the 113 participants.

Characteristic	Category	All	Placebo	VL	p Value	
Number of cases		113	57	56		
Age (years)		9.4 ± 1.5	9.5 ± 1.5	9.3 ± 1.5	0.478	†
Sex	boys	43 (38.1%)	22 (38.6%)	21 (37.5%)	1.000	††
	girls	70 (61.9%)	35 (61.4%)	35 (62.5%)		
Parental myopia	both parents	56 (51.9%)	24 (45.3%)	32 (58.2%)		
	only father	22 (20.4%)	10 (18.9%)	12 (21.8%)	0.196	††
	only mother	30 (17.4%)	19 (35.8%)	11 (20.0%)		
Height (cm)		135.3 ± 10.9	135.8 ± 9.9	134.7 ± 11.9	0.989	†
Weight (kg)		31.16 ± 7.35	31.15 ± 6.86	31.17 ± 7.88	0.629	†
Best corrected visual acuity (log MAR)	right eyes	−0.09 ± 0.03	−0.09 ± 0.03	−0.09 ± 0.03	0.985	
	left eyes	−0.08 ± 0.03	−0.08 ± 0.03	−0.09 ± 0.03	0.718	
Axial length (mm)	right eyes	24.49 ± 0.81	24.53 ± 0.67	24.45 ± 0.93	0.724	
	left eyes	24.50 ± 0.83	24.54 ± 0.67	24.45 ± 0.97	0.658	
SER (D)	right eyes	−2.74 ± 0.86	−2.66 ± 0.85	−2.82 ± 0.87	0.328	
	left eyes	−2.78 ± 0.90	−2.66 ± 0.87	−2.90 ± 0.92	0.156	
Number of participants with glasses at the first visit		59 (52.2%)	28 (49.1%)	31 (55.4%)	0.574	††
Environmental factors						
Near-work time (min/day)		193.45 ± 93.13	214.50 ± 104.11	172.02 ± 75.48	0.015	†
Sunlight exposure time (min/day)		58.75 ± 52.18	54.52 ± 47.34	63.03 ± 56.80	0.388	†
Sleeping hours (hours/day)		8.56 ± 0.67	8.57 ± 0.63	8.54 ± 0.72	0.841	†

Data represent means ± SDs; min: minutes; log MAR: logarithm of the minimum angle of resolution; SER: spherical equivalent refraction; D: diopter; VL group: violet light-transmitting eyeglasses group; †: t-test; ††: Fisher test; others: Mann–Whitney U test.

3.3. Adverse Events

No adverse effects associated with violet light exposure were reported during the 2-year-clinical study. All adverse events reported during the study were not associated with violet light exposure (Table S2).

3.4. Comparison of Myopia Progression after 24 Months

A total of 113 participants were enrolled and randomly dichotomized into two groups, of which 57 (mean age 9.5 ± 1.5 SD year old, 22 males and 35 females) belonged to the placebo group and 56 (mean age 9.3 ± 1.5 year old, 21 males, 35 females) to the VL group. Finally, 91 participants—46 in the placebo group and 45 in the VL group—were selected after application of exclusion criteria such as familial issues and protocol deviation from the research protocol. PPS is defined as cases excluding subjects who fell into the exclusion criteria. FAS is defined as all the cases included in this study. For example, PPS does not include those who did not spend more than 1 h outdoors (Table S1). In total, 113 subjects were analyzed as FAS and 91 were analyzed as PPS. It was confirmed that randomization was appropriate by analyzing statistics of the background in each group, and the balance of the background was judged to be appropriate. In PPS, the variation in axial length after 24 months was 0.758 mm (95% CI: 0.711–0.810) in the placebo group and 0.728 mm (95% CI: 0.682–0.775) in the VL group, while SER was −1.531 D (95% CI: −1.729−−1.330) in the placebo group and −1.421 D (95% CI: −1.617−−1.225) in the VL group. In the VL group, the average variation in axial length was as small as −0.030 (95% CI: −0.096, 0.037, $p = 0.381$), and that of the spherical equivalent was similarly small at 0.110 (95% CI: −0.168,

0.389, $p = 0.431$), without significant statistical difference by the mixed effect model with individual variation factors and repetition effects of the bilateral eyes (Table 2).

Table 2. Results of the mixed-effects model fitted to 24-month change for both eyes.

	Placebo PPS n = 46			VL PPS n = 45			Difference in Amount of Change from the Baseline		
	LS Mean	95% CI		LS Mean	95% CI		Difference	95% CI	p-Value
Axial length PPS									
first visit (baseline)	24.54	24.31	24.77	24.63	24.4	24.87			
24 months	25.30	25.07	25.53	25.36	25.13	25.59			
change from baseline	0.76	0.71	0.81	0.73	0.68	0.78	−0.03	−0.10 0.04	0.381
SER PPS									
first visit (baseline)	−2.73	−2.97	−2.49	−2.96	−3.2	−2.71			
24 months	−4.26	−4.56	−3.96	−4.38	−4.68	−4.08			
change from baseline	−1.53	−1.73	−1.33	−1.42	−1.62	−1.23	0.11	−0.17 0.39	0.434

VL group: violet light-transmitting eyeglasses group; LS mean: least squares mean; 95% CI: 95% confidence interval.; SER: spherical equivalent refraction under accommodative paralysis; PPS: per protocol set. Linear mixed model: variable factors are "individuals," repeated effects are left and right sides of the participants' eyes, intervention contents are groups wearing normal glasses and violet light-transmitting glasses, fixed effects are interactions of intervention contents and time.

Factors that contributed to deterioration of myopia were investigated by logistic analysis in this study. This approach suggested that risk factors of 1.2 mm or more of axial elongation were young age, having already worn eyeglasses at the baseline, small change in BMI, paternal myopia, and short sleeping duration (Table 3). Risk factors of −2.5 D or less for SER deterioration were young age, having already worn eyeglasses at the baseline, small change in BMI, and paternal myopia (Table 4). Besides, multivariate analysis was performed with adjustment by gender, "already wearing glasses at first visit", and parental myopia (Tables S3 and S4). The result of the analysis showed that the odds ratio of "already wearing glasses at first visit" for the deterioration of the axial length and the SER was kept at 4.0 even in the multivariate model. This result suggested that "already wearing glasses at first visit" can be considered to be a deteriorating factor.

When analyzing children limited to those who first started using eyeglasses, 11 children in each group, the change in axial length was 0.856 mm (95% CI: 0.856–1.057) in the placebo group and 0.751 mm (95% CI: 0.646–0.855) in the VL group, respectively, when near-work time was less than 180 min. The change in SER was −1.841D (95% CI: −2.056−−1.626) in the placebo group and −1.538D (95% CI: −1.860−−1.316) in the VL group, respectively. The mean change in axial length in the VL group was significantly small (difference: −0.206 mm; 95% CI: −0.351, 0.060; $p = 0.006$), whereas the mean change in SER in the VL group was small but not significant (difference 0.303, 95% CI: −0.006, 0.612, $p = 0.055$) using a mixed effect model (Table 5, Figure 2).

The results were obtained by linear mixed-effects model analysis. (A) The adjusted means of change in AL in the VL group were significantly ($p = 0.006$) smaller than those in the placebo group at 24 months. (B) The adjusted means of SER changes in the VL group were smaller than those in the placebo group at 24 months, which was not significant ($p = 0.055$). Orange lines show the VL group and blue lines show the placebo group. Error bars show 95% confidence intervals. ** $p < 0.01$. AL: axial length; SER: spherical equivalent refraction; VL group: violet light-transmitting eyeglasses group.

Table 3. Factors for increase in axial length of 1.2 mm or more.

	Univariate Logistic Regression			
	OR	95% CI		p-Value
Age (y)	0.28	0.16	0.51	<0.0001
Female	0.56	0.19	1.60	0.279
Change in BMI	0.54	0.30	0.98	0.044
Continuous near-work time (min)	1.00	0.99	1.02	0.643
Continuous near-work time (digital devices) (min)	1.00	0.99	1.02	0.556
Already wearing glasses at first visit	4.67	1.28	17.06	0.020
Near-work time (min)	1.00	0.99	1.00	0.617
Near-work time (digital devices) (min)	1.00	0.99	1.01	0.907
Near-work time (books) (min)	0.99	0.97	1.00	0.171
Outdoor activity time (min)	1.00	0.98	1.01	0.410
Birth weight (kg)	1.00	1.00	1.00	0.403
Birth height (cm)	1.05	0.84	1.32	0.648
Parental myopia				
Only father	1.00		ref	
Only mother	0.00	0.00		0.997
Both parents	0.17	0.05	0.55	0.003
Distance from the television (cm)	0.87	0.48	1.57	0.652
Near-working distance (cm)	1.00	0.93	1.09	0.930
Brightness of the bedroom while sleeping				
Bright	0.00	0.00		0.999
Dim	0.73	0.25	2.15	0.570
Dark	1.00		ref	
Bedtime (hr)	0.38	0.15	0.96	0.041
Sleeping hours (hr)	1.86	0.84	4.09	0.124
Extracurricular activities (outside) (min)	0.60	0.13	2.75	0.507

OR: odds ratio; 95% CI: 95% confidence interval; ref: reference standard; BMI: body mass index.

Table 4. Factors for decrease in spherical equivalent power of −2.5 D or less.

	Univariate Logistic Regression			
	OR	95% CI		p-Value
Age (y)	0.47	0.31	0.72	0.0004
Female	0.85	0.30	2.37	0.750
Change in BMI	0.35	0.18	0.70	0.003
Continuous near-work time (min)	1.00	0.99	1.02	0.718
Continuous near-work time (digital devices) (min)	1.01	0.99	1.02	0.496
Already wearing glasses at first visit	3.47	1.08	11.13	0.037
Near-work time (min)	1.00	1.00	1.01	0.539
Near-work time (digital devices) (min)	1.00	1.00	1.01	0.189
Near-work time (books) (min)	0.99	0.97	1.00	0.145
Outdoor activity time (min)	0.99	0.98	1.01	0.257
Birth weight (kg)	1.00	1.00	1.00	0.783
Birth height (cm)	1.07	0.85	1.33	0.573
Parental myopia				
Only father	1.00		ref	
Only mother	0.28	0.07	1.15	0.077
Both parents	0.28	0.09	0.90	0.033
Distance from the television (cm)	0.80	0.43	1.49	0.481
Near-working distance (cm)	0.98	0.90	1.06	0.583
Brightness of the bedroom while sleeping				
Bright	0.00	0.00		0.999
Dim	1.11	0.37	3.34	0.854
Dark	1.00		ref	
Bedtime (hr)	0.72	0.32	1.64	0.438
Sleeping hours (hr)	1.13	0.53	2.41	0.761
Extracurricular activities (outside) (min)	0.55	0.12	2.52	0.441

OR: odds ratio; 95% CI: 95% confidence interval; ref: reference standard; BMI: body mass index.

Table 5. Results of the mixed-effects model fitted to 24 months of change for both eyes under the limited condition in which near-work time is less than 180 min and there was no previous history of eyeglasses use.

	Placebo			VL			Difference in Amount of Change from the Baseline		
n	LS Mean	95% CI	n	LS Mean	95% CI		Difference	95% CI	p-Value
Axial length									
Change after wearing the eyeglasses for 24 months									
11	0.96	0.86 1.06	11	0.75	0.65	0.86	−0.21	−0.35 −0.06	0.006
SER									
Change after wearing the eyeglasses for 24 months									
11	−1.84	−2.06 −1.63	11	−1.54	−1.76	−1.32	0.30	−0.01 0.61	0.055

LS mean: least squares mean; 95% CI: 95% confidence interval; SER: spherical equivalent refraction under accommodative paralysis; VL group: violet light-transmitting eyeglasses group. Adjusted by group, time, interaction of group and time, both/left/right eyes.

4. Discussion

According to previous reports, VL has an effect on suppressing myopia progression [19,26,30]. Based on this research, the application of instruments that could distinguish the effective light to prevent myopia progression from harmful lights to protect the eyes was attempted. The VL glasses, which actually transmit VL and block detrimental constituent such as UV, were invented in our laboratory and were expected to exert potency in clinical situations. This 2-year randomized controlled study was designed to investigate the effectiveness of VL glasses in suppressing the progression of myopia, and it revealed that the mean change in axial length in the VL glasses group was significantly smaller than that in the placebo glasses group when time for near-work was less than 180 min and when the subjects were limited to those who had never used eyeglasses before this trial ($p < 0.01$). This is the first randomized controlled study of VL glasses that reflects their potency. However, this study could not attain statistical significance when no limitation regarding near-work time and eyeglasses histories of the subjects was applied. Because VL transmitting eyeglasses do not exert their effect until they transmit VL in an outdoor environment, it was inappropriate to perform analysis while including the cases who did not have enough time for outdoor activity; therefore, PPS was performed. Nevertheless, since there were unexpectedly many unregistered cases, and those of protocol deviation such as shortage of outdoor activity time, VL glasses were merely found to have a tendency to be effective, but they did not reach statistical significance, even by PPS. The subgroup analysis limited to the group with no history of eyeglasses before this study, and with less than 180 min of near-work time, eventually revealed that VL glasses significantly suppressed axial elongation. The suppressive rate of axial elongation in the VL glasses group for two years was 21.4%, which could be considered meaningful to some extent.

The reason why limiting the subjects with no history of wearing eyeglasses led to the result being significant regarding axial elongation was sought. This study also revealed that the speed of myopia progression in the subgroup that had already worn conventional eyeglasses was actually fast; this result is possibly due to genetic background and the development of myopia at the early stage of life (Tables 3 and 4). The excessive burden of near-work accelerates myopia progression and may cause attenuation of the effect of VL glasses. In addition, during a period of blocking VL transmission by wearing conventional eyeglasses, myopia progression could be facilitated.

As a prerequisite for a human study, there have been some reports concerning animal experimental models. Exposure to long-wavelength red light developed hyperopic responses in Rhesus monkeys and tree shrews [21,35], whereas red light was, in contrast, demonstrated to induce myopia response in chicks [22]. Meanwhile, short-wavelength light exposure led to hyperopia in chickens, fish and guinea pigs [22,23,25,36]. Furthermore, lens-induced myopia (LIM) models in chicks, mice and guinea pigs showed suppression of axial elongation and myopic shift of refractive error when exposed to VL [19,24,26,37]. Among visible lights, VL was the most effective wavelength for suppressing myopia progression in LIM [26].

VL is characteristic of the shortest wavelength and adjacent to ultraviolet waves. Because of this fact, it has often been considered whether VL is detrimental to the eyes. In this study, we did not find any adverse events during the two-years period through this study by regular examinations, including ocular surface, cataracts, allergy, and the fundus (Table S2). When VL glasses are worn, the amount of VL reaching the eye is more than that when conventional eyeglasses are worn. Furthermore, the amount of VL transmitted when VL glasses are worn is less than that when no glasses are worn. This fact may have contributed to no adverse effects being observed.

To date, there have been many types of eyeglasses sold to the public. In order to study the pure effectiveness of VL glasses, the subjects were limited to children who had never worn eyeglasses. Moreover, at the baseline, near-work time in the VL group was less than that in the placebo group, as shown in Table 1; it is well known that near-work time is an important factor for the progression of myopia. Therefore, subgroup analysis was performed and was limited to a group in which near-work time was less than 180 min. As a result, axial elongation was suppressed in the VL glasses group unless the time for near-work exceeded 180 min. The suppressive rate of the axial elongation with VL glasses for 2 years was 21.4% (Figure 3A). While this value does not surpass the suppressive rate of axial elongation with orthokeratology, multifocal contact lenses, or the defocus incorporated multiple segments (DIMS) eyeglasses [38,39], it is competitive with other methodologies such as progressive addition lenses (PAL), radial refractive gradient lenses, and positively aspherized PAL. The suppressive rate of axial elongation in PAL was 0–16%, that in radial refractive gradient lenses was not statistically significant, and that in positively aspherized PAL was 12% [31,40,41]. Additionally, the suppressive rate of axial elongation with 0.01% atropine drops, one of the current major standard remedies for myopia suppression, is reported to be 12% in Low-Concentration Atropine for Myopia Progression (LAMP) and 18% in Atropine for the Treatment of Myopia in Japan (ATOM-J) studies [42,43]. VL glasses, the suppressive rate of which is 21.4% under the limited condition regarding near-work time and the history of eyeglasses use, are demonstrated to be barely superior to atropine eye drops as a preventive measure against myopia progression.

This study includes some limitations. First, it was performed in a rural area in Japan where children spend much time outdoors; sufficient outdoor activities were an essential condition to demonstrate the myopia-suppressive effect of the VL glasses, as VL exists in the outdoor environment but not in the indoor environment. However, the result did not follow our expectations. The mean time for outdoor activities in a day did not reach 1 h; therefore, we could not analyze all the participants to judge the effectiveness of the VL glasses. Second, we established the necessary number of subjects by calculating sample sizes referring to previous research regarding MyoVision eyeglasses [31]. Despite our endeavors in recruiting the participants twice and extending the recruitment time, the number of subjects did not reach 140. This is probably because the subjects themselves judged they would waste 2 years when they were assigned to the placebo group, in spite of the existing methods of myopia prevention such as orthokeratology and atropine eyedrops. Moreover, there were many dropout cases during the research period, resulting in analyses of 91 participants as the final number. To make matters worse, the prevalence of COVID-19 disabled the participants in keeping their time for outdoor activities, which influenced the proper analysis regarding the effectiveness of VL glasses in all subjects. These obstacles may have affected the result of this study, not showing statistical significance upon comparing the two groups. Meanwhile, it was considered to be of much importance that subgroup analysis for the participants who had never used any types of eyeglasses before this research revealed the effectiveness of VL glasses on myopia suppression, especially on the suppression of axial elongation. The result of the analysis was not biased by the past usage of any type of eyeglasses, and it truly reflected the potential of the VL glasses. Furthermore, the suppressive effect on myopia of the VL glasses works especially when they are used in the outdoor environments, and therefore, whether the suppressive effect was owing to the

VL glasses or the outdoor environments is difficult to discern. However, the outdoor time in the placebo group and that in the VL group were not significantly different. The fact that the suppressive effect of the VL glasses exceeds that of the placebo glasses in the same outdoor time may suggest that myopia progression is due to the difference in whether the glasses transmit VL or not.

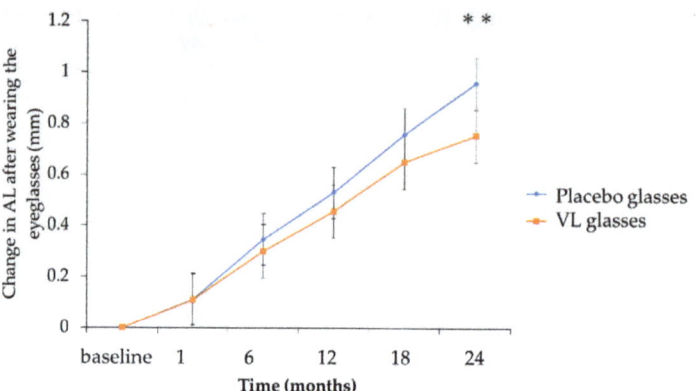

A

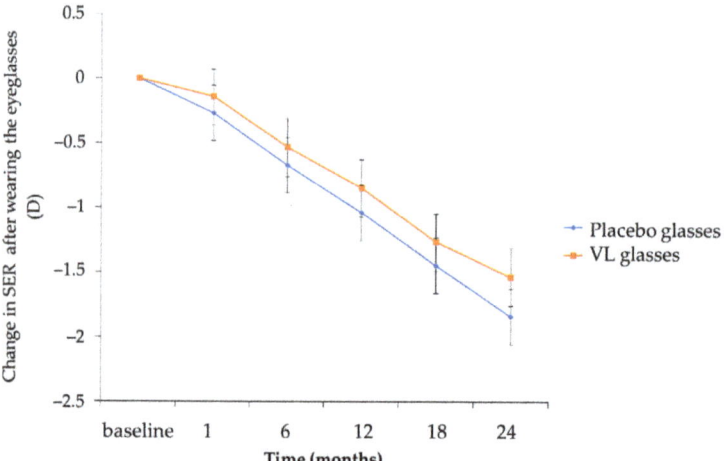

B

Figure 3. Time course of the adjusted mean axial elongation and SER change under the limited condition in which near-work time was less than 180 min and there was no previous history of eyeglasses use. (A) change in AL after wearing the eyeglasses, (B) change in SER after wearing the eyeglasses. AL: axial length, SER: spherical equivalent refraction ** $p < 0.01$.

5. Conclusions

Violet light-transmitting eyeglasses suppressed axial elongation without any adverse events and their suppressive rate was 21.4%.

6. Patent

A patent has been applied for the optical components internationally (Patent No. WO2017/090128) and registered in Japan (JP.6629343), US (US.10866433) and China (CN.108474888) by Tsubota Laboratory, Inc. and JINS HOLDINGS, Inc.

Supplementary Materials: The following are available online at https://www.mdpi.com/article/10.3390/jcm10225462/s1, Table S1: Details of the reasons for withdrawn and protocol deviation; Table S2: Safety; Table S3: Factors for increase in axial length of 1.2 mm or more; Table S4: Factors for decrease in spherical equivalent power of −2.5 D or less.

Author Contributions: Conceptualization, K.M., H.T., T.K. and K.T.; methodology, Y.H. and M.H.; investigation, K.M., Y.H. and M.H.; data curation, K.M.; project administration, K.M. and H.T.; writing—original draft preparation, K.M. and H.T.; writing—review and editing, K.M., H.T., Y.H., M.H., E.Y., A.H., K.N., T.K. and K.T.; supervision, K.N., T.K. and K.T. All authors made a substantial contribution in the revision of the manuscript. All authors have read and agreed to the published version of the manuscript.

Funding: The current study was financially supported from JINS HOLDINGS, Inc.

Institutional Review Board Statement: The study was performed in compliance with the Declaration of Helsinki, Ethical Guidelines for Medical and Health Research Involving Human Subjects, and local regulatory requirements, and was also conducted under the approval of all study institutional review boards (IRB) and ethics committees. This trial was approved by the Certified Review Board of Keio (Approval No. N20188004). This trial was also registered by Japan Registry of Clinical Trials with the registration number jRCTs032180418. This randomized control trial followed CONSORT guidelines.

Informed Consent Statement: Informed consent was obtained from all subjects involved in the study.

Data Availability Statement: All data underlying this article are available in the article and in its online supplementary material. We will willingly share our knowledge, protocol, and expertise when asked.

Acknowledgments: The authors thank T. Shimizu, K. Yamashita, Y. Tsuneyoshi, H. Kunimi, Y. Hirayama, H. Mochimaru, S. Hato, E. Inagaki, H. Mitamura and E. Kanemaru in Hara Eye Clinic. We are also grateful to A. Kaneko and T. Okano in Satt Co., Ltd., H. Yamakage in Satista, Inc. and S. Kondo in Tsubota Laboratory, Inc.

Conflicts of Interest: Tsubota laboratory, Inc., for which Kazuo Tsubota works as the Chief Executive Officer (CEO), receives distribution royalty fees for selling the lenses used in this study from JINS HOLDINGS, Inc., a sponsor of this research.

References

1. Enthoven, C.A.; Tidessman, J.W.L.; Polling, J.R.; Tedja, M.S.; Raat, H.; Iglesias, A.I.; Verhoeven, V.J.M.; Klaver, C.C.W. Interaction between lifestyle and genetic susceptibility in myopia: The Generation R study. *Eur. J. Epidemiol.* **2019**, *34*, 777–784. [PubMed]
2. Holden, B.A.; Jong, M.; Davis, S.; Wilson, D.; Fricke, T.; Resnikoff, S. Nearly 1 billion myopes at risk of myopia-related sight-threatening conditions by 2050–time to act now. *Clin. Exp. Optom.* **2015**, *98*, 491–493. [CrossRef] [PubMed]
3. Bikbov, M.M.; Gilmanshin, T.R.; Kazakbaeva, G.M.; Zainullin, R.M.; Rakhimova, E.M.; Rusakova, I.A.; Bolshakova, N.I.; Safiullina, K.R.; Zaynetdinov, A.F.; Zinatullin, A.A.; et al. Prevalence of Myopic Maculopathy Among Adults in a Russian Population. *JAMA Netw. Open* **2020**, *3*, e200567. [CrossRef] [PubMed]
4. Bikbov, M.M.; Kazakbaeva, G.M.; Rakhimova, E.M.; Rusakova, I.A.; Fakhretdinova, A.A.; Tuliakova, A.M.; Panda-Jonas, S.; Gilmanshin, T.R.; Zainullin, R.M.; Bolshakova, N.I.; et al. Prevalence Factors Associated With Vision Impairment and Blindness Among Individuals 85 Years and Older in Russia. *JAMA Netw. Open* **2021**, *4*, e2121138. [CrossRef] [PubMed]
5. Iwase, A.; Araie, M.; Tomidokoro, A.; Yamamoto, T.; Shimizu, H.; Kitazawa, Y. Prevalence and causes of low vision and blindness in a Japanese adult population: The Tajimi Study. *Ophthalmology* **2006**, *113*, 1354–1362. [CrossRef]
6. Bullimore, M.A.; Brennan, N.A. Myopia Control: Why Each Diopter Matters. *Optom. Vis. Sci.* **2019**, *96*, 463–465. [CrossRef] [PubMed]
7. Bullimore, M.A.; Richdale, K. Myopia Control 2020: Where are we and where are we heading? *Ophthalmic Physiol. Opt.* **2020**, *40*, 254–270. [CrossRef]
8. Saw, S.M.; Gazzard, G.; Shih-Yen, E.C.; Chua, W.H. Myopia and associated pathological complications. *Ophthalmic Physiol. Opt.* **2005**, *25*, 381–391. [CrossRef]

9. Mutti, D.O.; Mitchell, G.L.; Moeschberger, M.L.; Jones, L.A.; Zadnik, K. Parental myopia, near work, school achievement, and children's refractive error. *Investig. Ophthalmol. Vis. Sci.* **2002**, *43*, 3633–3640.
10. Saw, S.M.; Shankar, A.; Tan, S.B.; Taylor, H.; Tan, D.T.; Stone, R.A.; Wong, T.Y. A cohort study of incident myopia in Singaporean children. *Investig. Ophthalmol. Vis. Sci.* **2006**, *47*, 1839–1844. [CrossRef]
11. Ip, J.M.; Rose, K.A.; Morgan, I.G.; Burlutsky, G.; Mitchell, P. Myopia and the urban environment: Findings in a sample of 12-year-old Australian school children. *Investig. Ophthalmol. Vis. Sci.* **2008**, *49*, 3858–3863. [CrossRef] [PubMed]
12. Ip, J.M.; Saw, S.M.; Rose, K.A.; Morgan, I.G.; Kifley, A.; Wang, J.J.; Mitchell, P. Role of near work in myopia: Findings in a sample of Australian school children. *Investig. Ophthalmol. Vis. Sci.* **2008**, *49*, 2903–2910. [CrossRef]
13. Jones, L.A.; Sinnott, L.T.; Mutti, D.O.; Mitchell, G.L.; Moeschberger, M.L.; Zadnik, K. Parental history of myopia, sports and outdoor activities, and future myopia. *Investig. Ophthalmol. Vis. Sci.* **2007**, *48*, 3524–3532. [CrossRef] [PubMed]
14. Wu, P.C.; Chen, C.T.; Lin, K.K.; Sun, C.C.; Kuo, C.N.; Huang, H.M.; Poon, Y.C.; Yang, M.L.; Chen, C.Y.; Huang, J.C.; et al. Myopia Prevention and Outdoor Light Intensity in a School-Based Cluster Randomized Trial. *Ophthalmology* **2018**, *125*, 1239–1250. [CrossRef]
15. Cao, K.; Wan, Y.; Yusufu, M.; Wang, N. Significance of Outdoor Time for Myopia Prevention: A Systematic Review and Meta-Analysis Based on Randomized Controlled Trials. *Ophthalmic Res.* **2020**, *63*, 97–105. [CrossRef]
16. Jin, J.X.; Hua, W.J.; Jiang, X.; Wu, X.Y.; Yang, J.W.; Gao, G.P.; Fang, Y.; Pei, C.L.; Wang, S.; Zhang, J.Z.; et al. Effect of outdoor activity on myopia onset and progression in school-aged children in northeast China: The Sujiatun Eye Care Study. *BMC Ophthalmol.* **2015**, *15*, 73. [CrossRef]
17. He, M.; Xiang, F.; Zeng, Y.; Mai, J.; Chen, Q.; Zhang, J.; Smith, W.; Rose, K.; Morgan, I.G. Effect of Time Spent Outdoors at School on the Development of Myopia Among Children in China: A Randomized Clinical Trial. *JAMA* **2015**, *314*, 1142–1148. [CrossRef]
18. Wu, P.C.; Chen, C.T.; Chang, L.C.; Niu, Y.Z.; Chen, M.L.; Liao, L.L.; Rose, K.; Morgan, I.G. Increased Time Outdoors Is Followed by Reversal of the Long-Term Trend to Reduced Visual Acuity in Taiwan Primary School Students. *Ophthalmology* **2020**, *127*, 1462–1469. [CrossRef]
19. Torii, H.; Kurihara, T.; Seko, Y.; Negishi, K.; Ohnuma, K.; Inaba, T.; Kawashima, M.; Jiang, X.; Kondo, S.; Miyauchi, M.; et al. Violet Light Exposure Can Be a Preventive Strategy Against Myopia Progression. *EBioMedicine* **2017**, *15*, 210–219. [CrossRef] [PubMed]
20. Hung, L.F.; Arumugam, B.; She, Z.; Ostrin, L.; Smith, E.L., 3rd. Narrow-band, long-wavelength lighting promotes hyperopia and retards vision-induced myopia in infant rhesus monkeys. *Exp. Eye Res.* **2018**, *176*, 147–160.
21. Gawne, T.J.; Ward, A.H.; Norton, T.T. Long-wavelength (red) light produces hyperopia in juvenile and adolescent tree shrews. *Vis. Res.* **2017**, *140*, 55–65. [CrossRef]
22. Foulds, W.S.; Barathi, V.A.; Luu, C.D. Progressive myopia or hyperopia can be induced in chicks and reversed by manipulation of the chromaticity of ambient light. *Investig. Ophthalmol. Vis. Sci.* **2013**, *54*, 8004–8012. [CrossRef]
23. Kröger, R.H.; Fernald, R.D. Regulation of eye growth in the African cichlid fish Haplochromis burtoni. *Vis. Res.* **1994**, *34*, 1807–1814. [CrossRef]
24. Strickland, R.; Landis, E.G.; Pardue, M.T. Short-Wavelength (Violet) Light Protects Mice From Myopia Through Cone Signaling. *Investig. Ophthalmol. Vis. Sci.* **2020**, *61*, 13. [CrossRef]
25. Zou, L.; Zhu, X.; Liu, R.; Ma, F.; Yu, M.; Liu, H.; Dai, J. Effect of Altered Retinal Cones/Opsins on Refractive Development under Monochromatic Lights in Guinea Pigs. *J. Ophthalmol.* **2018**, *2018*, 9197631. [CrossRef]
26. Jiang, X.; Pardue, M.T.; Mori, K.; Ikeda, S.I.; Torii, H.; D'Souza, S.; Lang, R.A.; Kurihara, T.; Tsubota, K. Violet light suppresses lens-induced myopia via neuropsin (OPN5) in mice. *Proc. Natl. Acad. Sci. USA* **2021**, *118*, e2018840118. [CrossRef]
27. Nguyen, M.T.; Vemaraju, S.; Nayak, G.; Odaka, Y.; Buhr, E.D.; Alonzo, N.; Tran, U.; Batie, M.; Upton, B.A.; Darvas, M.; et al. An opsin 5-dopamine pathway mediates light-dependent vascular development in the eye. *Nat. Cell Biol.* **2019**, *21*, 420–429. [CrossRef] [PubMed]
28. Torii, H.; Ohnuma, K.; Kurihara, T.; Tsubota, K.; Negishi, K. Violet Light Transmission is Related to Myopia Progression in Adult High Myopia. *Sci. Rep.* **2017**, *7*, 14523. [CrossRef]
29. Tarttelin, E.E.; Bellingham, J.; Hankins, M.W.; Foster, R.G.; Lucas, R.J. Neuropsin (Opn5): A novel opsin identified in mammalian neural tissue. *FEBS Lett.* **2003**, *554*, 410–416. [CrossRef]
30. Zhang, K.X.; D'Souza, S.; Upton, B.A.; Kernodle, S.; Vemaraju, S.; Nayak, G.; Gaitonde, K.D.; Holt, A.L.; Linne, C.D.; Smith, A.N.; et al. Violet-light suppression of thermogenesis by opsin 5 hypothalamic neurons. *Nature* **2020**, *585*, 420–425. [CrossRef]
31. Kanda, H.; Oshika, T.; Hiraoka, T.; Hasebe, S.; Ohno-Matsui, K.; Ishiko, S.; Hieda, O.; Torii, H.; Varnas, S.R.; Fujikado, T. Effect of spectacle lenses designed to reduce relative peripheral hyperopia on myopia progression in Japanese children: A 2-year multicenter randomized controlled trial. *Jpn. J. Ophthalmol.* **2018**, *62*, 537–543. [CrossRef] [PubMed]
32. Li, S.M.; Wu, S.S.; Kang, M.T.; Liu, Y.; Jia, S.M.; Li, S.Y.; Zhan, S.Y.; Liu, L.R.; Li, H.; Chen, W.; et al. Atropine slows myopia progression more in Asian than white children by meta-analysis. *Optom. Vis. Sci.* **2014**, *91*, 342–350. [CrossRef]
33. Hsu, C.C.; Huang, N.; Lin, P.Y.; Fang, S.Y.; Tsai, D.C.; Chen, S.Y.; Tsai, C.Y.; Woung, L.C.; Chiou, S.H.; Liu, C.J. Risk factors for myopia progression in second-grade primary school children in Taipei: A population-based cohort study. *Br. J. Ophthalmol.* **2017**, *101*, 1611–1617. [CrossRef]

34. Matsumura, S.; Lanca, C.; Htoon, H.M.; Brennan, N.; Tan, C.S.; Kathrani, B.; Chia, A.; Tan, D.; Sabanayagam, C.; Saw, S.M. Annual Myopia Progression and Subsequent 2-Year Myopia Progression in Singaporean Children. *Transl. Vis. Sci. Technol.* **2020**, *9*, 12. [CrossRef] [PubMed]
35. Smith, E.L., 3rd; Hung, L.F.; Arumugam, B.; Holden, B.A.; Neitz, M.; Neitz, J. Effects of Long-Wavelength Lighting on Refractive Development in Infant Rhesus Monkeys. *Investig. Ophthalmol. Vis. Sci.* **2015**, *56*, 6490–6500. [CrossRef]
36. Liu, R.; Qian, Y.F.; He, J.C.; Hu, M.; Zhou, X.T.; Dai, J.H.; Qu, X.M.; Chu, R.Y. Effects of different monochromatic lights on refractive development and eye growth in guinea pigs. *Exp. Eye Res.* **2011**, *92*, 447–453. [CrossRef]
37. Jiang, L.; Zhang, S.; Schaeffel, F.; Xiong, S.; Zheng, Y.; Zhou, X.; Lu, F.; Qu, J. Interactions of chromatic and lens-induced defocus during visual control of eye growth in guinea pigs (Cavia porcellus). *Vis. Res.* **2014**, *94*, 24–32. [CrossRef] [PubMed]
38. Fujikado, T.; Ninomiya, S.; Kobayashi, T.; Suzaki, A.; Nakada, M.; Nishida, K. Effect of low-addition soft contact lenses with decentered optical design on myopia progression in children: A pilot study. *Clin. Ophthalmol.* **2014**, *8*, 1947–1956. [CrossRef]
39. Lam, C.S.Y.; Tang, W.C.; Tse, D.Y.; Lee, R.P.K.; Chun, R.K.M.; Hasegawa, K.; Qi, H.; Hatanaka, T.; To, C.H. Defocus Incorporated Multiple Segments (DIMS) spectacle lenses slow myopia progression: A 2-year randomised clinical trial. *Br. J. Ophthalmol.* **2020**, *104*, 363–368. [CrossRef]
40. Hasebe, S.; Jun, J.; Varnas, S.R. Myopia control with positively aspherized progressive addition lenses: A 2-year, multicenter, randomized, controlled trial. *Investig. Ophthalmol. Vis. Sci.* **2014**, *55*, 7177–7188. [CrossRef]
41. Yang, Z.; Lan, W.; Ge, J.; Liu, W.; Chen, X.; Chen, L.; Yu, M. The effectiveness of progressive addition lenses on the progression of myopia in Chinese children. *Ophthalmic Physiol. Opt.* **2009**, *29*, 41–48. [PubMed]
42. Yam, J.C.; Jiang, Y.; Tang, S.M.; Law, A.K.P.; Chan, J.J.; Wong, E.; Ko, S.T.; Young, A.L.; Tham, C.C.; Chen, L.J.; et al. Low-Concentration Atropine for Myopia Progression (LAMP) Study: A Randomized, Double-Blinded, Placebo-Controlled Trial of 0.05%, 0.025%, and 0.01% Atropine Eye Drops in Myopia Control. *Ophthalmology* **2019**, *126*, 113–124. [CrossRef] [PubMed]
43. Hieda, O.; Hiraoka, T.; Fujikado, T.; Ishiko, S.; Hasebe, S.; Torii, H.; Takahashi, H.; Nakamura, Y.; Sotozono, C.; Oshika, T.; et al. Efficacy and safety of 0.01% atropine for prevention of childhood myopia in a 2-year randomized placebo-controlled study. *Jpn. J. Ophthalmol.* **2021**, *65*, 315–325. [CrossRef] [PubMed]

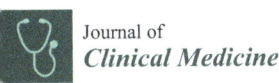

Article

Effects of 0.01% Atropine Instillation Assessed Using Swept-Source Anterior Segment Optical Coherence Tomography

Tadahiro Mitsukawa, Yumi Suzuki *, Yosuke Momota, Shun Suzuki and Masakazu Yamada

Department of Ophthalmology, Kyorin University School of Medicine, 6-20-2 Shinkawa, Mitaka, Tokyo 181-8611, Japan; mitsukawa@ks.kyorin-u.ac.jp (T.M.); momota@ks.kyorin-u.ac.jp (Y.M.); suzuki-s@ks.kyorin-u.ac.jp (S.S.); yamadamasakazu@ks.kyorin-u.ac.jp (M.Y.)
* Correspondence: yumis@ks.kyorin-u.ac.jp; Tel.: +81-422-47-5511; Fax: +81-422-46-9309

Abstract: In this paper, we assessed the short-term effects of 0.01% atropine eye drops on anterior segment parameters by performing ocular biometry using a swept-source anterior segment optical coherence tomography system (AS-OCT). We recruited 17 healthy volunteers (10 men and 7 women aged 24–35 years) with no history of eye disease. Participants without accommodative demand demonstrated significant mydriasis 1 h after the atropine instillation (4.58 ± 0.77 to 5.41 ± 0.83 mm). Pupil diameters with a 5 diopter (D) accommodative stimulus at 1 h (4.70 ± 1.13 mm) and 24 h (4.05 ± 1.06 mm) after atropine instillation were significantly larger than those at baseline (3.71 ± 0.84 mm). Barring pupil diameter, no other biometric parameters significantly changed at any point in time after atropine instillation without accommodative demand. However, with an accommodative stimulus, anterior chamber depth (ACD) at 1 h and posterior curvature of the lens at 1 and 24 h were both significantly larger than those before atropine instillation. Using AS-OCT, we detected a slight decrease in the accommodation response of ocular biometric components evoked by 0.01% atropine instillation. Morphologically, our measurements suggested a change in the ACD and horizontal radius of the lens' posterior surface curvatures due to the subtle reduction of accommodation.

Keywords: accommodation; anterior segment optical coherence tomography; low-concentration atropine; myopia; ocular biometric components

1. Introduction

Myopia is the leading cause of preventable visual impairment in childhood and adolescence [1,2]. An increasing prevalence of myopia has been reported in East and Southeast Asia, including China, Korea, and Japan [1–6]. In addition, the number of patients with myopia has increased in the United States and Europe, mainly among school-aged children and young adults [2,7,8]. As a result, the global prevalence of myopia, including pathologic myopia, is increasing, and has gained prominent attention as a social health problem. Complications resulting from myopia can incur large social and economic costs [9]. Therefore, the prevention of myopia progression has become increasingly important.

Myopia is generally present at the school-going age in patients. However, with the use of appropriate treatment modalities targeting children with myopia, it is possible to reduce the lifetime risk of retinal complications by reducing the severity of final myopia [10]. Several methods for the prevention of myopia progression have been reported to date, and they are broadly classified into nonpharmacological and pharmacological treatments. The former includes optical approaches such as the use of special spectacles, contact lenses, and orthokeratology [11–15]. The latter relies on the use of atropine eye drops, which are an established pharmacotherapy for the prevention of myopia progression [16–18].

Owing to its antimuscarinic action, atropine has long been used in ophthalmology in the form of 1% atropine eye drops for accommodation paralysis, and as an anti-inflammatory agent for conditions such as keratitis and iritis [19]. A study in 2006, Atropine for the Treatment of Myopia (ATOM-1), reported that the use of 1% atropine was effective in halting the progression of myopia [16]. However, over a 2 year period, the researchers observed photophobia resulting from dilated pupils and impaired near vision due to accommodation paralysis in eyes treated with 1% atropine. These side effects greatly interfered with the daily lives of patients. In addition to the rapid progression of myopia after discontinuation of the eye drops, a 1% concentration was considered inappropriate for myopia control [20]. As a result of this, that same research group subsequently conducted a study using various low-concentration atropine treatments. In 2012, they reported the results of a clinical study that assessed the inhibitory effect of atropine on myopia progression (ATOM-2), using 0.5%, 0.1%, and 0.01% atropine eye drops [17]. In their survey of the prevention of 2 year myopia progression, the researchers found that the group that received the lowest concentration of atropine (0.01%) achieved approximately half the inhibitory effect of the placebo group (−0.49 diopters (D) compared with −1.20 D). Furthermore, the instillation of 0.01% atropine resulted in minimal adverse reactions when compared with the instillation of 0.1% and 0.5% atropine [17]. Consequently, the use of low-concentration atropine to reduce myopia progression has garnered attention because of its limited effect on visual function. However, in the ATOM-2 study, Chia et al. [17] reported that a small proportion (6%) of the patients required combined photochromatic progressive glasses because they developed impaired near vision and photophobia. In a study of the use of low-concentration atropine for preventing myopia progression, Yam et al. [18] assessed patients using a visual function questionnaire and found that atropine instillation had no effect on general vision, near vision activities, social functioning, or color vision. Although the instillation of 0.01% atropine eye drops only has a subtle effect on the pupil diameter and accommodative amplitude, concerns remain regarding the undesirable effects of atropine on patients' daily life [17].

Nonetheless, there are limited data regarding the short-term effects of low-concentration atropine instillation on pupil diameter and accommodative function in young adult subjects [21]. In our previous study, we successfully analyzed ocular biometric components (OBCs), including changes in the crystalline lens during accommodation, and the effects of cycloplegics, using a commercially available anterior segment optical coherence tomography (AS-OCT) system [22]. In recent years, AS-OCT has been used for in vivo studies of ocular lens behavior during accommodation. A newly developed swept-source AS-OCT system (CASIA 2, Tomey Corp., Nagoya, Japan) has enabled detailed biometry measurements to be obtained from the corneal surface to the posterior surface of the lens by elongating the range of the imaging depth and increasing the sensitivity [23,24]. In the present study, we used the AS-OCT system to quantitatively evaluate the effects of 0.01% atropine eye drops on OBCs in the anterior segment of the eye.

The current study aims to determine how the instillation of 0.01% atropine produces morphological changes in the eye by assessing ocular biometric components (OBCs) before and after instillation, using anterior-segment optical coherence tomography.

2. Subjects and Methods

2.1. Participants

This study followed the guidelines outlined in the Declaration of Helsinki from the World Medical Association. All participants received a full explanation of the procedures and they provided written informed consent before they agreed to participate in the study. The study protocol was approved by the Institutional Review Board of Kyorin University School of Medicine (Project H30-099).

In this study, we examined young adults rather than children, as low-concentration atropine eyedrops for myopia have not been approved for children in Japan.

The study participants included 17 healthy volunteers (10 men and 7 women) aged 24–35 years (mean ± standard deviation: 28.9 ± 3.6 years). None of the participants had a history of eye disease, except for refractive errors, and all had a best-corrected visual acuity of 20/20 or better. The exclusion criteria were a history of any ocular disease, ophthalmic surgery, or laser treatment. We also excluded participants who were taking systemic medications that could affect accommodation.

We examined each participant's noncycloplegic refraction using an ARK-1 autorefractor (NIDEK Co. Ltd., Gamagori, Japan). We considered the effect that the degree of refractive error would give to accommodation factors, as 17 participants had refractive errors from approximately -11 D to 0 D [25]. However, in this study, to ensure participants' ability to accommodate 5 D or greater, we also examined the accommodation of the participants using the ARK-1 autorefractor.

2.2. Procedures and Assessments

We examined both eyes of all participants using the CASIA 2 swept-source AS-OCT system. The AS-OCT device has a swept-source laser that operates at a central wavelength of 1310 nm and a scan rate of 50,000 A-scans per second. The maximum imaging area is 16.0 mm × 16.0 mm, and the maximum imaging depth is 11.0 mm. This device enables simultaneous biometry measurements to be obtained for all anterior segment structures, including the cornea, anterior chamber, and crystalline lens.

All OCT images were obtained in a dimly lit examination room. During the measurements, the participants were instructed to fixate on the coaxial accommodative target image present in the OCT device. The negative or positive lens was set to compensate for the participant's spherical ametropia for near-equivalent spherical refractive correction. Next, we added a -5.0 D lens to stimulate physiological accommodation using an optical system in the OCT system. The active eye tracker of the OCT system was centered on the participant's eye. Two experienced operators (M.Y. and S.S.) collected all images.

Measurements were performed with and without a single instillation of 0.01% atropine eye drops. To prepare the 0.01% atropine eye drops, commercial 1% atropine sulfate hydrate (Nitten ATROPINE Ophthalmic Solution 1%; Nitten Pharmaceutical Co. Ltd., Nagoya, Japan) was diluted with saline. OCT images of the eye were obtained before instillation, and at 1, 24, and 48 h after instillation. The OBCs measured using AS-OCT included pupil diameter, anterior chamber depth (ACD), lens thickness (LT), and the horizontal radii of the lens' anterior curvature (LAC) and lens' posterior surface curvature (LPC). The boundaries of both the cornea and lens were outlined for anterior segment biometry. The positioning of the anterior and posterior surfaces of the lens on the horizontal meridian was traced, and the radius of the crystalline lens was determined using measurements that permitted circular fitting to the anterior and posterior lens surfaces.

The participants' accommodative amplitude was measured using the ARK-1 autorefractor before instillation, and at 1, 24, and 48 h after instillation of the 0.01% atropine eye drops.

Objective measurement of accommodation was performed with the participant focusing on a target that moved to a near point from a distance. Additionally, we conducted the measurement of participants' axial length using an optical axial length measuring device (OPTICAL BIOMETER OA-2000, Tomey Corp., Nagoya, Japan)

The participants were also instructed to answer questionnaires 1, 24, and 48 h after atropine administration about the difficulties they experienced with near vision and photophobia, separately, in which they rated their symptoms on a scale ranging from 0 (none) to 10 (inability to perform daily tasks).

2.3. Statistical Analysis

The Statistical Package for the Social Sciences version 27.0 for Windows (IBM Armonk, NY, USA) was used for all statistical analyses. The Mann–Whitney U test and Wilcoxon signed-rank test were used to perform comparisons. p-Values < 0.05 were considered to indicate statistical significance.

3. Results

3.1. Baseline Characteristics of the Participants

Table 1 presents the baseline biometric parameters of both eyes before the instillation of 0.01% atropine eye drops. The noncycloplegic refraction of the right eye ranged from −0.38 to −10.88 D, and that of the left eye ranged from +0.38 to −11.25 D; there was no significant difference in refraction between the right and left eyes ($p = 0.691$, Mann–Whitney U test). There was also no significant difference in accommodation between the right and left eyes, and both eyes were able to accommodate more than 5 D. We did not find any significant differences in any baseline biometric parameters between the right and left eyes before the instillation of 0.01% atropine eye drops (Mann–Whitney U test). Therefore, we present the findings of only the right eyes.

Table 1. Baseline biometric parameters of both eyes before instillation of 0.01% atropine eye drops.

	Right Eye		Left Eye		p-Value *
	Median	IQR	Median	IQR	
Baseline biometric parameter					
Spherical equivalent (D)	−5.88	6.50	−5.37	6.94	0.69
Axial length (mm)	25.39	2.37	25.45	2.52	0.95
Accommodation amplitude (D)	6.48	1.49	6.53	1.07	0.95
Central corneal thickness (μm)	537	42	527	42	0.97
Anterior chamber depth (mm)	3.28	0.35	3.33	0.31	0.62
Pupil diameter (mm)	4.38	1.26	4.59	0.79	0.55
Lens thickness (mm)	3.61	0.25	3.61	0.27	0.96
Radius of the lens' anterior surface curvature (mm)	11.65	1.97	12.04	3.39	0.57
Radius of the lens' posterior surface curvature (mm)	5.73	0.60	5.81	0.67	0.86

IQR, interquartile range; D, diopters; * Mann–Whitney U test.

3.2. Effects of 0.01% Atropine on Pupil Diameter

Figure 1a presents a comparison of pupil diameters in the relaxed state, and those with the 5 D accommodative stimulus, before and 1, 24, and 48 h after instillation of 0.01% atropine eye drops. The pupil diameter was significantly larger 1 h after atropine instillation than before the atropine instillation (from 4.58 ± 0.77 to 5.41 ± 0.83 mm) in the relaxed state ($p < 0.05$, Wilcoxon signed-rank test). With the 5 D accommodative stimulus, the pupil diameter at 1 and 24 h was significantly larger than that before atropine instillation (from 3.71 ± 0.84 mm to 4.70 ± 1.13 and 4.05 ± 1.06 mm, respectively, $p < 0.05$, Wilcoxon signed-rank test). In contrast, there was no significant difference in the pupil diameter 24 and 48 h after atropine instillation compared with that before atropine instillation in the relaxed state, or in the pupil diameter 48 h after atropine instillation compared to before atropine instillation with the 5 D accommodative stimulus.

3.3. Effects of Atropine on Other Biometric Parameters Measured Using AS-OCT

Figure 1b–e shows a comparison of biometric parameters (ACD, LT, LAC, LPC) between before and 1, 24, and 48 h after the instillation of 0.01% atropine eye drops in the relaxed state and with the 5 D accommodative stimulus. Other than pupil diameter, none of the biometric parameters showed changes in the relaxed state at any point in time when compared to before the instillation.

However, with the 5 D accommodative stimulus, ACD at 1 h was significantly larger than that before the instillation (from 3.08 ± 0.16 mm to 3.10 ± 0.18 mm, $p < 0.05$). LPC at 1 and 24 h was significantly larger than that before the instillation (from 5.21 ± 0.43 mm to 5.36 ± 0.35 and 5.50 ± 0.50 mm, respectively, $p < 0.05$).

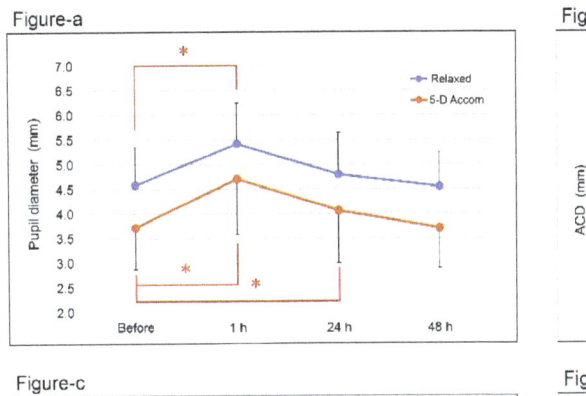
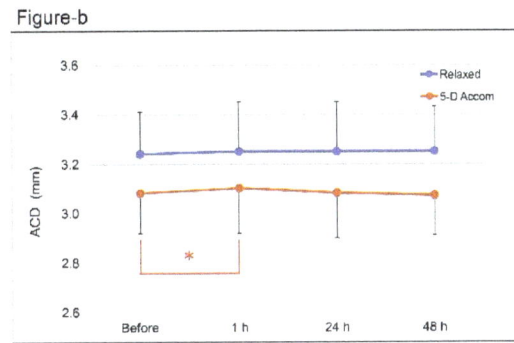
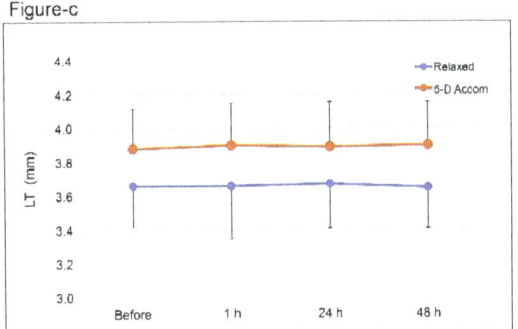
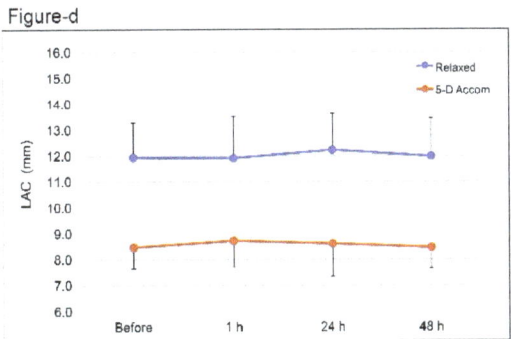
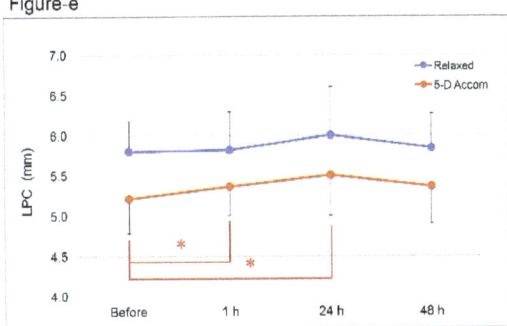

* $P < 0.05$ (Wilcoxon signed-rank test)

Figure 1. Change in biometric parameters after the instillation of 0.01% atropine eye drops. Shown is a comparison of the biometric parameters in the relaxed state (Relaxed) and with the 5 D accommodative stimulus (5-D Accom) before and 1, 24, and 48 h after instillation of 0.01% atropine eye drops. (**a**) The pupil diameter increased significantly 1 h after instillation in the relaxed state but returned to the pre-instillation level at 24 h. With the 5 D accommodative stimulus, the pupil diameter significantly increased at 1 and 24 h but returned to the pre-instillation level at 48 h. (**b**–**e**) In the non-accommodative eyes, none of the assessed biometric parameters (ACD, LT, LAC, LPC), with the exception of pupil diameter, showed changes at any time point when compared to that before the instillation. However, with the 5 D accommodative stimulus, ACD significantly increased at 1 h (**b**) and LPC significantly increased at 1 and 24 h (**e**) after atropine instillation when compared with that before instillation ($p < 0.05$). D, diopter; ACD, anterior chamber depth; LT, lens thickness; LAC, horizontal radius of the lens' anterior surface curvature; LPC, horizontal radius of the lens' posterior surface curvature. * $p < 0.05$, Wilcoxon signed-rank test.

3.4. Effects of Atropine on Refraction, Accommodation Amplitude, and Subjective Symptoms

Table 2 shows the spherical equivalent 1, 24, and 48 h after the instillation of 0.01% atropine eye drops. There were no significant changes in the mean spherical equivalent from the values before the instillation ($p = 0.10$, $p = 0.86$, and $p = 0.55$, respectively).

Table 2. Change in refraction, accommodation amplitude, and subjective symptoms after the instillation of 0.01% atropine eye drops.

	Pre-Instillation		1 h after Ocular Instillation		24 h after Ocular Instillation		48 h after Ocular Instillation	
	Median	IQR	Median	IQR	Median	IQR	Median	IQR
Spherical equivalent (D)	−5.88	6.50	−6.25 (p, 0.10)	6.44	−6.13 (p, 0.86)	6.13	−6.13 (p, 0.55)	6.19
Accommodation amplitude (D)	6.48	1.49	6.49 (p, 0.76)	1.38	6.40 (p, 0.50)	1.09	6.59 (p, 0.07)	1.00
Subjective symptoms	0.00	0.00	0.00 (p, 0.11)	0.00	0.00	0.00	0.00	0.00

D, diopters; h, hour; p, p-value (Wilcoxon signed-rank test).

Table 2 shows the accommodative amplitudes 1, 24, and 48 h after the instillation of 0.01% atropine eye drops. There were no significant changes in the mean accommodative amplitude at any point in time when compared with that before the instillation ($p = 0.76$, $p = 0.50$, and $p = 0.07$, respectively).

In terms of the two subjective symptoms, we found no serious adverse events related to atropine. None of the participants reported photophobic sensation, although three participants reported mild difficulty with near vision (rated as 1/10 and 3/10 in one and two participants, respectively) 1 h after the atropine instillation.

4. Discussion

Recent studies have shown that atropine effectively inhibits the progression of myopia and axial elongation [16–18,26,27]. Treatment guidelines for the inhibition of myopia progression, developed by Wu et al. [27], ranked low-concentration atropine eye drops as the key component to successful inhibition. The reported side effects of low-concentration atropine eye drops were limited to photophobia due to mydriasis and impaired near vision resulting from the impairment of accommodative amplitude [17,18,21]. Although these adverse events were rare and mild, objective measurements of changes in OBCs after 0.01% atropine instillation might be important. With this background in mind, we assessed the effects of low-concentration atropine eye drops on OBCs using AS-OCT. Our results revealed significant but subtle changes in OBCs.

In our previous study, we used a commercially available AS-OCT system (CASIA 2) to measure the OBCs, including lens parameters [22]. This system enables detailed biometric measurements to be obtained from the corneal surface to the posterior lens surface by increasing the range of the imaging depth and improving performance sensitivity [23,24]. Our prior study revealed an increase in LT and a decrease in ACD, LAC, and LPC with accommodation, which suggested that steepening and anterior movement of the lens during accommodation occurred. After the application of cycloplegics (cyclopentolate), there was a decrease in LT, which resulted in an equivalent increase in ACD [22]. Therefore, the CASIA 2 swept-source AS-OCT system could detect changes in OBCs during accommodation.

Accordingly, we used the same technique in this study to assess OBCs before and 1, 24, and 48 h after the instillation of 0.01% atropine. Although no participants reported photophobic sensations, 0.01% atropine had a minor effect on pupil diameter. While the pupil diameter increased significantly 1 h after instillation in a relaxed pupil state, it returned to the pre-instillation level at 24 h. The pupil diameters at 1 and 24 h were significantly larger with a 5 D accommodative stimulus, but they returned to the pre-instillation level at 48 h. Kaymak et al. [21] reported the short-term effects of 0.01% atropine instillation on pupil diameter and accommodation amplitude in 14 young adults. The reported pupil diameters before and 24 h after instillation were 3.3 ± 0.5 and 3.9 ± 0.8 mm, respectively, which indicated a significant increase ($p < 0.02$). Our study also confirmed that instillation of 0.01% atropine caused a slight and transient increase in pupil diameter.

In the relaxed state, none of the assessed OBCs (ACD, LT, LAC, and LPC), other than pupil diameter, showed significant changes at any of the assessed points in time compared to before the instillation. In contrast, with the 5 D accommodative stimulus, ACD 1 h and LPC 1 and 24 h after atropine instillation were significantly larger than those before the treatment ($p < 0.05$). However, there were no differences in either LT or LAC. Therefore, we confirmed that the cycloplegic effect following the instillation of 0.01% atropine eye drops was marginal. Our results suggest that measuring OBCs using the AS-OCT system is useful for detecting subtle changes that result from low-concentration atropine instillation. The AS-OCT results corresponded with the measurement of the accommodation amplitude. In our study, we found no decrease in the accommodation amplitude as a result of the instillation of 0.01% atropine. Only a few participants reported experiencing some difficulties with near vision 1 h after atropine instillation. Similarly, Kaymak et al. [21] reported no difference in the accommodation amplitude before and 24 h after 0.01% atropine instillation ($p = 0.06$).

Our study has some limitations. First, the participants were young adults rather than school-aged children, which could have influenced the results. Low-concentration atropine instillation has been used to inhibit myopia progression in school- and preschool-aged children to address the trend of early-onset myopia and the increase in the number of preschool- and school-aged patients with myopia. In this respect, the ocular permeability of atropine and its pharmacokinetics might differ between children and adults. The accommodation amplitude also differs between school-aged children and young adults. Hence, as the participants were young adults aged 24-35 years, the results might not be directly applicable to school-aged children. Second, we observed only the short-term effects of a single instillation of 0.01% atropine. Our study showed that at a dose of 0.01% atropine, short-term effects included a slight increase in pupil diameter and minor accommodation paralysis. However, the long-term effects of low-concentration atropine instillation are not clear, and further studies are needed to clarify this issue. Third, similar to most other studies using AS-OCT, we were unable to analyze the entire lens shape through the pupil [28–33]. Because of the variability in the measurements and the asphericity of the lens, the curvature radius obtained by fitting the circular curve might not precisely express the shape of the lens. Finally, although the effect of atropine eye drops on vergence reactions should have been evaluated, we did not examine this in the present study.

In conclusion, we assessed the effects of 0.01% atropine eye drops by performing ocular biometry using the CASIA 2 AS-OCT system. Similar to the findings in previous reports, we did not observe significant photophobia or subjective difficulty in near vision. However, our measurements did suggest a change in the pupil diameter, ACD, and LPC, which are part of the assessed OBCs, which resulted from a subtle reduction in accommodation. In other words, morphologically, we were able to confirm an increase in the pupil diameter and a decrease in the accommodation response of OBCs with a 5 D accommodative stimulus following the instillation of 0.01% atropine. Moreover, we demonstrated that AS-OCT could evaluate subtle changes evoked by low-concentration atropine administration.

Author Contributions: Conceptualization, Y.S. and M.Y.; methodology, T.M., Y.S. and M.Y.; software, Y.M.; validation, Y.S. and M.Y.; formal analysis, Y.S.; investigation, S.S. and Y.M.; resources, M.Y.; data curation, Y.S.; writing—original draft preparation, Y.S.; writing—review and editing, T.M., Y.S. and M.Y.; visualization, T.M. and Y.S.; supervision, M.Y.; project administration, T.M., Y.S. and M.Y.; funding acquisition, M.Y. All authors have read and agreed to the published version of the manuscript.

Funding: This research was supported by a grant from the Ministry of Health, Labour and Welfare, Japan (Grant number 19FA1010).

Institutional Review Board Statement: This study followed the guidelines outlined by the Declaration of Helsinki of the World Medical Association. The study protocol was approved by the Institutional Review Board of Kyorin University School of Medicine (project H30-099).

Informed Consent Statement: All participants received a full explanation of the procedures and provided written informed consent before agreeing to participate in the study.

Data Availability Statement: All data relevant to this study were included in the article.

Conflicts of Interest: The authors declare no conflict of interest. The funders had no role in the design of the study; in the collection, analysis, or interpretation of data; in the writing of the manuscript; or in the decision to publish the results.

References

1. Morgan, I.; Ohno Matsui, K.; Saw, S. Myopia. *Lancet* **2012**, *379*, 1739–1748. [CrossRef]
2. Holden, B.A.; Jong, M.; Davis, S.; Wilson, D.; Fricke, T.; Resnikoff, S. Nearly 1 billion myopes at risk of myopia-related sight-threatening conditions by 2050—Time to act now. *Clin. Exp. Optom.* **2015**, *98*, 491–493. [CrossRef]
3. Jung, S.; Lee, J.; Kakizaki, H.; Jee, D. Prevalence of myopia and its association with body stature and educational level in 19-year-old male conscripts in seoul, south korea. *Investig. Ophthalmol. Vis. Sci.* **2012**, *53*, 5579–5583. [CrossRef] [PubMed]
4. Lee, Y.; Lo, C.; Sheu, S.; Lin, J. What factors are associated with myopia in young adults? A survey study in taiwan military conscripts. *Investig. Ophthalmol. Vis. Sci.* **2013**, *54*, 1026–1033. [CrossRef]
5. Sun, J.; Zhou, J.; Zhao, P.; Lian, J.; Zhu, H.; Zhou, Y.; Sun, Y.; Wang, Y.; Zhao, L.; Wei, Y.; et al. High prevalence of myopia and high myopia in 5060 chinese university students in shanghai. *Investig. Ophthalmol. Vis. Sci.* **2012**, *53*, 7504–7509. [CrossRef] [PubMed]
6. Wu, J.F.; Bi, H.S.; Wang, S.M.; Hu, Y.Y.; Wu, H.; Sun, W.; Lu, T.L.; Wang, X.R.; Jonas, J.B. Refractive error, visual acuity and causes of vision loss in children in shandong, china. the shandong children eye study. *PLoS ONE* **2013**, *8*, e82763. [CrossRef] [PubMed]
7. Vitale, S.; Sperduto, R.D.; Ferris, F.L. Increased prevalence of myopia in the united states between 1971–1972 and 1999–2004. *Arch. Ophthalmol.* **2009**, *127*, 1632–1639. [CrossRef] [PubMed]
8. Dayan, Y.B.; Levin, A.; Morad, Y.; Grotto, I.; Ben-David, R.; Goldberg, A.; Onn, E.; Avni, I.; Levi, Y.; Benyamini, O.G. The changing prevalence of myopia in young adults: A 13-year series of population-based prevalence surveys. *Investig. Ophthalmol. Vis. Sci.* **2005**, *46*, 2760–2765. [CrossRef] [PubMed]
9. Rudnicka, A.R.; Kapetanakis, V.V.; Wathern, A.K.; Logan, N.S.; Gilmartin, B.; Whincup, P.H.; Cook, D.G.; Owen, C.G. Global variations and time trends in the prevalence of childhood myopia, a systematic review and quantitative meta-analysis: Implications for aetiology and early prevention. *Br. J. Ophthalmol.* **2016**, *100*, 882–890. [CrossRef]
10. Dolgin, E. The myopia boom. *Nature* **2015**, *519*, 276–278. [CrossRef]
11. Gwiazda, J.; Hyman, L.; Hussein, M.; Everett, D.; Norton, T.T.; Kurtz, D.; Leske, M.C.; Manny, R.; Marsh-Tootle, W.; Scheiman, M.; et al. A randomized clinical trial of progressive addition lenses versus single vision lenses on the progression of myopia in children. *Investig. Ophthalmol. Vis. Sci.* **2003**, *44*, 1492–1500. [CrossRef]
12. Zhu, Q.; Liu, Y.; Tighe, S.; Zhu, Y.; Su, X.; Lu, F.; Hu, M. Retardation of myopia progression by multifocal soft contact lenses. *Int. J. Med. Sci.* **2019**, *16*, 198–202. [CrossRef]
13. Hiraoka, T.; Sekine, Y.; Okamoto, F.; Mihashi, T.; Oshika, T. Safety and efficacy following 10-years of overnight orthokeratology for myopia control. *Ophthalmic Physiol. Opt.* **2018**, *38*, 281–289. [CrossRef]
14. VanderVeen, D.K.; Kraker, R.T.; Pineles, S.L.; Hutchinson, A.K.; Wilson, L.B.; Galvin, J.A.; Lambert, S.R. Use of orthokeratology for the prevention of myopic progression in children: A report by the american academy of ophthalmology. *Ophthalmology* **2019**, *126*, 623–636. [CrossRef] [PubMed]
15. Prousali, E.; Haidich, A.B.; Fontalis, A.; Ziakas, N.; Brazitikos, P.; Mataftsi, A. Efficacy and safety of interventions to control myopia progression in children: An overview of systematic reviews and meta-analyses. *BMC Ophthalmol.* **2019**, *19*, 106. [CrossRef] [PubMed]
16. Chua, W.H.; Balakrishnan, V.; Chan, Y.H.; Tong, L.; Ling, Y.; Quah, B.L.; Tan, D. Atropine for the treatment of childhood myopia. *Ophthalmology* **2006**, *113*, 2285–2291. [CrossRef] [PubMed]
17. Chia, A.; Chua, W.H.; Cheung, Y.B.; Wong, W.L.; Lingham, A.; Fong, A.; Tan, D. Atropine for the treatment of childhood myopia: Safety and efficacy of 0.5%, 0.1%, and 0.01% doses (atropine for the treatment of myopia 2). *Ophthalmology* **2012**, *119*, 347–354. [CrossRef]
18. Yam, J.C.; Jiang, Y.; Tang, S.M.; Law, A.K.; Chan, J.J.; Wong, E.; Ko, S.T.; Young, A.L.; Tham, C.C.; Chen, L.J.; et al. Low-concentration atropine for myopia progression (LAMP) study: A randomized, double-blinded, placebo-controlled trial of 0.05%, 0.025%, and 0.01% atropine eye drops in myopia control. *Ophthalmology* **2019**, *126*, 113–124. [CrossRef]
19. Mauger, T.F.; Craig, E.L.; Havener, W.H. *Havener's Ocular Pharmacology*, 6th ed.; Mosby-Year Book: St. Louis, MI, USA, 1994; pp. 140–146.
20. Tong, L.; Huang, X.L.; Koh, A.L.; Zhang, X.; Tan, D.T.; Chua, W.H. Atropine for the treatment of childhood myopia: Effect on myopia progression after cessation of atropine. *Ophthalmology* **2009**, *116*, 572–579. [CrossRef] [PubMed]

21. Kaymak, H.; Fricke, A.; Mauritz, Y.; Löwinger, A.; Klabe, K.; Breyer, D.; Lagenbucher, A.; Seitz, B.; Schaeffel, F. Short-term effects of low-concentration atropine eye drops on pupil size and accommodation in young adult subjects. *Graefes Arch. Clin. Exp. Ophthalmol.* **2018**, *256*, 2211–2217. [CrossRef]
22. Mitsukawa, T.; Suzuki, Y.; Momota, Y.; Suzuki, S.; Yamada, M. Anterior segment biometry during accommodation and effects of cycloplegics by swept-source optical coherence tomography. *Clin. Ophthalmol.* **2020**, *14*, 1237–1243. [CrossRef]
23. Shoji, T.; Kato, N.; Ishikawa, S.; Ibuki, H.; Yamada, N.; Kimura, I.; Shinoda, K. In vivo crystalline lens measurements with novel swept-source optical coherent tomography: An investigation on variability of measurement. *BMJ Open Ophthalmol.* **2017**, *1*, e000058. [CrossRef]
24. Shoji, T.; Kato, N.; Ishikawa, S.; Ibuki, H.; Yamada, N.; Kimura, I.; Shinoda, K. Association between axial length and in vivo human crystalline lens biometry during accommodation: A swept-source optical coherence tomography study. *Jpn. J. Ophthalmol.* **2020**, *64*, 93–101. [CrossRef]
25. Millodot, M. The effect of refractive error on the accommodative response gradient: A summary and update. *Ophthalmic Physiol.Opt.* **2015**, *35*, 607–612. [CrossRef]
26. Li, F.; Yam, J. Low-concentration atropine eye drops for myopia progression. *Asia-Pac. J. Ophthalmol. (Phila)* **2019**, *8*, 360–365. [CrossRef]
27. Wu, P.C.; Chuang, M.N.; Choi, J.; Chen, H.; Wu, G.; Ohno-Matsui, K.; Jonas, J.B.; Cheung, C.M.G. Update in myopia and treatment strategy of atropine use in myopia control. *Eye* **2019**, *33*, 3–13. [CrossRef] [PubMed]
28. Du, C.; Shen, M.; Li, M.; Zhu, D.; Wang, M.R.; Wang, J. Anterior segment biometry during accommodation imaged with ultralong scan depth optical coherence tomography. *Ophthalmology* **2012**, *119*, 2479–2485. [CrossRef] [PubMed]
29. Gambra, E.; Ortiz, S.; Perez-Merino, P.; Gora, M.; Wojtkowski, M.; Marcos, S. Static and dynamic crystalline lens accommodation evaluated using quantitative 3-D OCT. *Biomed. Opt. Express* **2013**, *4*, 1595–1609. [CrossRef] [PubMed]
30. Zhong, J.; Tao, A.; Xu, Z.; Jiang, H.; Shao, Y.; Zhang, H.; Liu, C.; Wang, J. Whole eye axial biometry during accommodation using ultra-long scan depth optical coherence tomography. *Am. J. Ophthalmol.* **2014**, *157*, 1064–1069. [CrossRef] [PubMed]
31. Sun, Y.; Fan, S.; Zheng, H.; Dai, C.; Ren, Q.; Zhou, C. Noninvasive imaging and measurement of accommodation using dual-channel SD-OCT. *Curr. Eye Res.* **2014**, *39*, 611–619. [CrossRef]
32. Zhang, J.; Ni, Y.; Li, P.; Sun, W.; Liu, M.; Guo, D.; Du, C. Anterior segment biometry with phenylephrine and tropicamide during accommodation imaged with ultralong scan depth optical coherence tomography. *J. Ophthalmol.* **2019**, *2019*, 6827215. [CrossRef] [PubMed]
33. Neri, A.; Ruggeri, M.; Protti, A.; Leaci, R.; Gandolfi, S.A.; Macaluso, C. Dynamic imaging of accommodation by swept-source anterior segment optical coherence tomography. *J. Cataract. Refract. Surg.* **2015**, *41*, 501–510. [CrossRef] [PubMed]

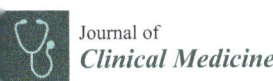

Journal of
Clinical Medicine

Article

Impact of the Pressure-Free Yutori Education Program on Myopia in Japan

Satoshi Ishiko [1,*], Hiroyuki Kagokawa [2], Noriko Nishikawa [3], Youngseok Song [3], Kazuhiro Sugawara [3], Hiroaki Nakagawa [3], Yuichiro Kawamura [4] and Akitoshi Yoshida [3]

[1] Department of Medicine and Engineering Combined Research Institute, Asahikawa Medical University, Asahikawa 078-8510, Hokkaido, Japan
[2] Asahikawa Red Cross Hospital, Asahikawa 070-8530, Hokkaido, Japan; hkago@asahikawa-rch.gr.jp
[3] Department of Ophthalmology, Asahikawa Medical University, Asahikawa 078-8510, Hokkaido, Japan; nnori@asahikawa-med.ac.jp (N.N.); ysong@asahikawa-med.ac.jp (Y.S.); k-sugawara@asahikawa-med.ac.jp (K.S.); nakagawa@asahikawa-med.ac.jp (H.N.); pyoshida@asahikawa-med.ac.jp (A.Y.)
[4] Health Administration Center, Asahikawa Medical University, Asahikawa 078-8510, Hokkaido, Japan; yk5610@asahikawa-med.ac.jp
* Correspondence: ishiko@asahikawa-med.ac.jp

Abstract: This study aimed to investigate the influence of educational pressure on myopia. A less-intense school curriculum was introduced nationally in Japan beginning in 2012 based on a pressure-free education policy. In this retrospective observational study, a total of 1025 Japanese medical students of Asahikawa Medical University underwent measurements of the cycloplegic refractive error and axial length (AL), from 2011 to 2020. The spherical equivalent (SE) and AL were correlated significantly with the fiscal year of births ($p = 0.004$ and $p = 0.034$, respectively) only during enforcement of the system of high-pressure education. The SE and AL regression rates during the two educational approaches differed significantly ($p = 0.004$ and $p = 0.037$, respectively). The prevalence of high myopia was correlated significantly ($p < 0.001$) only during the system of high-pressure education. The regression of the prevalence rate of high myopia during the two education approaches differed significantly ($p = 0.010$). The progression rates of myopia and increased prevalence of high myopia were observed only during high-pressure education, suggesting that not only ophthalmologists but also educators and the government should work on together to control the progression of myopia.

Keywords: prevalence of myopia; degree of myopia; high-pressure education; pressure-free education; Yutori education

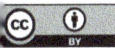

1. Introduction

The prevalence rates of myopia and high myopia have increased dramatically in the past 50 to 60 years, especially in developed countries in east and southeast Asia [1–5]. Recently, the coronavirus disease (COVID-19) had led to an unprecedented global pandemic. To contain COVID-19, strict containment measures were imposed internationally, including social-distancing regulations, limited outdoor gatherings, school closures, and switching from in-person education to online, home-based learning. With the implementation of these measures, citizens spent more time using digital devices for entertainment and education. The rapid increase in digital screen time may potentially lead to a rise of myopia rates worldwide, especially in Asia. A meta-analysis suggested that myopia and high myopia would develop in, respectively, 50% and 10% of the world's population by 2050 [6]. High myopia increases the risk of ocular conditions with serious visual impairment, such as retinal detachments, macular holes, glaucoma, and myopia macular degeneration [7–9]. In addition, early onset of myopia is associated with higher final myopia [10–12]. Therefore, prevention of myopia progression needs to begin at younger ages. Although the etiology of the onset and progression of myopia remains unclarified, education as one of the environmental factors has been reported to be correlated with them [13–15], and school curriculum consisting of greater amounts of near work is associated with a higher rate of myopia [15–17].

In Japan, graduating from a good university is a guarantee of joining a good company, and this has driven the "education-background society" and "exam hell". The university entrance examinations have been the dominant factor in Japanese education. Therefore, the educational system in Japan had been characterized by cramming, e.g., rote learning, drilling, testing, etc., the so-called high-pressure educational practices. However, these have resulted in school dropout, bullying, school absenteeism, violence, and classroom collapse. To solve these educational problems, a less-intense school curriculum for the first nine years of compulsory education was introduced nationally based on a pressure-free or relaxed education policy, the so-called "Yutori" educational policy in Japan, from fiscal year (FY) 2002 [18,19]. This approach sought to create a relaxed learning environment for children by reducing classroom hours and learning content. The classroom hours gradually decreased from 8935 h to 8307 h during elementary school and junior high school until FY 2012.

Furthermore, Japan also adopted a five-day school week, with cessation of Saturday classes. Unexpectedly, this educational reform provided an opportunity to conduct a nationwide social experiment in Japan to study the impact of education on myopia.

To analyze the association between educational pressure and myopia, we investigated the refractive error, axial length (AL), and the prevalence rates of myopia and high myopia before and after the introduction of the Yutori educational policy in Japan.

2. Materials and Methods

2.1. Study Population

A total of 1025 Japanese medical students of Asahikawa Medical University participated. The students underwent ophthalmic examinations to measure the refractive error and AL and determine the status of the fundus during the clinical clerkship for ophthalmology, conducted over 10 years from April 2011 to February 2020. All investigations in this study adhered to the tenets of the Declaration of Helsinki; Institutional Review Board/Ethics Committee of Asahikawa Medical University approval was obtained. All participants provided informed consent before the examination.

In Japan, the FY runs from 2 April to 1 April of the following year. The FYs of the student births ranged from 1961 to 1997. The Yutori educational approach started from FY 2002, which corresponded to the FY of birth 1987. Additionally, the new educational system introduced from FY 2012, which corresponded to FY of birth 1997. Therefore, we excluded nine students who were born in or later than FY 1997.

Students who had undergone laser in-situ keratomileusis ($n = 9$), an eye surgery ($n = 2$), or had a history of wearing orthokeratology contact lens ($n = 1$) were excluded. We also excluded students if there were only one or two born in a particular FY ($n = 9$). After excluding these students, 995 (97.1%) were included in this study (Figure 1).

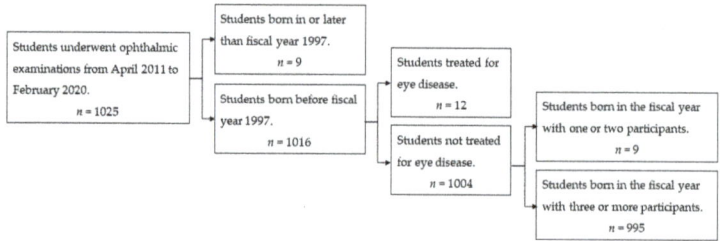

Figure 1. Study flowchart.

2.2. Measures

Sixty minutes after instillation of 0.5% tropicamide and 0.5% phenylephrine hydrochloride in the left eyes, students underwent the refractive error measurement using an autorefractometer (TONOREF RKT-7700, Nidek, Japan) with cycloplegic refraction and the axial length (AL) measurement using a partial coherence interferometry (IOL MASTER 500, Carl Zeiss Meditec, Oberkochen, Germany). The accuracy of the measurement for the autorefractometer was set at 0.01 diopter (D). For autorefraction measurements, the results were converted to the spherical equivalent (SE) (half the amount of cylinder plus the spherical component). Myopia was defined as a SE refractive error of −0.5 D or lower. High myopia was defined as a SE refractive error of −6.0 D or lower. All examinations were performed using the same device throughout the 10-year study period.

2.3. Statistical Methods

Gender differences in age, SE, and AL were evaluated using the unpaired t-test, and differences in the prevalence rates were compared using the chi-square test. We used regression analysis and analysis of covariance to compare the regression by FY of birth between before 1987 and after 1987. Statistical analysis was performed using SPSS software, version 24.0 (IBM Corp., Armonk, New York, NY, USA). p-Values less than 0.05 were statistically significant.

3. Results

A total of 995 students (317 women; 678 men; mean ± standard deviation, 24.8 ± 3.8 years) were included; the FYs of birth ranged from 1967 to 1996. The women were significantly (p = 0.016) younger than the men. The mean spherical equivalent (SE) and the mean AL, respectively, were −4.3 D and 25.59 mm (95% confidence interval (CI); −4.49 D to −4.12 D and 25.51 mm to 25.68 mm, respectively). The mean SE values in women and men did not differ significantly, while the mean AL in women was significantly (p < 0.001) shorter than in men. There were no significant gender differences in the prevalence rates of myopia (p = 0.635) and those of high myopia (p = 0.800) (Table 1). The SE was correlated significantly (r = 0.829, p < 0.001) with the AL (Figure 2).

Table 1. Prevalence rates of myopia and high myopia. * Unpaired t-test; † chi-square test. SE, spherical equivalent; D, diopters.

	Total (n = 995)	Female (n = 317)	Male (n = 678)	p Value
Age (years)	24.8 ± 3.8	24.4 ± 3.8	25.0 ± 3.8	0.016 *
Range	21 to 52	21 to 52	21 to 45	
SE (D)	−4.30 ± 2.96	−4.35 ± 2.94	−4.28 ± 2.97	0.733 *
Range	+4.62 to −14.73	+2.44 to −13.37	+4.62 to −14.73	
Axial length (mm)	25.59 ± 1.35	25.22 ± 1.28	25.77 ± 1.36	<0.001 *
Range	22.16 to 29.69	22.16 to 29.25	22.25 to 29.69	
Prevalence rate (%)				
Myopia (≤−0.5 D)	89.5	90.2	89.2	0.635 †
High Myopia (≤−6.0 D)	27.2	27.8	27.0	0.800 †

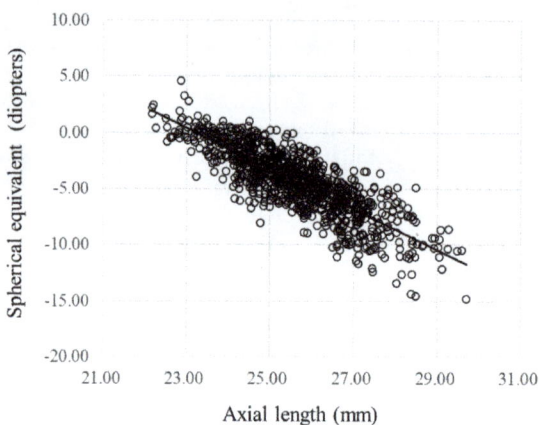

Figure 2. Spherical equivalent and axial length. y = 42.07 − 1.81x, r^2 = 0.687, p < 0.001. ○, data of eyes in each student.

When we divided the FYs of birth into two groups, i.e., before 1987 and 1987 and after, the SEs were correlated significantly with the FYs of birth (r = −0.213, p = 0.004) and decreased about 0.16 D annually during the FYs of birth before 1987. However, the SEs were not correlated significantly with the FYs of birth (p = 0.441) from 1987 and after. The SE regression rates based on the FYs of birth before 1987 and after differed significantly (p = 0.004) (Figure 3).

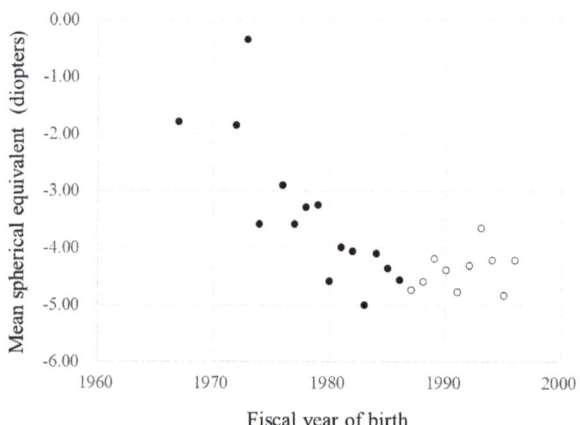

Figure 3. The fiscal year (FY) of birth and mean spherical equivalent. ●, data during the FYs of birth before 1987. ○, data during the FYs of birth of 1987 and after. During the FYs of birth before 1987, y = 310.0 − 0.158x, r = 0.213, p = 0·004. During the FYs of birth of 1987 and after, p =0.441. The regression of spherical equivalent by FYs of birth before 1987 and after, p = 0.004 (analysis of covariance (ANCOVA)).

The ALs were correlated significantly with the FYs of birth (r = 0.157, p = 0.034) and increased about 0.05 mm annually during the FYs of birth before 1987. However, the ALs were not correlated significantly with the FYs of birth (p = 0.599) from 1987 and after. The AL regression rates based on the FYs of birth before 1987 and after differed significantly (p = 0.037) (Figure 4).

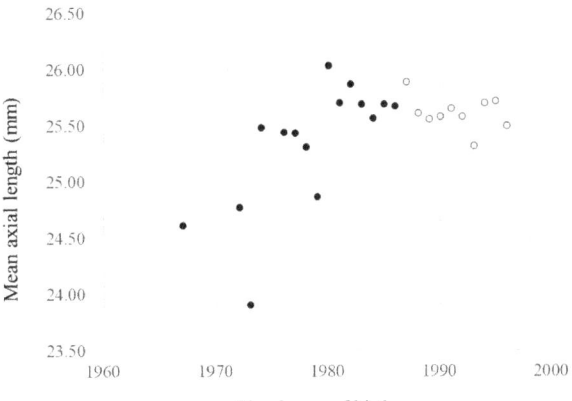

Figure 4. The fiscal year (FY) of birth and mean axial length. ●, data during the FYs of birth before 1987. ○, data during the FYs of birth of 1987 and after. During the FYs of birth before 1987, y = −78.9 + 0.0527x, r = 0.157, p = 0.034. During the FYs of birth of 1987 and after, p = 0.599. The regression of spherical equivalent by FYs of birth before 1987 and after, p = 0.004 (ANCOVA).

The myopia prevalence rates were not correlated significantly with the FYs of birth before and after 1987 (p = 0.428, p = 0.080, respectively). In contrast, the prevalence rates of high myopia were correlated significantly with the FYs of birth (r = 0.851, p < 0.001) and increased about 2.4% annually during the FYs of birth before 1987. However, the high myopia prevalence rate was not correlated significantly with the FYs of birth (p = 0.692) from 1987 and after. The regression rates of the prevalence of high myopia by FY of birth before 1987 and after differed significantly (p = 0.010) (Figure 5). The mean prevalence rates of myopia and high myopia during FYs of birth before 1987 were 82.5% and 18.1% (95% CI; 73.3% to 91.7% and 10.3% to 25.9%, respectively), and those of 1987 and after were 90.2% and 28.6% (95% CI; 88.2% to 92.2% and 24.1% to 33.1%, respectively).

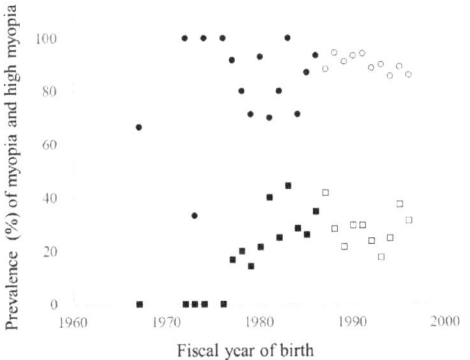

Figure 5. The fiscal years (FYs) of birth and prevalence of myopia and high myopia. ●, the prevalence of myopia during the FYs of birth before 1987. ○, the prevalence of myopia during the FYs of birth of 1987 and after. ■, the prevalence of high myopia during the FYs of birth before 1987. □, the prevalence of high myopia during the FYs of birth of 1987 and after. The prevalence of myopia: during the FYs of birth before 1987, p = 0.428; during the FYs of birth of 1987 and after, p = 0.080. The prevalence of high myopia: during the FYs of birth before 1987, y = −4826 + 2.45x, r = 0.851, p < 0.001; and during the FYs of birth of 1987 and after, p = 0.692. The regressions of the spherical equivalent by FYs of birth before 1987 and after, p = 0.010 (analysis of covariance).

4. Discussion

In the current study, we investigated the degree of myopia and the prevalence rates of myopia and high myopia before and after the introduction of the Yutori educational system in Japan. During high-pressure education, the degree of myopia and the prevalence of high myopia increased with the passage of the FY of birth; however, no myopia progression was observed after implementation of Yutori education. Because the pressure-free education policy reduced myopia progression, it would be interesting to understand the etiology of myopia.

A significant correlation was observed between the SE with AL. During high-pressure education, the SE decreased about 0.16 D annually, and the AL increased about 0.05 mm annually, which corresponded to about 3.0 D/mm. Therefore, the refractive change toward myopia was accompanied by AL elongation. In longitudinal studies among university students and medical students, the mean refractive changes were −0.11 D and −0.17 D annually [20,21]. The refractive difference followed by the birth year in the current study was similar to the individual refractive changes annually in those studies. Therefore, the difference in the refractive component among the different birth years should receive attention when myopia is investigated in cross-sectional studies.

In the current study, the prevalence of myopia was 90.2% after the introduction of Yutori education, which was independent of the FY of birth. High prevalence rates of myopia, i.e., about 90% or more, had been reported among medical or university students in Asia [4,21,22], which would result from a ceiling effect. In contrast, the prevalence of high myopia increased up to about 28.6% with the FY of birth during high-pressure education but stabilized after the introduction of Yutori education. This might have resulted from reduced educational pressure, but it also might have been the result of a ceiling effect, as the prevalence had been sufficiently high and was similar to 28.7% in medical students in Singapore [22].

A higher level of education has been associated with more myopia [14,15,23]. However, the level of education in the current study was the same because the participants were the same medical students in the same university. The time spent engaged in educational activities and the intensity of education also are important factors in myopia [24,25]. In Yutori education, the total number of classroom hours during the first nine years of compulsory education, starting from the age of seven years, was reduced gradually from 8935 h (until FY 1986) to 8307 h (in FY 1995). However, according to the survey on time use and leisure activities conducted by the Ministry of Internal Affairs and Communications in Japan (https://www.e-stat.go.jp/stat-search/files?page=1&toukei=00200533&result_page=1, accessed on 10 May 2020), the daily average time spent on schoolwork including classroom hours during elementary school and junior high school were almost the same or slightly increased from 281 and 326 min in FYs 2001 to 281 and 335 min in FY 2006, respectively. This suggests that the time after school increased, which might have been caused by the increased time spent doing homework and "cramming" or in private tutorial classes. Therefore, the length of time for education itself would be unrelated to the different tendency of myopia progression observed in this study. Further, both the study time and learning content were reduced during Yutori education. The time spent on the primary subjects, i.e., mathematics, science, social study, and Japanese language, were reduced, and integrated learning lessons, i.e., problem-solving or experiential learning to develop the ability to think and learn independently, were introduced. This reduced the time needed for cramming or rote learning and near work, such as reading and writing, even with the same classroom hours based on the curriculum. More time spent on near-work activities had been reported to increase the risk of myopia [24,25]. Therefore, the intensity of education and near work would be related to myopia progression during high-pressure education. In addition, Saturday became a holiday in the Yutori system, and students had more chances to play outdoors during the day. The effect of increased time spent outdoors on myopia prevention and slowing myopia progression had been reported [26–29]. Introduction of the Yutori education system might be related to prevention of myopia progression.

In previous birth cohort studies [2,30], an increase was reported in the prevalence of myopia in the population with a more recent birth year. The increase was widely considered to be driven by environmental factors, such as decreased time outdoors and increased near-work activities, among other factors. As societies develop, there have been systematic increases in education, but there have been parallel changes in the number of other parameters, such as living environments, including changes in population density, style of housing, pollution, diet, and lifestyle [1,6]. Recently, use of computers, smart phones, and tablets are suggested to play a role [2]. Our data demonstrated that the progression of myopia was similar to a previous report [2,6], but that occurred only during high-pressure education. Therefore, these data indicated that educational pressure is related to myopia progression. Although other environmental factors that continuously affect myopia progression would increase the myopia progression year by year, myopia did not progress after the high-pressure education was stopped. Because the Yutori education system started from FY 2002 and gradually reduced the classroom hours to FY 2010, the degree of high-pressure education would decrease year by year. Other environmental factors and the degree of high-pressure education might have been counterbalanced and resulted in stabilization of the degree of myopia after the introduction of Yutori education. Our study focused on adults; therefore, if we focused on children, who are at greater risk of developing myopia, the result might have been different. Additionally, our data showed the influence of the environmental factor in childhood. Such kinds of observational studies not only for children but also for adult should be done to help monitor the prevalence of myopia. The COVID-19 pandemic has changed educational institutions across the world, compelling to adopt and use the available technologies to enable remote learning for students. This recent rapidly increased screen time may potentially accelerate the high myopia-prevalence rate in Asia and worldwide [31]. It would be important to study the prevalence of myopia in children during the COVID-19 pandemic, but it would also be important to conduct a follow-up study on same population as they grow up.

During the compulsory education period, children would not have a choice to select their educational environment, as the school curriculum has been determined by the government. As the educational environment can influence the myopia progression, the government should appoint an ophthalmologist to the committee for the educational system assessment. However, the environment for daily life cannot be fully controlled. To control the progression of myopia, it would be important to inform parents and educators about the harmful effect of prolonged hours of near work and the beneficial effect of outdoor activities.

The Organization of Economic Cooperation and Development (OECD) Programme for International Student Assessment (PISA) measures 15-year-olds' ability to use their reading, mathematics, and science knowledge and skills to meet real-life challenges (https://www.oecd.org/pisa/, accessed on 6 May 2020). The OECD PISA was first performed in 2000 and repeated every three years. Both countries with a high prevalence rate of myopia and those with lower prevalence rates of myopia had significant international rankings of educational performance, suggesting that high educational outcomes in PISA are not necessarily associated with an epidemic of myopia [1,2]. However, the OECD PISA results in Japanese students in 2003 and 2007 during Yutori education fell dramatically compared with those in 2000 during high-pressure education. Japan dropped from first to sixth and then to tenth place (in 2003 and 2006, respectively) in mathematical literacy, from eight to fourteenth and then fifteenth place in reading literacy, and from second to second and sixth place in science literacy. There were few racial differences, and the same language is spoken in Japan; only the educational system differed among these periods. The Japanese nation was shocked by this turndown of students' academic abilities resulting from Yutori education. Therefore, pressure-free education might contribute to both preventing myopia progression and decreasing the educational standing. To solve this problem, a new school curriculum was introduced that abandoned the pressure-free education policy from FY

2012 after a one-year transition period in Japan. Further study is needed to clarify the effect of educational pressure on myopia progression after cessation of pressure-free education.

The current study had some limitations. First, the current study was not completely reflective of the population in Japan because medical students who were at a higher education level were evaluated. However, we excluded the possibility of the effect of the educational level on myopia progression, as all were medical students in the same university. Second, the study population had twice the number of men compared with women in the current study. Therefore, the ratio of men to women differed between the participants in the current study and the Japanese population. Because no gender difference was observed regarding the SE, the prevalence rates of myopia and high myopia would not be affected by gender differences. Third, we studied only left eyes, although many previous studies used data from right eyes. However, no refractive difference between the left and right eyes has been reported previously. Therefore, this likely did not affect the current results.

5. Conclusions

In conclusion, we investigated the degree and prevalence of myopia before and after the introduction of free-pressure education in Japan. This study indicated that the program policy for compulsory education appeared to be associated with the progression of myopia. It is important to prevent myopia progression without compromising the education level. In order to control the progression of myopia, not only ophthalmologists but also educators and the government should work on together.

Author Contributions: Conceptualization, S.I. and A.Y.; methodology, S.I.; validation, H.K., N.N., Y.S., K.S., H.N., Y.K. and A.Y.; formal analysis, S.I.; investigation, S.I.; data curation, K.S. and H.N.; writing—original draft preparation, S.I.; writing—review and editing, H.K., N.N., Y.S., Y.K. and A.Y.; supervision, A.Y.; project administration, S.I. All authors have read and agreed to the published version of the manuscript.

Funding: This research received no external funding.

Institutional Review Board Statement: The study was conducted according to the guidelines of the Declaration of Helsinki and approved by the Institutional Review Board of Asahikawa Medical University (No. 696, 2010.3.31).

Informed Consent Statement: Informed consent was obtained from all subjects involved in the study.

Data Availability Statement: The data presented in this study are available on request from the corresponding author.

Acknowledgments: We thank Norio Sugimoto, Sugimoto Data Analysis Service, for the advice related to statistical analysis.

Conflicts of Interest: The authors declare no conflict of interest.

References

1. Morgan, I.; Ohno-Matsui, K.; Saw, S.M. Myopia. *Lancet* **2012**, *5*, 1739–1748. [CrossRef]
2. Morgan, I.G.; French, A.N.; Ashby, R.S.; Guo, X.; Ding, X.; He, M.; Rose, K.A. The epidemics of myopia: Aetiology and prevention. *Prog. Retin. Eye Res.* **2018**, *62*, 134–149. [CrossRef]
3. Jung, S.K.; Lee, J.H.; Kakizaki, H.; Je, D. Pevalence of myopia and its association with body stature and education level in 19-year-old male conscripts in Seoul, South Korea. *Investig. Ophthalmol. Vis. Sci.* **2012**, *53*, 5579–5583. [CrossRef]
4. Sun, J.; Zhou, J.; Zhao, P.; Lian, J.; Zhu, H.; Zhou, Y.; Sun, Y.; Wang, Y.; Zhao, L.-Q.; Wei, Y.; et al. High Prevalence of Myopia and High Myopia in 5060 Chinese University Students in Shanghai. *Investig. Opthalmol. Vis. Sci.* **2012**, *53*, 7504–7509. [CrossRef] [PubMed]
5. Singh, N.K.; James, R.; Yadav, A.; Kumar, R.; Asthana, S.; Labani, S. Prevalence of myopia and associated risk factors in schoolchildres in North India. *Optom. Vis. Sci.* **2019**, *96*, 200–205. [CrossRef] [PubMed]
6. Holden, B.A.; Fricke, T.R.; Wilson, D.A.; Jong, M.; Naidoo, K.S.; Sankaridurg, P.; Wong, T.Y.; Naduvilath, T.; Resnikoff, S. Global Prevalence of Myopia and High Myopia and Temporal Trends from 2000 through 2050. *Ophthalmology* **2016**, *123*, 1036–1042. [CrossRef] [PubMed]
7. Ikuno, Y. Overview of the Complications of High Myopia. *Retina* **2017**, *37*, 2347–2351. [CrossRef] [PubMed]

8. Saw, S.-M.; Gazzard, G.; Shih-Yen, E.C.; Chua, W.-H. Myopia and associated pathological complications. *Ophthalmic Physiol. Opt.* **2005**, *25*, 381–391. [CrossRef] [PubMed]
9. Ohno-Matsui, K.; Lai, T.; Lai, C.-C.; Cheung, C.M.G. Updates of pathologic myopia. *Prog. Retin. Eye Res.* **2016**, *52*, 156–187. [CrossRef]
10. Liang, C.-L.; Yen, E.; Su, J.-Y.; Liu, C.; Chang, T.-Y.; Park, N.; Wu, M.-J.; Lee, S.; Flynn, J.T.; Juo, S.-H.H. Impact of Family History of High Myopia on Level and Onset of Myopia. *Investig. Opthalmol. Vis. Sci.* **2004**, *45*, 3446–3452. [CrossRef] [PubMed]
11. Iribarren, R.; Cortinez, M.F.; Chiappe, J.P. Age of First Distance Prescription and Final Myopic Refractive Error. *Ophthalmic Epidemiol.* **2009**, *16*, 84–89. [CrossRef]
12. Chua, S.Y.L.; Sabanayagam, C.; Cheung, Y.; Chia, A.; Valenzuela, R.K.; Tan, D.; Wong, T.; Cheng, C.-Y.; Saw, S. Age of onset of myopia predicts risk of high myopia in later childhood in myopic Singapore children. *Ophthalmic Physiol. Opt.* **2016**, *36*, 388–394. [CrossRef] [PubMed]
13. Quek, T.P.L.; Chua, C.G.; Chong, C.S.; Chong, J.H.; Hey, H.W.D.; Lee, J.; Lim, Y.F.; Saw, S.-M. Prevalence of refractive errors in teenage high school students in Singapore. *Ophthalmic Physiol. Opt.* **2004**, *24*, 47–55. [CrossRef] [PubMed]
14. Rose, K.A.; French, A.N.; Morgan, I.G. Environmental Factors and Myopia. *Asia-Pac. J. Ophthalmol.* **2016**, *5*, 403–410. [CrossRef]
15. Mountjoy, E.; Davies, N.M.; Plotnikov, D.; Smith, G.D.; Rodriguez, S.; Williams, C.E.; Guggenheim, J.A.; Atan, D. Education and myopia: Assessing the direction of causality by mendelian randomisation. *BMJ* **2018**, *361*, k2022. [CrossRef]
16. Gifford, K.; Richdale, K.; Kang, P.; Aller, T.A.; Lam, C.S.; Liu, Y.M.; Michaud, L.; Mulder, J.; Orr, J.B.; Rose, K.A.; et al. IMI–clinical management guidelines report. *Investig. Ophthalmol. Vis. Sci.* **2019**, *60*, M184–M203. [CrossRef]
17. Zylbermann, R.; Landau, D.; Berson, D. The Influence of Study Habits on Myopia in Jewish Teenagers. *J. Pediatr. Ophthalmol. Strabismus* **1993**, *30*, 319–322. [CrossRef]
18. Wada, M.; Brunet Brunet, B. Yutori Kyoiku and the uncertainty of recent neo-liberal reforms in Japanese higher education. *Bull. Cent. Res. Support Educ. Pract.* **2011**, *7*, 69–78.
19. Takayama, K. A Nation at Risk Crosses the Pacific: Transnational Borrowing of the US Crisis Discourse in the Debate on Education Reform in Japan. *Comp. Educ. Rev.* **2007**, *51*, 423–446. [CrossRef]
20. Kinge, B.; Midelfart, A.; Jacobsen, G.; Rystad, J. Biometric changes in the eyes of Norwegian university students—A three-year longitudinal study. *Acta Ophthalmol. Scand.* **1999**, *77*, 648–652. [CrossRef]
21. Lin, L.L.-K.; Shih, Y.-F.; Lee, Y.-C.; Hung, P.-T.; Hou, P.-K. Changes in Ocular Refraction and Its Components Among Medical Students???A 5-Year Longitudinal Study. *Optom. Vis. Sci.* **1996**, *73*, 495–498. [CrossRef]
22. Woo, W.W.; Lim, K.A.; Yang, H.; Lim, X.Y.; Liew, F.; Lee, Y.S.; Saw, S.M. Refractive errors in medical students in Singapore. *Singap. Med. J.* **2004**, *45*, 470–474.
23. Mirshahi, A.; Ponto, K.A.; Hoehn, R.; Zwiener, I.; Zeller, T.; Lackner, K.; Beutel, M.E.; Pfeiffer, N. Myopia and level of education: Results from the Gutenberg Health Study. *Ophthalmology* **2014**, *121*, 2047–2052. [CrossRef]
24. Saw, S.-M.; Chua, W.-H.; Hong, C.-Y.; Wu, H.-M.; Chan, W.-Y.; Chia, K.-S.; Stone, R.A.; Tan, D. Nearwork in early-onset myopia. *Investig. Ophthalmol. Vis. Sci.* **2002**, *43*, 332–339.
25. Huang, H.-M.; Chang, D.S.-T.; Wu, P.-C. The Association between Near Work Activities and Myopia in Children—A Systematic Review and Meta-Analysis. *PLoS ONE* **2015**, *10*, e0140419. [CrossRef] [PubMed]
26. Wu, P.-C.; Tsai, C.-L.; Wu, H.-L.; Yang, Y.-H.; Kuo, H.-K. Outdoor Activity during Class Recess Reduces Myopia Onset and Progression in School Children. *Ophthalmology* **2013**, *120*, 1080–1085. [CrossRef] [PubMed]
27. Jin, J.-X.; Hua, W.-J.; Jiang, X.; Wu, X.-Y.; Yang, J.-W.; Gao, G.-P.; Fang, Y.; Pei, C.-L.; Wang, S.; Zhang, J.-Z.; et al. Effect of outdoor activity on myopia onset and progression in school-aged children in northeast China: The Sujiatun Eye Care Study. *BMC Ophthalmol.* **2015**, *15*, 73. [CrossRef] [PubMed]
28. He, M.; Xiang, F.; Zeng, Y.; Mai, J.; Chen, Q.; Zhang, J.; Smith, W.; Rose, K.; Morgan, I.G. Effect of time spent outdoors at school on the development of myopia among children in China: A randomized clinical trial. *JAMA* **2015**, *314*, 1142–1148. [CrossRef] [PubMed]
29. Williams, K.M.; Bertelsen, G.; Cumberland, P.; Wolfram, C.; Verhoeven, V.; Anastasopoulos, E.; Buitendijk, G.H.; Cougnard-Grégoire, A.; Creuzot-Garcher, C.; Erke, M.G.; et al. Increasing Prevalence of Myopia in Europe and the Impact of Education. *Ophthalmology* **2015**, *122*, 1489–1497. [CrossRef] [PubMed]
30. Wu, P.C.; Chen, C.T.; Lin, K.K.; Su, C.C.; Kuo, C.N.; Huang, H.M.; Poon, Y.C.; Yang, M.L.; Chen, C.Y.; Huanget, G.C.; et al. Myopia prevention and outdoor light intensity in a school-based cluster randomized trial. *Ophthalmology* **2018**, *125*, 1239–1250. [CrossRef]
31. Singh, N.K. Letter to the editor: Myopia epidemic post-coonavirus disease 2019. *Optom. Vis. Sci.* **2020**, *97*, 911. [CrossRef] [PubMed]

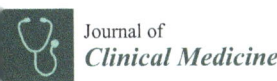

Article

Determination of the Standard Visual Criterion for Diagnosing and Treating Presbyopia According to Subjective Patient Symptoms

Yukari Tsuneyoshi [1], Sachiko Masui [1], Hiroyuki Arai [2], Ikuko Toda [3], Miyuki Kubota [4], Shunsuke Kubota [4], Kazuo Tsubota [1], Masahiko Ayaki [1,5,*] and Kazuno Negishi [1,*]

1. Department of Ophthalmology, Keio University School of Medicine, Tokyo 160-8582, Japan; yukari.a7@keio.jp (Y.T.); m.sac@a7.keio.jp (S.M.); tsubota@z3.keio.jp (K.T.)
2. Queen's Eye Clinic, Yokohama 220-6204, Japan; arai@minatomiraieye.jp
3. Minamiaoyama Eye Clinic, Tokyo 107-0061, Japan; toda@minamiaoyama.or.jp
4. Department of Ophthalmology, Shonan Keiiku Hospital, Fujisawa 252-0816, Japan; myu.kubota@gmail.com (M.K.); shun_kubota@live.jp (S.K.)
5. Otake Clinic Moon View Eye Center, Yamato 242-0001, Japan
* Correspondence: mayaki@olive.ocn.ne.jp (M.A.); kazunonegishi@keio.jp (K.N.)

Citation: Tsuneyoshi, Y.; Masui, S.; Arai, H.; Toda, I.; Kubota, M.; Kubota, S.; Tsubota, K.; Ayaki, M.; Negishi, K. Determination of the Standard Visual Criterion for Diagnosing and Treating Presbyopia According to Subjective Patient Symptoms. *J. Clin. Med.* **2021**, *10*, 3942. https://doi.org/10.3390/jcm10173942

Academic Editor: António Queirós Pereira

Received: 23 June 2021
Accepted: 30 August 2021
Published: 31 August 2021

Publisher's Note: MDPI stays neutral with regard to jurisdictional claims in published maps and institutional affiliations.

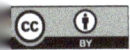

Copyright: © 2021 by the authors. Licensee MDPI, Basel, Switzerland. This article is an open access article distributed under the terms and conditions of the Creative Commons Attribution (CC BY) license (https://creativecommons.org/licenses/by/4.0/).

Abstract: Presbyopia treatments using various modalities have been developed recently; however, no standard criteria exist for the diagnosis and treatment endpoint. This study assessed the relationship between the near visual acuity (NVA) and the subjective symptoms of phakic presbyopia and determined the numerical NVA threshold to diagnose phakic presbyopia and evaluate the effectiveness of presbyopia treatment. The binocular distance, NVA with habitual correction, and monocular conventional VA were measured. Patients were asked about their awareness of presbyopia and difficulty performing near tasks. This prospective observational study included 70 patients (mean age, 56 years; range, 32–77). Most patients became aware of presbyopia in their late forties, although some had difficulty with vision-related near tasks before becoming aware of presbyopia. Eighty three percent of patients (20/24) experienced difficulty with near vision-related tasks even with excellent NVA at 40 cm with habitual correction of 0.0 logMAR (20/20 in Snellen VA). In conclusion, the current study showed that patients became aware of presbyopia in their late forties, although some had difficulty with near vision-related tasks before becoming aware of presbyopia. Further investigation should include the proposal of appropriate diagnostic criteria for presbyopia and better management for patients with presbyopia.

Keywords: presbyopia; near visual acuity; standard criterion; diagnosis

1. Introduction

Presbyopia is a global problem that affects about one quarter of the world's population [1]. The number of people with impaired near vision due to presbyopia is estimated to decrease by about 20% by 2050 because of the increasing myopia prevalence [1]. However, presbyopia remains an important health problem that may affect the quality of life of individuals not only in developing countries without awareness of presbyopia or accessibility to affordable treatment [1,2] but also in developed countries where people tend to be engaged in near tasks because of the increasing use of digital technology.

Several definitions of presbyopia have been used historically, and most were functional or qualitative [1,2]. Previous studies of presbyopia treatment using various treatment modalities [3] used arbitrary numerical criteria to determine treatment efficacy because of the absence of standardized criteria. The patient-reported outcome measures have also been used in clinical trials and quality-of-life studies for presbyopia treatment [3,4]. Among them, the Near Activity Visual Questionnaire was identified as the most appropriate for assessing near-vision functioning in presbyopia, although the measure was not validated in a purely phakic presbyopia sample [4]. Considering recent developments of presbyopia treatments using various modalities [3,5–9], simple and easily accessible standardized criteria for diagnosis and endpoints of treatment are necessary.

The purpose of this study was to assess the relationship between the near visual acuity (NVA) and the subjective symptoms of phakic presbyopia and to determine the numerical NVA threshold to diagnose phakic presbyopia and evaluate the effectiveness of presbyopia correction according to subjective patient symptoms.

2. Materials and Methods

2.1. Study Design and Patients

This study was a clinic-based prospective observational study conducted at four eye clinics: Minamiaoyama Eye Clinic (Tokyo, Japan), Queen's Eye Clinic (Kanagawa, Japan), Shonan Keiiku Hospital (Kanagawa, Japan), and Keio University Hospital (Tokyo, Japan). All patients provided written informed consent before participating in this study. The institutional review boards of each institution approved the study (approval numbers, 20181025-2, Minamiaoyama Eye Clinic; 20181025-2, Queen's Eye Clinic; 18-002, Shonan Keiiku Hospital; and 20150280, Keio University Hospital), which followed the tenets of the Declaration of Helsinki. The protocol for this study was registered with the University Hospital Medical Information Network Clinical Trial Registry (UMIN000021587).

2.2. Inclusion and Exclusion Criteria

The inclusion criteria were age 20 years and older, phakia because of the need to measure the refraction and undergo VA tests for diagnosis or treatments, and a binocular distance visual acuity (DVA) of 0.10 logMAR (16/20 in Snellen acuity) and over. The exclusion criteria were a history of refractive surgery and decreased cognitive function.

2.3. Ophthalmic Examinations and Questionnaire

Experienced examiners performed all examinations. The ophthalmologic evaluation of the participants included measurement of the monocular corrected DVA (CDVA) and monocular distance-corrected NVA (DCNVA), binocular DVA with habitual correction (DVAHC), and binocular NVA at 40 cm with habitual correction (NVAHC). If a patient did not use any corrective lens for near visual tasks, the binocular NVA was measured without correction. All distance and near VA charts followed the Japanese industrial standards (JIS) T7309 (http://kikakurui.com/t7/T7309-2002-01.html, accessed on 29 August 2021), which is based on International Organization for Standardization (ISO) 8596: 1994, Ophthalmic optics: Visual acuity testing—Standard optotype and its presentation; and ISO 8597: 1994, Optics and optical instruments: Visual acuity testing—Method of correlating optotypes. It was reported that the VA charts that adhere to the JIS are consistent with the ones that adhere to the international standard (http://kikakurui.com/t7/T7309-2002-01.html, accessed on 29 August 2021). When the VA was measured using a decimal VA chart, the measured decimal VA was converted to logarithm of the minimum angle of resolution (logMAR) units according to the VA conversion chart [10]. Using an interview sheet, patients were asked to determine the presence or absence of presbyopic symptoms and the age at which they heard or realized by themselves for the first time that the symptoms they had had for a while represented presbyopia. Patients also were asked about the degree of difficulty while reading a newspaper and reading a book for an extended time. The degrees of difficulty were divided into no difficulty, slight difficulty, and great difficulty.

2.4. Statistical Analysis

All statistical analyses were conducted using commercially available statistical software (IBM SPSS Statistics, version 25, Armonk, NY, USA). The Mann-Whitney U test was used to compare the VA and subjective refraction when the data were not normally distributed. The χ^2 test was used to compare the proportions of patients who were male and female. All tests of statistical significance were two-sided, and $p < 0.05$ was considered statistically significant.

3. Results

3.1. Patient Profile

The study included 70 patients (30 male and 40 female patients). The mean age was 56.0 ± 13.0 (standard deviation: SD) years old (range: 32–77). The mean monocular subjective refraction (spherical equivalent) of all eyes was −2.78 ± 3.70 (SD) dioptors, and the mean corrected distance visual acuity (CDVA) and DCNVA (distance corrected near visual acuity) at 40 cm were −0.09 ± 0.09 (SD) and 0.28 ± 0.33 (SD), respectively for all 140 eyes of 70 patients. The binocular distance visual acuity with habitual correction (DVAHC) and the near visual acuity with habitual correction (NVAHC) were −0.03 ± 0.12 (SD) and 0.05 ± 0.16 (SD), respectively. In our data, the monocular CDVA of all patients was 0.10 logMAR (16/20 Snellen acuity) and better except for one patient whose CDVA was 0.22 logMAR (12/20) in the right eye and 0.15 logMAR (14/20) in the left eye. However, the binocular DVA with habitual correction (DVAHC) of this patient was 0.2 logMAR (12/20), which was relatively good without being affected by the reduced CDVA.

Figure 1 is a histogram of the patients' ages.

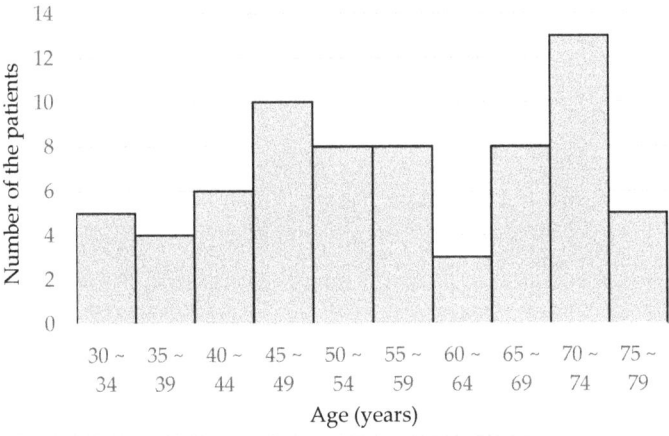

Figure 1. Distribution of patient age (N = 70).

In some cases, multiple ocular complications developed that included cataract (22 cases), dry eye (20 cases), vitreous macular traction (13 cases), chorioretinal atrophy (13 cases), optic disc cupping (12 cases), age-related macular degeneration (7 cases), conjunctivitis (6 cases), epiretinal membrane (3 cases), and corneal opacity, keratoconus, pterygium, uveitis (1 case each). Those patients with multiple complications developed were asthma and hypertension (3 cases each), hay fever (2 cases), and allergic sinusitis, atopic dermatitis, breast cancer, chronic nephritis, diabetes mellites, endometriosis, fatty liver, heart disease, hypothyroidism, Parkinson's disease, rheumatic disease, and sarcoidosis (1 case each). No patient had complications that severely affected visual function, meaning 0.40 logMAR (20/40 in Snellen acuity) and worse in CDVA.

3.2. Questionnaire Results

The questionnaire showed that 65.7% (46/70) of patients replied that they had presbyopic symptoms. The percentages of patients who were aware of presbyopia by age are shown in Figure 2.

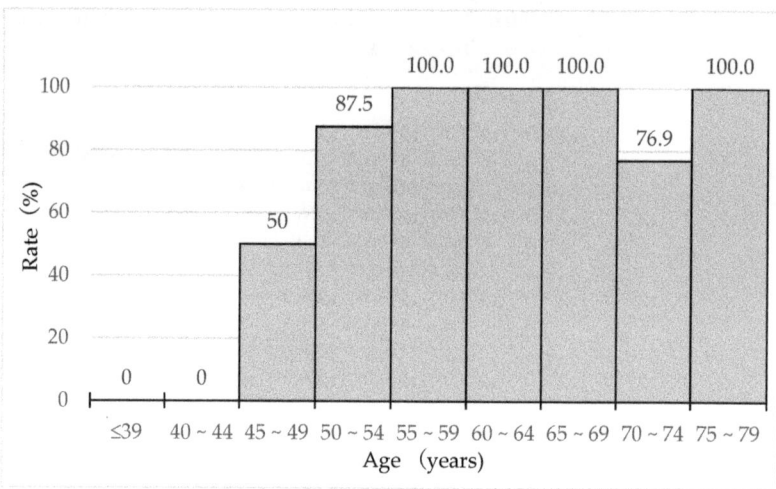

Figure 2. Rate of the patients with awareness of presbyopia.

No one was aware of presbyopia before reaching 45 years of age, and the percentages of patients with subjective presbyopia increased dramatically over 45 years of age and plateaued after 55 years. The mean initial age of the patients with subjective presbyopia was 50.9 (standard deviation 7.1; range, 38–70) years. Figure 3 shows the relationship between the level of difficulty when performing near tasks and the percentages of patients 45 years old and over with subjective presbyopia.

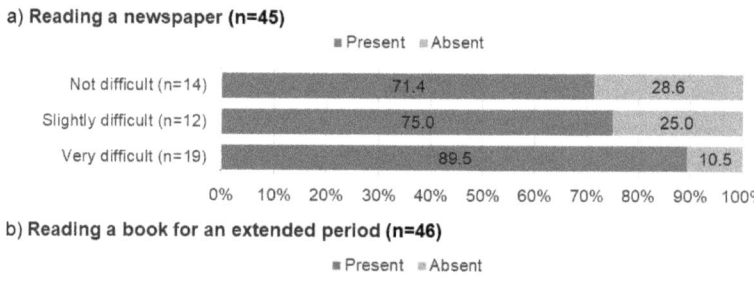

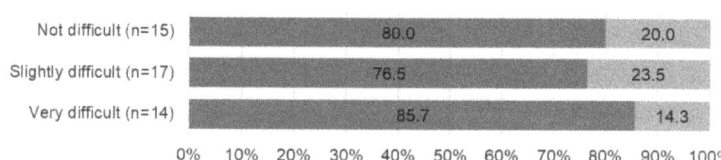

Figure 3. Awareness of presbyopia and subjective symptoms for near tasks in patients aged 45 years and older ($n = 55$).

The percentage of patients who were aware of presbyopia increased when they considered it very difficult to read a newspaper or book for an extended period compared with those who described no or slight difficulty. However, around 25% of the patients were unaware of presbyopia despite having slight difficulty performing near tasks.

3.3. Differences in Subjective Refraction and VAs between Patients with/without Awareness of Presbyopia

Table 1 shows the differences in the subjective refraction and VAs between patients with and without an awareness of presbyopia.

Table 1. Comparisons of the clinical data between the awareness and absence of awareness of presbyopia.

	Aware (n = 46)	Unaware (n = 24)	p Value
Age (years)	62.2 ± 9.7	44.2 ± 12.0	0.000
Sex (male/female)	16/30	14/10	0.059
Monocular examination			
Subjective refraction (SE) of the relatively hyperopic eye (D)	−1.58 ± 3.48	−4.13 ± 3.37	0.005
Subjective refraction (SE) of the relatively myopic eye (D)	−2.21 ± 3.80	−4.80 ± 3.11	0.006
CDVA (logMAR) of the better eye	−0.10 ± 0.08	−0.12 ± 0.08	0.118
CDVA (logMAR) of the worse eye	−0.06 ± 0.09	−0.11 ± 0.10	0.013
DCNVA (logMAR) at 40 cm of the better eye	0.37 ± 0.22	−0.03 ± 0.23	0.000
DCNVA (logMAR) at 40 cm of the worse eye	0.49 ± 0.27	−0.00 ± 0.25	0.000
Binocular examination			
DVAHC (logMAR)	−0.28 ± 0.11	−0.04 ± 0.15	0.434
Binocular NVAHC at 40 cm (logMAR)	0.11 ± 0.15	−0.05 ± 0.13	0.000

D—diopters; CDVA—corrected distance visual acuity; logMAR—logarithm of the minimum angle of resolution; DCNVA—distance corrected near visual acuity; DVAHC—distance visual acuity with habitual correction; NVAHC—near visual acuity with habitual correction.

The subjective refraction of the patients who were unaware of presbyopia was significantly more myopic than those who were unaware of presbyopia. Naturally, the binocular NVA with habitual correction was significantly worse in patients who were aware of presbyopia, although there was no significant difference in the binocular DVA with habitual correction.

3.4. Relationship between Binocular NVA and Subjective Symptoms

Figure 4 shows the percentages of patients who were aware of presbyopia, those who had difficulty reading a newspaper, and those who had difficulty reading a book for an extended period based on the NVA with habitual correction.

All of the percentages of patients who were aware of presbyopia and who had difficulty reading a newspaper and difficulty reading a book for an extended period increased dramatically when the binocular NVDAC at 40 cm decreased to 0.0 (20/20).

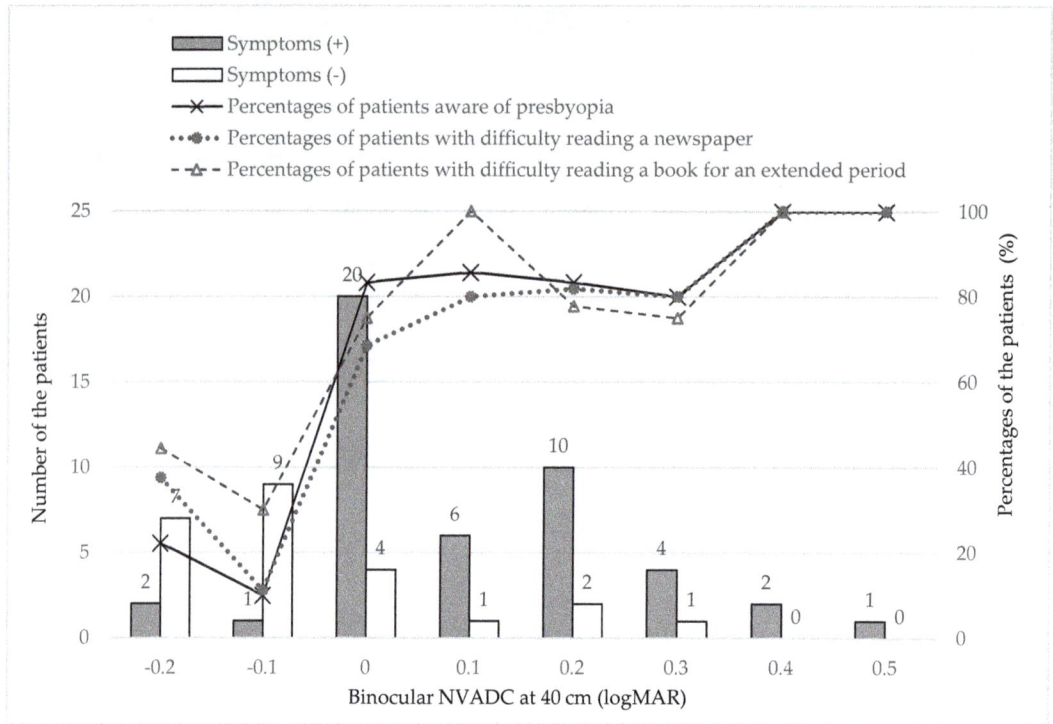

Figure 4. Binocular NVAHC and the rates of the patients with awareness of presbyopia, difficulty in checking a newspaper, and difficulty in reading a book for a long time (N = 70).

4. Discussion

Several methods can evaluate the visual function in presbyopia including measurement of the NVA, defocus curves, accommodative amplitude, and reading speed. Among them, the NVA test at 40 cm is the most common clinical examination, although the test distances are not standardized.

Holden defined functional presbyopia as the need for addition of a significant optical correction to the presenting distance refractive correction to achieve a NVA absolute (such as N8 or J1) or relative (such as 1 line of acuity improvement) criteria [11]. Other epidemiologic studies have reported that presbyopia is the inability of individuals aged 35 years or older to read binocularly N8 (or 6/12) at 40 cm or their habitual working distance; in some studies, presbyopia was limited to those patients whose NVA improved with the addition of corrective lenses [12–15]. The Japanese Society of Presbyopia determined two different criteria for diagnosing presbyopia, i.e., medical presbyopia and clinical presbyopia [16]. According to the definition, medical presbyopia is an ocular condition with an accommodative amplitude less than 2.5 diopters (D) regardless of presbyopic symptoms, and clinical presbyopia is an ocular condition in which the NVA is less than 20/50 with habitual correction in addition to the presence of presbyopic symptoms.

Regarding the endpoints for presbyopia treatments, the number of primary eyes with a DCNVA at 40 cm achieving 20/40 or better and a gain of at least 10 letters was adopted in clinical trials of the treatment modality for presbyopia [17–19].

According to our results, the percentages of patients who had difficulty with near tasks (reading a newspaper and reading a book for an extended period) and the rate of awareness of presbyopia dramatically increased when the binocular NVA decreased to 20/20. In addition, 83% (20/24) of patients reported difficulty with near vision-related tasks even with an excellent logMAR NVAHC of 0.0 (20/20 in Snellen VA). This indicates that a NVA over 20/20 is necessary for comfortable near vision, and the most common threshold for presbyopia treatment to read binocularly N8 (or 20/40) at 40 cm might be too low as an endpoint of presbyopia correction. Other aspects of vision, such as insufficient accommodation amplitude (for example, less than 4 D), contrast sensitivity, and/or stability of the ocular surface, also may play an important role in determining difficulty performing near visual tasks, and we should pay more attention more to these factors to predict patients' need of intervention for presbyopia.

It is difficult to diagnose degraded near visual function in subjects with early presbyopia with good conventional VA clinically and quantitatively. We reported previously that the near functional VA (FVA) test detected early presbyopia better than the conventional VA test [20]. The FVA Measurement System, which is commercially available, can calculate the mean VA over 60 s from the VA data measured continuously for 60 s. The near FVA was negatively and significantly linearly correlated with the accommodative amplitude, and the decrease in the near FVA for a reduction of 1.00 D of accommodative power was greater than that of the DCNVA, which means that the near FVA may be a good option for diagnosing presbyopia [20].

Our results showed that the subjective refraction of patients unaware of presbyopia was significantly more myopic than those aware of the presbyopia. Myopic eyes need less accommodative efforts due to the difference between the ocular and spectacle accommodation [21]. Moreover, myopic subjects can use the effect of the forward spectacle shift [21]. These advantages for near vision in myopic eyes might affect the awareness of presbyopia.

Our study also showed that there were many presbyopic patients who were unaware of the presbyopia. Among patients aged 45 years and older, between 15% and 20% were unaware of presbyopia despite difficulty performing near tasks.

Uncorrected presbyopia resulted in significant decreases in productivity and quality of life in the poorest communities [3,12,13,15,22–25]. Even in developed countries, presbyopia may cause severe health problems due to eye strain and asthenopia [26,27] because of the dramatically increasing use of digital devices. The results of our study implied the presence of considerable uncorrected presbyopia in developed countries, where it is easy to access treatment, due to the lack of awareness of presbyopia. We should enlighten patients regarding the onset, symptoms, effects, and corrective methods to minimize its impact. Establishing a universal, precise diagnostic criteria for presbyopia can result in an appropriate understanding of the burden of presbyopia and need for correction.

The current study had some limitations. First, this study included a small number of cases and, second, we measured only the conventional distance and NVAs. Several important parameters, such as the near point distance, the deviation of the habitual refraction from the best subjective refraction, and the habitual reading distance, were not recorded.

This warrants further investigation that considers potentially relevant factors such as age and pupillary size in more cases with other detailed visual function tests such as the FVA test. However, the conventional near visual test is one of the most common and easily accessible tests to evaluate near visual function. In addition, the use of the NVA with habitual correction is the strength of the current study to investigate the relationship between visual function and subjective symptoms compared with an evaluation using the arbitrary standard correction. Therefore, we believe our results are useful to determine the threshold visual function to diagnose presbyopia, especially in developed countries.

In conclusion, the current study showed that patients became aware of presbyopia in their late forties, although some had difficulty with near vision-related tasks before becoming aware of presbyopia. Surprisingly, 83% (20/24) of patients experienced difficulty with near vision-related tasks even with an excellent logMAR NVAHC of 0.0 (20/20 in Snellen VA). This means that a visual acuity of 20/20 at near distances is not correlated with the level of comfort when performing near tasks for an extended time. This is probably due to accommodative fatigue that occurs more often as accommodative amplitude decreases. Considering the current results, the vision threshold for intervening in presbyopia may have to be set at a stricter level than the present one and we may have to reconsider the goal of the treatment of presbyopia much more than the current criteria, at least in developed countries.

Author Contributions: Conceptualization, Y.T. and K.N.; data curation, S.M., H.A., I.T., M.K., S.K. and M.A.; formal analysis, S.M. and K.N.; investigation, S.M., H.A., I.T., M.K., S.K., M.A. and K.N.; methodology, Y.T., S.M. and K.N.; project administration, K.N.; resources, H.A., I.T., M.K., S.K., M.A. and K.N.; supervision, K.T.; validation, S.M. and K.N.; visualization, S.M. and K.N.; writing—original draft, Y.T., S.M. and K.N.; writing—review and editing, Y.T., S.M., H.A., I.T., M.K., S.K., K.T., M.A. and K.N. All authors have read and agreed to the published version of the manuscript.

Funding: This research received no external funding.

Institutional Review Board Statement: The study was conducted according to the guidelines of the Declaration of Helsinki, and approved by the Institutional Review Board of each institution (approval numbers, 20181025-2, Minamiaoyama Eye Clinic; 20181025-2, Queen's Eye Clinic; 18-002, Shonan Keiiku Hospital; and 20150280, Keio University School of Medicine).

Informed Consent Statement: Informed consent was obtained from all subjects involved in the study.

Data Availability Statement: Supporting data are not available because consent for sharing data was not obtained.

Conflicts of Interest: Kazuo Tsubota holds the patent rights to the method and apparatus used to measure the FVA (US patent no.: 255 7470026) and is Chief Executive Officer of Tsubota Laboratory, Inc., Tokyo, Japan. Hiroyuki Arai is the director of the Queen's Eye Clinic, Kanagawa, Japan; Ikuko Toda is the director of the Minamiaoyama Eye Clinic, Tokyo, Japan. The remaining authors have no commercial relationships to disclose.

References

1. Fricke, T.R.; Tahhan, N.; Resnikoff, S.; Papas, E.; Burnett, A.; Ho, S.M.; Naduvilath, T.; Naidoo, K.S. Global Prevalence of Presbyopia and Vision Impairment from Uncorrected Presbyopia: Systematic Review, Meta-analysis, and Modelling. *Ophthalmology* **2018**, *125*, 1492–1499. [CrossRef]
2. Frick, K.D.; Joy, S.M.; Wilson, D.A.; Naidoo, K.S.; Holden, B.A. The Global Burden of Potential Productivity Loss from Uncorrected Presbyopia. *Ophthalmology* **2015**, *122*, 1706–1710. [CrossRef]
3. Wolffsohn, J.S.; Davies, L.N. Presbyopia: Effectiveness of correction strategies. *Prog. Retin. Eye Res.* **2019**, *68*, 124–143. [CrossRef]
4. Sharma, G.; Chiva-Razavi, S.; Viriato, D.; Naujoks, C.; Patalano, F.; Bentley, S.; Findley, A.; Johnson, C.; Arbuckle, R.; Wolffsohn, J. Patient-reported outcome measures in presbyopia: A literature review. *BMJ Open Ophthalmol.* **2020**, *5*, e000453. [CrossRef] [PubMed]
5. Bennett, E.S. Contact lens correction of presbyopia. *Clin. Exp. Optom.* **2008**, *91*, 265–278. [CrossRef] [PubMed]
6. Grzybowski, A.; Markeviciute, A.; Zemaitiene, R. A Review of Pharmacological Presbyopia Treatment. *Asia Pac. J. Ophthalmol.* **2020**, *9*, 226–233. [CrossRef]
7. Hipsley, A.; Hall, B.; Rocha, K.M. Scleral surgery for the treatment of presbyopia: Where are we today? *Eye Vis.* **2018**, *5*, 4. [CrossRef]
8. Moarefi, M.A.; Bafna, S.; Wiley, W. A Review of Presbyopia Treatment with Corneal Inlays. *Ophthalmol. Ther.* **2017**, *6*, 55–65. [CrossRef]
9. Renna, A.; Alió, J.L.; Vejarano, L.F. Pharmacological treatments of presbyopia: A review of modern perspectives. *Eye Vis.* **2017**, *4*, 3. [CrossRef] [PubMed]
10. Holladay, J.T. Visual acuity measurements. *J. Cataract. Refract. Surg.* **2004**, *30*, 287–290. [CrossRef] [PubMed]
11. Holden, B.A. Global Vision Impairment Due to Uncorrected Presbyopia. *Arch. Ophthalmol.* **2008**, *126*, 1731. [CrossRef]
12. Cheng, F.; Shan, L.; Song, W.; Fan, P.; Yuan, H. Distance-and near-visual impairment in rural Chinese adults in Kailu, Inner Mongolia. *Acta Ophthalmol.* **2016**, *94*, 407–413. [CrossRef]
13. Girum, M.; Desalegn Gudeta, A.; Shiferaw Alemu, D. Determinants of high unmet need for presbyopia correction: A community-based study in northwest Ethiopia. *Clin. Optom.* **2017**, *9*, 25–31. [CrossRef]
14. Muhit, M.; Minto, H.; Parvin, A.; Jadoon, M.Z.; Islam, J.; Yasmin, S.; Khandaker, G. Prevalence of refractive error, presbyopia, and unmet need of spectacle coverage in a northern district of Bangladesh: Rapid Assessment of Refractive Error study. *Ophthalmic Epidemiol.* **2018**, *25*, 126–132. [CrossRef]
15. Nsubuga, N.; Ramson, P.; Govender, P.; Chan, V.F.; Wepo, M.; Naidoo, K.S. Uncorrected refractive errors, presbyopia and spectacle coverage in Kamuli District, Uganda. *Afr. Vis. Eye Health J.* **2016**, *75*, 1–6. [CrossRef]
16. Ide, T.; Fujikado, T.; Maeda, N.; Oshika, T.; Bissen-Miyajima, H.; Kurosaka, D.; Toda, I.; Arai, H.; Okamoto, S.; Hieda, O.; et al. Definition and diagnostic criteria of presbyopia 2010. *Atarasii Ganka* **2011**, *28*, 985–988.

17. A Clinical Trial of the VisAbility Micro Insert System for Presbyopic Patients. Available online: https://clinicaltrials.gov/ct2/show/NCT02374671 (accessed on 29 August 2021).
18. Korenfeld, M.S.; Robertson, S.M.; Stein, J.M.; Evans, D.G.; Rauchman, S.H.; Sall, K.N.; Venkataraman, S.; Chen, B.-L.; Wuttke, M.; Burns, W. Topical lipoic acid choline ester eye drop for improvement of near visual acuity in subjects with presbyopia: A safety and preliminary efficacy trial. *Eye* **2021**, 1–10. [CrossRef]
19. Vukich, J.A.; Durrie, D.S.; Pepose, J.S.; Thompson, V.; Van De Pol, C.; Lin, L. Evaluation of the small-aperture intracorneal inlay: Three-year results from the cohort of the U.S. Food and Drug Administration clinical trial. *J. Cataract. Refract. Surg.* **2018**, *44*, 541–556. [CrossRef]
20. Katada, Y.; Negishi, K.; Watanabe, K.; Shigeno, Y.; Saiki, M.; Torii, H.; Kaido, M.; Tsubota, K. Functional Visual Acuity of Early Presbyopia. *PLoS ONE* **2016**, *11*, e0151094. [CrossRef]
21. Rabbetts, R.B. *Accommodation and Near Vision. The Inadequate-Stimulus Myopias*; Butterworth-Heinemann: Oxford, UK; Woburn, MA, USA, 1998; pp. 114–116.
22. Berdahl, J.; Bala, C.; Dhariwal, M.; Lemp-Hull, J.; Thakker, D.; Jawla, S. Patient and Economic Burden of Presbyopia: A Systematic Literature Review. *Clin. Ophthalmol.* **2020**, *14*, 3439–3450. [CrossRef]
23. Hookway, L.A.; Frazier, M.; Rivera, N.; Ramson, P.; Carballo, L.; Naidoo, K. Population-based study of presbyopia in Nicaragua. *Clin. Exp. Optom.* **2016**, *99*, 559–563. [CrossRef] [PubMed]
24. Naidoo, K.S.; Jaggernath, J.; Ramson, P.; Chinanayi, F.; Zhuwau, T.; Øverland, L. The prevalence of self-reported vision difficulty in economically disadvantaged regions of South Africa. *Afr. J. Disabil.* **2015**, *4*, 1–11. [CrossRef] [PubMed]
25. Schellini, S.; Ferraz, F.; Opromolla, P.; Oliveira, L.; Padovani, C. Main visual symptoms associated to refractive errors and spectacle need in a Brazilian population. *Int. J. Ophthalmol.* **2016**, *9*, 1657–1662. [PubMed]
26. Coles-Brennan, C.; Sulley, A.; Young, G. Management of digital eye strain. *Clin. Exp. Optom.* **2019**, *102*, 18–29. [CrossRef]
27. Reindel, W.; Zhang, L.N.; Chinn, J.; Rah, M. Evaluation of binocular function among pre-and early-presbyopes with asthenopia. *Clin. Optom.* **2018**, *10*, 1–8. [CrossRef] [PubMed]

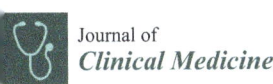

Short-Term Efficacy and Safety of Cataract Surgery Combined with Iris-Fixated Phakic Intraocular Lens Explantation: A Multicentre Study

Miki Kamikawatoko Omoto [1], Hidemasa Torii [1], Sachiko Masui [1], Masahiko Ayaki [1], Ikuko Toda [2], Hiroyuki Arai [3,4], Tomoaki Nakamura [5], Kazuo Tsubota [1] and Kazuno Negishi [1,*]

1. Department of Ophthalmology, Keio University School of Medicine, Tokyo 160-8582, Japan; m.toko.tkm@keio.jp (M.K.O.); hidemasatorii@yahoo.co.jp (H.T.); m.sac@a7.keio.jp (S.M.); mayaki@olive.ocn.ne.jp (M.A.); tsubota@z3.keio.jp (K.T.)
2. Minamiaoyama Eye Clinic, Tokyo 107-0061, Japan; toda@minamiaoyama.or.jp
3. Minatomirai Eye Clinic, Kanagawa 220-6208, Japan; arai@minatomiraieye.jp
4. Queen's Eye Clinic, Kanagawa 220-6204, Japan
5. Nagoya Eye Clinic, Aichi 456-0003, Japan; nic@bc5.so-net.ne.jp
* Correspondence: kazunonegishi@keio.jp; Tel.: +81-3-3353-1211

Abstract: The purpose of this study was to evaluate the short-term efficacy and safety of cataract surgery for patients with iris-fixated phakic intraocular lenses (pIOLs). This study included 96 eyes of 91 patients. The changes in the logMAR uncorrected visual acuity (UCVA), best-corrected visual acuity (BCVA), subjective spherical equivalent (SE), astigmatism, and endothelial cell density (ECD) were collected retrospectively. The intraoperative and postoperative complications also were investigated to assess the surgical safety. The preoperative UCVA and BCVA improved significantly at month 1 postoperatively, respectively ($p < 0.001$ for both comparisons). The efficacy and safety index at month 1 postoperatively were 1.02 ± 0.56 and 1.31 ± 0.64, respectively. The SE at month 1 postoperatively was significantly ($p < 0.001$) higher compared to preoperatively, whereas the subjective astigmatism did not differ significantly ($p = 0.078$). The ECD significantly decreased at month 1 ($p < 0.001$). The most common postoperative complication was intraocular pressure elevation exceeding 25 mmHg in 10.4% of eyes, which was controlled with medications in all cases until month 1 postoperatively. No intraoperative complications developed. Cataract surgeries for patients with iris-fixated pIOLs were performed safely with good visual outcomes.

Keywords: cataract; phakic intraocular lens; multicentre study

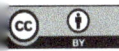

1. Introduction

Uncorrected refractive error is a major cause of visual impairment worldwide [1], and the prevalence of myopia is reported to be growing, especially in Asian countries [2–4]. Implantation of phakic intraocular lens (pIOL) is an option to correct myopia [5,6]. The reversibility when necessary should be an advantage of pIOL implantation compared to laser corneal refractive surgery, such as laser in situ keratomileusis (LASIK). Some studies have reported good long-term outcomes up to 10 years [7–9]. However, some cases need pIOL explantation due to cataract formation or decreased endothelial cell density (ECD) [10–12]. Some studies have reported the safety and efficacy of combined cataract surgery/pIOL explantation; however, small case series [13–17] or case reports of new surgical techniques [18,19], except for the study by Vargas et al., investigated 87 eyes of 55 patients [20]. Furthermore, including the study of Vargas et al., most of these studies focused on posterior-chamber pIOLs. Anterior-chamber pIOLs are associated with a lower rate of cataract formation and pigment dispersion compared to posterior-chamber pIOL [5,21]. However, few studies have investigated pIOL explantation and cataract surgeries for eyes with iris-fixated pIOL. We report the short-term efficacy and safety of cataract surgery with iris-fixated pIOL explantation.

2. Materials and Methods

2.1. Study Institutions and Institutional Review Board Approval

This was a multicentre (Keio University Hospital, Minamiaoyama Eye Clinic, Minatomirai Eye Clinic, Queen's Eye Clinic, and Nagoya Eye Clinic), retrospective, observational study. The Research Ethics Committee of the Keio University School of Medicine (approval number: 20190278) approved the study, and the other eye clinics participating in the study were described as collaborators in the ethics committee document and were thus covered under the approval granted by the Keio University School of Medicine. This study was conducted according to the tenets of the Declaration of Helsinki. Patients or the public were not involved in the design, conduct, reporting, or dissemination plans of our research.

2.2. Participants

One hundred and fifty-nine eyes of 139 patients were enrolled in the study; all had undergone pIOL explantation followed by phacoemulsification and IOL implantation at one of the five hospitals between December 2010 and April 2020. The inclusion criteria were eyes with an iris-fixated pIOL. The exclusion criteria were eyes with a vision-threatening disease except cataract, i.e., keratoconus, retinal detachment, central serous chorioretinopathy, macular edema, glaucoma, and choroidal neovascularization; or eyes that had undergone a previous ophthalmic surgery except pIOL implantation, i.e., LASIK, vitrectomy, and glaucoma surgeries. Therefore, 96 eyes of 91 patients were included in the final analysis.

2.3. Surgical Technique

Five surgeons performed all of the surgeries. A pIOL was explanted through a temporal or superior sclerocorneal incision (range, 2.4–7.0 mm), the size of which was determined based on the material from which the implanted pIOL was made, i.e., polymethyl methacrylate (PMMA) (Artisan® or Artisan Toric®, Ophtec BV, Groningen, The Netherlands) or silicone (Artiflex®, Ophtec BV). The nylon suture was set when the PMMA lens was explanted, which was left at the site until the end of the study period. Standard phacoemulsification and IOL implantation then were performed through a temporal or superior corneal incision (range, 2.3–2.4 mm). The surgeon chose the type of IOL based on the patient's request. The implanted IOLs are summarized in supplemental Table S1. The IOL power was calculated using Barrett Universal II Formula with the preoperative measurements of axial length, keratometry, and anterior chamber depth. The anterior chamber depth was manually measured and verified for accuracy because the participants had pIOLs. A topical antibiotic (moxifloxacin hydrochloride) and a corticosteroid (betamethasone sodium phosphate) were administered 3 times daily for one week and a non-steroidal anti-inflammatory agent (diclofenac sodium) for 3 months postoperatively. Drug doses were tapered over the postoperative course.

2.4. Ophthalmologic Examinations

The uncorrected visual acuity (UCVA) was measured preoperatively and on day 1, week 1, and month 1 postoperatively. The best-corrected VA (BCVA) was measured at the same time points; however, in about half of the cases, this examination was omitted on postoperative day 1. These VAs were calculated in logarithm of the minimum angle of resolution (logMAR) units. The subjective spherical equivalent (SE) and astigmatism were also collected at the same time points. The safety and efficacy index were calculated as the month 1 postoperative BCVA/preoperative BCVA and postoperative UCVA/preoperative BCVA. We calculated these indices because the current surgeries reported in this study were performed on patients without visual impairment in many cases. The decimal VA was used only for these calculations. The ECD was measured preoperatively and month 1 postoperatively using a specular microscope (EM-3000 (TOMEY, Tokyo, Japan) and CellChek SL, Noncon Robo II, or XII (Konan Medical, Hyogo, Japan). The axial length was measured using the IOLMaster 500 or IOLMaster 700 (Carl Zeiss Meditec AG, Jena, Germany).

2.5. Statistical Analysis

To reduce the possible bias of including both eyes of a patient, the values between the baseline and each time point were compared using a linear mixed model in which the random effect was the subjects. The linear mixed model adjusts for the hierarchical structure of the data, modeling in a way in which measurements are grouped within subjects [22,23]. This was followed by Dunnett's test for multiple comparisons when comparing the values between the baseline and each time point [24]. Statistical significance was set at 0.05. All analyses were performed using R 4.0.4 (R Foundation for Statistical Computing, Vienna, Austria).

3. Results

The mean ± standard deviation age of the patients at the time of cataract surgery was 55.0 ± 7.5 years. The duration between the cataract surgery and pIOL implantation was 9.7 ± 3.6 years. Fifty-three eyes received a PMMA phakic IOL and 43 eyes a silicone IOL. The UCVA and BCVA before the cataract surgery were 0.29 ± 0.34 and −0.01 ± 0.17 logMAR, respectively. The ECD was 1,986 ± 732 cells/mm^2. The detailed information is summarized in Table 1.

Table 1. Demographic data of the study participants.

Variable	Value
No. eyes	96 eyes/91 patients
Right/left eyes	48/48
Women/men	69/27
Age at cataract surgery (years)	55.0 ± 7.5
Age at pIOL implantation (years)	45.3 ± 7.4
Duration between surgeries (years)	9.7 ± 3.6
Emery-Little classification of nuclear cataract (eyes)	Grade I (16), grade II (46), grade III (31), grade IV (3)
pIOL material (eyes)	PMMA (53), silicone (43)
UCVA (logMAR)	0.29 ± 0.34
BCVA (logMAR)	−0.01 ± 0.17
Target refraction (D)	−0.17 ± 0.49
Spherical equivalent (D)	−1.43 ± 1.59
Cylinder (D)	−0.82 ± 0.73
Endothelial cell density (cells/mm^2)	1986 ± 732
Axial length (mm)	28.39 ± 1.94

Values are expressed as the mean ± standard deviation. The date of previous pIOL implantation was unknown in seven eyes and the UCVA before the cataract surgery in one eye. The age at pIOL implantation and duration between the surgeries were calculated without these eyes and the UCVA without the one eye. pIOL, phakic intraocular lens; PMMA, polymethyl methacrylate; UCVA, uncorrected visual acuity; BCVA, best-corrected visual acuity; D, diopters.

Figure 1A and Table 2 show the changes in the UCVA. The preoperative value significantly improved at day 1, week 1, and month 1 postoperatively ($p < 0.001$ for all comparisons by a linear mixed effect model followed by Dunnett's test). Similarly, the postoperative BCVA improved significantly at week 1 and month 1 ($p < 0.001$ for both comparisons) but not on day 1 ($p = 1.0$, Figure 1B, Table 2). The efficacy and safety indices on postoperative month 1 were 1.02 ± 0.56 and 1.31 ± 0.64, respectively.

The subjective SE was significantly larger (closer to 0) at all time points ($p < 0.001$ for all comparisons) (Figure 1C, Table 2), whereas the subjective astigmatism was greater on day 1 ($p = 0.0060$) but did not differ significantly at week 1 and month ($p = 1.0$ and $p = 0.078$, respectively) (Figure 1D, Table 2). The preoperative subjective astigmatism was significantly different between the patients with PMMA pIOLs and those with silicone IOLs

(p = 0.022, supplemental Figure S1). However, this difference was not found postoperatively. The ECD significantly decreased at month 1 ($p < 0.001$) (Figure 1E, Table 2).

The most common postoperative complication was an intraocular pressure (IOP) elevation exceeding 25 mmHg, which occurred in 10.4% of cases on day 1. With the exception of one case, no elevations were observed at postoperative week 1. Including this case, the IOP of all cases were controlled with medications. Corneal edema was observed in 8.3% of cases on day 1, which were not observed on day 7. No intraoperative complications developed. Other postoperative complications are summarized in Table 3.

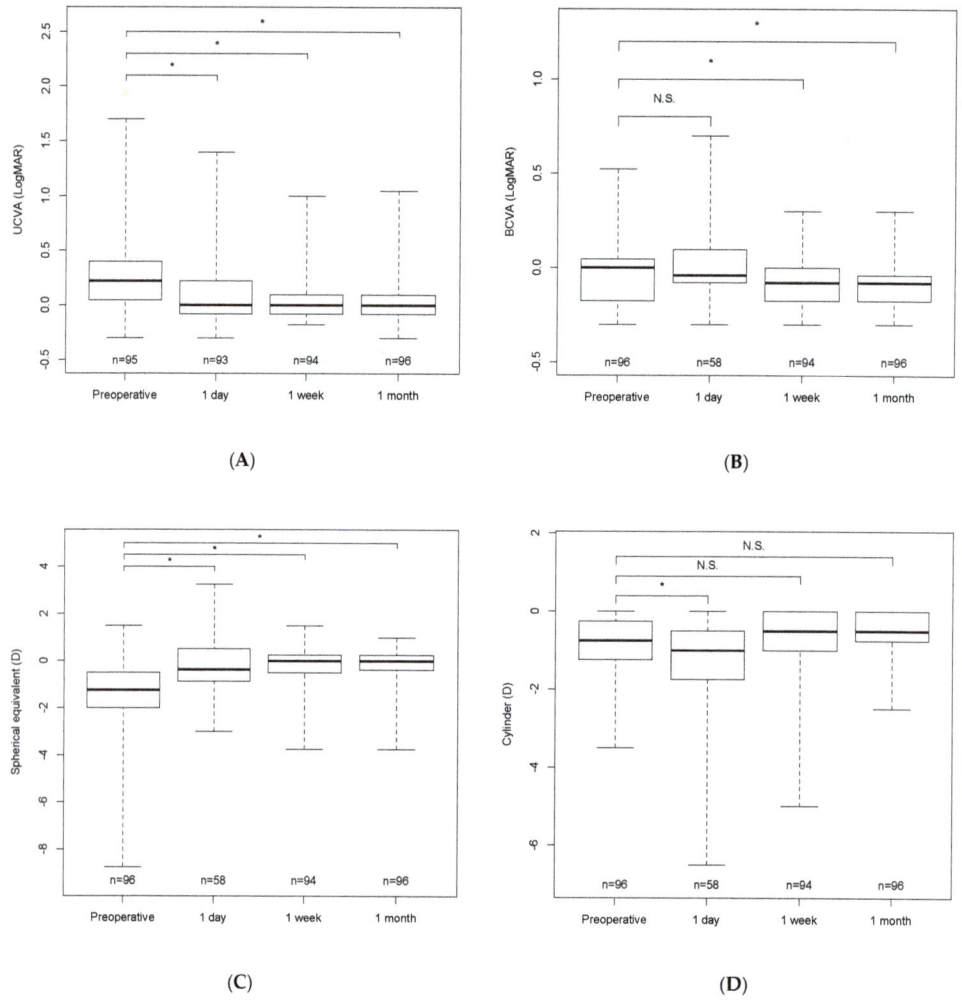

Figure 1. Cont.

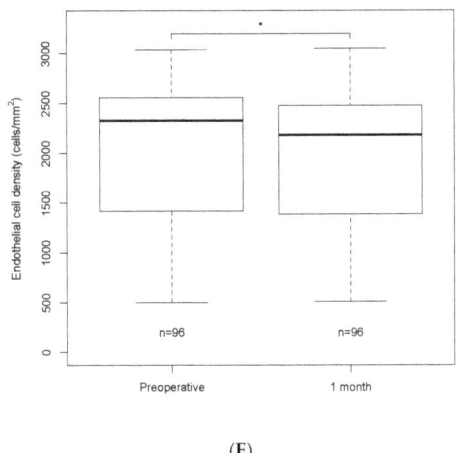

(E)

Figure 1. Box plots of each variable. (**A**) Changes in the uncorrected visual acuity (UCVA), (**B**) best-corrected visual acuity (BCVA), (**C**) spherical equivalent, (**D**) astigmatism, and (**E**) endothelial cell density. * indicates a significant difference between baseline and each time point. N.S., not significant; D, diopters; logMAR, logarithm of the minimum angle of resolution.

Table 2. Changes in each variable.

	UCVA (logMAR)			BCVA (logMAR)			SE (D)			Cylinder (D)			ECD (cells/mm²)		
	N	Variable	p Value	N	Variable	p Value	N	Variable	p Value	N	Variable	p Value	N	Variable	p Value
Preoperative	95	0.29 ± 0.34		96	−0.01 ± 0.17		96	−1.43 ± 1.59		96	−0.82 ± 0.73		96	1986 ± 732	
Day 1	93	0.11 ± 0.30	<0.001 *	58	0.01 ± 0.17	1.0	58	−0.32 ± 1.12	<0.001 *	58	−1.33 ± 1.45	0.0060 *			
Week 1	94	0.06 ± 0.23	<0.001 *	94	−0.08 ± 0.12	<0.001 *	94	−0.18 ± 0.78	<0.001 *	94	−0.82 ± 0.97	1.0			
Month 1	96	0.03 ± 0.19	<0.001 *	96	−0.09 ± 0.10	<0.001 *	96	−0.17 ± 0.84	<0.001 *	96	−0.57 ± 0.59	0.078	96	1897 ± 725	<0.001 *

The values are expressed as the mean ± standard deviation. * Statistically significant difference between baseline and each time point. UCVA, uncorrected visual acuity; BCVA, best-corrected visual acuity; SE, spherical equivalent; ECD: endothelial cell density; D, diopters.

Table 3. Postoperative complications.

Complication	% (eyes)
IOP elevation exceeding 25 mmHg	10.4% (10)
Corneal edema	8.3% (8)
Iritis	3.1% (3)
Corneal epithelial defect	2.1% (2)
Hyphema	2.1% (2)

IOP, intraocular pressure.

4. Discussion

In the current study, the efficacy and safety of cataract surgery combined with pIOL explantation were investigated in 96 eyes of 91 patients with an iris-fixated pIOL. This study included the largest number of cataract surgeries with pIOL explantation and was the largest study investigating patients with a iris-fixated pIOL. In a previous study with fewer cases, de Vries et al. [14] reported that the BCVA improved from 0.21 ± 0.21 to 0.17 ± 0.18. In the current study, the BCVA improved significantly from −0.01 ± 0.17 to −0.09 ± 0.10. A simple comparison of the studies was not possible because the baseline values differed in the study of de Vries et al., which included eyes with vision-threatening diseases, such as retinal detachment or myopic degeneration of the posterior pole. We excluded vision-threatening diseases; however, the improvements in the UCVA and BCVA were significant, with favorable efficacy and safety indices (1.02 ± 0.56 and 1.31 ± 0.64, respectively) at postoperative month 1, in light of the refractive correction.

In the current study, 10.4% of cases had a postoperative IOP elevation, despite the exclusion of glaucomatous eyes. A recent study by Vargas et al. [20] that included 87 eyes did not report IOP elevations. Meire et al. reported that two of 38 cases had ocular hypertension [16], one of which with steroid-induced ocular hypertension resulted in the need for an additional trabeculectomy because the steroids could not be discontinued due to systemic oncologic treatment. This rate was relatively high compared to uncomplicated cataract surgeries [25–27]. The exact reason is unclear; however, more intense inflammation that resulted from iris manipulation to remove the pIOL may be a reason. In the current study, the IOPs of all the cases were controlled safely only with medications until postoperative month 1; however, surgeons must be alert to IOP elevation postoperatively.

The current study had some limitations, one of which was the absence of a control group. Considering the baseline ECD (1986 ± 732 cells/mm^2) with an average patient age of 55.0 ± 7.5 years, the corneal endothelial damage was probably an important reason for the surgery. Therefore, other surgeries, such as standard cataract surgery or cataract surgeries for eyes with a posterior-chamber pIOL, were not considered as suitable controls because the indications differed. Despite this, we believe our data, comprised of the largest sample size of cataract surgery for eyes with pIOL, are valuable.

In the current study, the UCVA improved significantly from 0.29 ± 0.34 to 0.03 ± 0.19 at postoperative at month 1. The value at day 1 (0.11 ± 0.30) improved significantly from the preoperative level. However, the differences between the targeted and postoperative refractive errors were not assessed in this study. Although it was reported that the preoperative biometric measures were generally accurate [28], some miscalculations in the axial length were found along with the subsequent hyperopic change [29]. Furthermore, the types of inserted lens varied and included toric and multifocal IOLs because of the multicentre study. The targeted refractive error in most current cases was emmetropia or weak myopia (mean targeted refractive error, −0.17 ± 0.49) and the postoperative SE was −0.17 ± 0.84. Therefore, satisfactory outcomes were achieved in most cases; however, the specific analysis, such as the optimal IOL calculation formula to be used, will be addressed in our next study.

Our follow-up period was short. Although the recovery from the surgery was favorable despite this short follow-up period, the information about the clinical outcomes and safety with longer follow-up is essential for clinicians. In particular, the ECD significantly decreased at 1 month after surgery. The explantation of pIOL was carefully performed through sclerocorneal incision in order to not touch the endothelium. This procedure specific to the surgery might have had an effect. However, the ordinary cataract surgery with phacoemulsification and IOL implantation is well known to have an effect on ECD. The ECD change in our study was, on average, 4.5%. This was comparable to the past study of ordinary cataract surgery [30,31]. Thus, the ECD change was relatively small, but the early endothelial cell change cannot be fully evaluated by ECD [32]. Although the number of cases will be limited due to the retrospective design, careful and longer follow-up is needed. This will be discussed in the near future.

In conclusion, cataract surgeries for patients with iris-fixated pIOL were performed safely with good visual outcomes. We believe this option may be considered for patients with a pIOL who have visual impairment and endothelial cell loss.

Supplementary Materials: The following are available online at https://www.mdpi.com/article/10.3390/jcm10163672/s1, Figure S1: Comparison of subjective astigmatism between the pIOL materials, Table S1: Intraocular lenses implanted during cataract surgery.

Author Contributions: Conceptualization, M.K.O., I.T., H.A., T.N. and K.N.; Data Curation, M.K.O., S.M., I.T., H.A., T.N. and K.N.; Formal analysis, M.K.O.; Investigation, M.K.O. and K.N.; Methodology, M.K.O. and K.N.; Profect administration, K.N.; Resources, H.T., S.M., I.T., T.N. and K.N.; Supervision, S.M., M.A., I.T., H.A., T.N., K.T. and K.N.; Visualization, M.K.O.; Writing—original draft, M.K.O.; Writing—review and editing, H.T., S.M., M.A., I.T., H.A., T.N., K.T. and K.N. All authors will be informed about each step of manuscript processing including submission, revision, revision reminder, etc. via emails from our system or assigned Assistant Editor. All authors have read and agreed to the published version of the manuscript.

Funding: This research received no external funding.

Institutional Review Board Statement: The study was conducted according to the guidelines of the Declaration of Helsinki and approved by the Institutional Review Board of Keio University (Protocol code; 20190278, date of approval; 2 February 2020).

Informed Consent Statement: All patients read and signed the written informed consent form at each institute before the surgery. Patient consent for participating in this study was waived and the opt-out approach was used according to the Ethical Guidelines for Medical and Health Research Involving Human Subjects presented by the Ministry of Education, Culture, Sports, Science and Technology in Japan.

Data Availability Statement: The data presented in this study are available on request from the corresponding author with the permission of the Keio University Ethics Committee. The data is stored, and it will be discarded after the approved period by Ethics Committee.

Conflicts of Interest: The authors declare no conflict of interest.

References

1. Pascolini, D.; Mariotti, S.P. Global estimates of visual impairment: 2010. *Br. J. Ophthalmol.* **2012**, *96*, 614–618. [CrossRef] [PubMed]
2. Dolgin, E. The myopia boom. *Nature* **2015**, *519*, 276–278. [CrossRef] [PubMed]
3. Morgan, I.G.; French, A.N.; Ashby, R.S.; Guo, X.; Ding, X.; He, M.; Rose, K.A. The epidemics of myopia: Aetiology and prevention. *Prog. Retin. Eye Res.* **2018**, *62*, 134–149. [CrossRef] [PubMed]
4. Morgan, I.G.; Ohno-Matsui, K.; Saw, S.-M. Myopia. *Lancet* **2012**, *379*, 1739–1748. [CrossRef]
5. Guell, J.L.; Morral, M.; Kook, D.; Kohnen, T. Phakic intraocular lenses part 1: Historical overview, current models, selection criteria, and surgical techniques. *J. Cataract Refract. Surg.* **2010**, *36*, 1976–1993. [CrossRef] [PubMed]
6. Kohnen, T.; Kook, D.; Morral, M.; Guell, J.L. Phakic intraocular lenses: Part 2: Results and complications. *J. Cataract Refract. Surg.* **2010**, *36*, 2168–2194. [CrossRef] [PubMed]
7. Choi, J.H.; Lim, D.H.; Nam, S.W.; Yang, C.M.; Chung, E.S.; Chung, T.Y. Ten-year clinical outcomes after implantation of a posterior chamber phakic intraocular lens for myopia. *J. Cataract Refract. Surg.* **2019**, *45*, 1555–1561. [CrossRef]
8. Nakamura, T.; Isogai, N.; Kojima, T.; Yoshida, Y.; Sugiyama, Y. Posterior Chamber Phakic Intraocular Lens Implantation for the Correction of Myopia and Myopic Astigmatism: A Retrospective 10-Year Follow-up Study. *Am. J. Ophthalmol.* **2019**, *206*, 1–10. [CrossRef]

9. Tahzib, N.G.; Nuijts, R.M.; Wu, W.Y.; Budo, C.J. Long-term study of Artisan phakic intraocular lens implantation for the correction of moderate to high myopia: Ten-year follow-up results. *Ophthalmology* **2007**, *114*, 1133–1142. [CrossRef]
10. Alio, J.L.; Abdelrahman, A.M.; Javaloy, J.; Iradier, M.T.; Ortuno, V. Angle-supported anterior chamber phakic intraocular lens explantation causes and outcome. *Ophthalmology* **2006**, *113*, 2213–2220. [CrossRef]
11. Alio, J.L.; Toffaha, B.T.; Pena-Garcia, P.; Sadaba, L.M.; Barraquer, R.I. Phakic intraocular lens explantation: Causes in 240 cases. *J. Refract. Surg.* **2015**, *31*, 30–35. [CrossRef]
12. Sucu, M.E.; Cakmak, S.; Yildirim, Y.; Yildiz, B.K.; Yalcinkaya, G.; Besek, N.K.; Yasar, T. Explantation of phakic intraocular lenses: Causes and outcomes. *Int. Ophthalmol.* **2021**, *41*, 265–271. [CrossRef]
13. Bleckmann, H.; Keuch, R.J. Results of cataract extraction after implantable contact lens removal. *J. Cataract Refract. Surg.* **2005**, *31*, 2329–2333. [CrossRef]
14. de Vries, N.E.; Tahzib, N.G.; Budo, C.J.; Webers, C.A.; de Boer, R.; Hendrikse, F.; Nuijts, R.M. Results of cataract surgery after implantation of an iris-fixated phakic intraocular lens. *J. Cataract Refract. Surg.* **2009**, *35*, 121–126. [CrossRef]
15. Kamiya, K.; Shimizu, K.; Igarashi, A.; Aizawa, D.; Ikeda, T. Clinical outcomes and patient satisfaction after Visian Implantable Collamer Lens removal and phacoemulsification with intraocular lens implantation in eyes with induced cataract. *Eye* **2010**, *24*, 304–309. [CrossRef]
16. Meier, P.G.; Majo, F.; Othenin-Girard, P.; Bergin, C.; Guber, I. Refractive outcomes and complications after combined copolymer phakic intraocular lens explantation and phacoemulsification with intraocular lens implantation. *J. Cataract Refract. Surg.* **2017**, *43*, 748–753. [CrossRef]
17. Morales, A.J.; Zadok, D.; Tardio, E.; Anzoulatous, G., Jr.; Litwak, S.; Mora, R.; Martinez, E.; Chayet, A.S. Outcome of simultaneous phakic implantable contact lens removal with cataract extraction and pseudophakic intraocular lens implantation. *J. Cataract Refract. Surg.* **2006**, *32*, 595–598. [CrossRef]
18. Agarwal, P.; Navon, S.E.; Mithal, N. Novel technique of explantation of rigid phakic iris-claw lens and cataract extraction by sutureless manual small-incision surgery. *BMJ Case Rep.* **2019**, *12*, e233128. [CrossRef]
19. Khokhar, S.; Mahabir, M. Phacoemulsification in phakic iris-claw lens with cataract. *Indian J. Ophthalmol.* **2018**, *66*, 1609–1610.
20. Vargas, V.; Alio, J.L.; Barraquer, R.I.; D'Antin, J.C.; Garcia, C.; Duch, F.; Balgos, J.; Alio Del Barrio, J.L. Safety and visual outcomes following posterior chamber phakic intraocular lens bilensectomy. *Eye Vis.* **2020**, *7*, 34. [CrossRef]
21. van Rijn, G.A.; Gaurisankar, Z.S.; Ilgenfritz, A.P.; Lima, J.E.E.; Haasnoot, G.W.; Beenakker, J.M.; Cheng, Y.Y.Y.; Luyten, G.P.M. Middle-and long-term results after iris-fixated phakic intraocular lens implantation in myopic and hyperopic patients: A meta-analysis. *J. Cataract Refract. Surg.* **2020**, *46*, 125–137. [CrossRef] [PubMed]
22. Baayen, R.H.; Davidson, D.J.; Bates, D.M. Mixed-effects modeling with crossed random effects for subjects and items. *J. Mem. Lang.* **2008**, *59*, 390–412. [CrossRef]
23. Bates, D.; Mächler, M.; Bolker, B.; Walker, S. Fitting Linear Mixed-Effects Models Using lme4. *J. Stat. Softw.* **2015**, *67*. [CrossRef]
24. Dunnett, C.W. A multiple comparison procedure for comparing several treatments with a control. *Am. Stat. Assoc.* **1955**, *50*, 1096–1211. [CrossRef]
25. Grzybowski, A.; Kanclerz, P. Early postoperative intraocular pressure elevation following cataract surgery. *Curr. Opin. Ophthalmol.* **2019**, *30*, 56–62. [CrossRef]
26. Levkovitch-Verbin, H.; Habot-Wilner, Z.; Burla, N.; Melamed, S.; Goldenfeld, M.; Bar-Sela, S.M.; Sachs, D. Intraocular pressure elevation within the first 24 hours after cataract surgery in patients with glaucoma or exfoliation syndrome. *Ophthalmology* **2008**, *115*, 104–108. [CrossRef]
27. Syed, Z.A.; Moayedi, J.; Mohamedi, M.; Tashter, J.; Anthony, T.; Celiker, C.; Khazen, G.; Melki, S.A. Cataract surgery outcomes at a UK independent sector treatment centre. *Br. J. Ophthalmol.* **2015**, *99*, 1460–1465. [CrossRef]
28. Amro, M.; Chanbour, W.; Arej, N.; Jarade, E. Third- and fourth-generation formulas for intraocular lens power calculation before and after phakic intraocular lens insertion in high myopia. *J. Cataract Refract. Surg.* **2018**, *44*, 1321–1325. [CrossRef]
29. Yasa, D.; Kose, B.; Sucu, M.E.; Agca, A. Intraocular lens power calculation in a posterior chamber phakic intraocular lens implanted eye. *Int. Ophthalmol.* **2020**, *40*, 2017–2022. [CrossRef]
30. Goles, N.; Nerancic, M.; Konjik, S.; Pajic-Eggspuehler, B.; Pajic, B.; Cvejic, Z. Phacoemulsification and IOL-Implantation without Using Viscoelastics: Combined Modeling of Thermo Fluid Dynamics, Clinical Outcomes, and Endothelial Cell Density. *Sensors* **2021**, *21*, 2399. [CrossRef]
31. Hayashi, K.; Yoshida, M.; Manabe, S.; Hirata, A. Cataract surgery in eyes with low corneal endothelial cell density. *J. Cataract Refract. Surg.* **2011**, *37*, 1419–1425. [CrossRef]
32. Kim, D.H.; Wee, W.R.; Hyon, J.Y. The pattern of early corneal endothelial cell recovery following cataract surgery: Cellular migration or enlargement? *Graefes Arch. Clin. Exp. Ophthalmol.* **2015**, *253*, 2211–2216. [CrossRef]

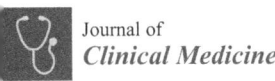

Article

The Effect of Ametropia on Glaucomatous Visual Field Loss

Eun Young Choi [1,2,3,†], Raymond C. S. Wong [1,2,†], Thuzar Thein [1,2], Louis R. Pasquale [4], Lucy Q. Shen [5], Mengyu Wang [1,2], Dian Li [1,2], Qingying Jin [1,6], Hui Wang [1,7], Neda Baniasadi [1], Michael V. Boland [8], Siamak Yousefi [9], Sarah R. Wellik [10], Carlos G. De Moraes [11], Jonathan S. Myers [12], Peter J. Bex [13] and Tobias Elze [1,2,*]

1. Schepens Eye Research Institute of Massachusetts Eye and Ear, Boston, MA 02114, USA; eunyoung.choi@duke.edu (E.Y.C.); ray_wong@meei.harvard.edu (R.C.S.W.); Thuzar.thein@mah.harvard.edu (T.T.); mengyu_wang@meei.harvard.edu (M.W.); dianli@ds.dfci.harvard.edu (D.L.); jljinqy@jlu.edu.cn (Q.J.); 108014@jlufe.edu.cn (H.W.); nbaniasa@bidmc.harvard.edu (N.B.)
2. Department of Ophthalmology, Harvard Medical School, Boston, MA 02114, USA
3. Department of Ophthalmology, Duke University Medical Center, Durham, NC 27705, USA
4. Department of Ophthalmology, Icahn School of Medicine at Mount Sinai, New York, NY 10029, USA; louis.pasquale@mssm.edu
5. Massachusetts Eye and Ear, Harvard Medical School, Boston, MA 02115, USA; lucy_shen@meei.harvard.edu
6. Department of Psychology, Jilin University, Changchun 130012, China
7. Jilin University of Finance and Economics, Changchun 130117, China
8. Wilmer Eye Institute, Johns Hopkins University School of Medicine, Baltimore, MD 21287, USA; michael_boland@meei.harvard.edu
9. Hamilton Eye Institute, University of Tennessee Health Science Center, Memphis, TN 38103, USA; siamak.yousefi@uthsc.edu
10. Bascom Palmer Eye Institute, University of Miami School of Medicine, Miami, FL 33136, USA; swellik@med.miami.edu
11. Edward S. Harkness Eye Institute, Columbia University, New York, NY 10032, USA; cvd2109@columbia.edu
12. Wills Eye Hospital, Thomas Jefferson University, Philadelphia, PA 19107, USA; jmyers@willseye.org
13. Department of Psychology, Northeastern University, Boston, MA 02115, USA; p.bex@neu.edu
* Correspondence: tobias_elze@meei.harvard.edu; Tel.: +1-(617)-912-0100
† These authors contributed equally to this work.

Abstract: Myopia has been discussed as a risk factor for glaucoma. In this study, we characterized the relationship between ametropia and patterns of visual field (VF) loss in glaucoma. Reliable automated VFs (SITA Standard 24-2) of 120,019 eyes from 70,495 patients were selected from five academic institutions. The pattern deviation (PD) at each VF location was modeled by linear regression with ametropia (defined as spherical equivalent (SE) starting from extreme high myopia), mean deviation (MD), and their interaction (SE × MD) as regressors. Myopia was associated with decreased PD at the paracentral and temporal VF locations, whereas hyperopia was associated with decreased PD at the Bjerrum and nasal step locations. The severity of VF loss modulated the effect of ametropia: with decreasing MD and SE, paracentral/nasal step regions became more depressed and Bjerrum/temporal regions less depressed. Increasing degree of myopia was positively correlated with VF depression at four central points, and the correlation became stronger with increasing VF loss severity. With worsening VF loss, myopes have increased VF depressions at the paracentral and nasal step regions, while hyperopes have increased depressions at the Bjerrum and temporal locations. Clinicians should be aware of these effects of ametropia when interpreting VF loss.

Keywords: glaucoma; ametropia; myopia; hyperopia; visual field; OCT; SITA standard 24-2; pattern deviation; mean deviation; spherical equivalent

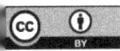

1. Introduction

Glaucoma is an optic neuropathy characterized by progressive loss of retinal ganglion cells, resulting in optic nerve damage and eventual visual field (VF) loss. Since glaucoma tends to produce specific VF defects, the pattern deviation (PD) plot, which shows relative light sensitivity normalized by age-matched controls at each VF location, is crucial for the diagnosis of this optic neuropathy. Standard automated perimetry, particularly the Swedish interactive thresholding algorithm (SITA) standard 24-2 [1,2] is a widely used tool to characterize and monitor functional vision loss from glaucoma [3,4].

High myopia is considered a risk factor for glaucoma in several studies [5–7]. It is well-known that refractive error is associated with ocular biometric features. In general, myopic eyes tend to have a longer axial length and are more prolate than emmetropic eyes, while hyperopic eyes tend to have a shorter axial length and are more oblate (Figure 1A) [8,9]. In addition, the superior and inferior arcuate retinal nerve fiber bundles lie closer to the fovea in myopes compared to emmetropes or hyperopes (Figure 1B), resulting in a thicker temporal peripapillary retinal nerve fiber layer (RNFL) in myopic eyes [10–13]. Previous studies have shown the association between the spherical equivalent (SE) of refractive error and various anatomical parameters of the optic nerve head (ONH), which serve as important diagnostic criteria for glaucoma [12,14,15]. For example, increasing myopia is associated with greater optic disc torsion and tilt [14,15]. Furthermore, we have previously shown that the central retinal vessel trunks (CRVT), where retinal vessels enter and exit the optic disc, are located more nasally in myopes compared to hyperopes [15]. The nasalization of CRVTs, in turn, has been correlated with a central pattern of VF loss [16–18]. These findings suggest that myopes and hyperopes, with their varying structural parameters, may also have different patterns of light sensitivity. Previous works show myopia to be a risk factor for paracentral VF defects in glaucomatous eyes [19–22], while others report a high incidence of temporal VF defects in highly myopic eyes without known glaucoma [23]. We sought to build upon these studies by systematically examining the interaction effect of the full range of ametropia and VF loss severity on global VF patterns. Our goal is to understand how functional vision is affected by ametropia in patients with glaucoma.

In this study, we investigate the relationship between ametropia and VF patterns utilizing a large VF dataset from 5 academic institutions. Furthermore, we study the role of VF loss severity in modulating this relationship. We hypothesize that (A) given the structural differences in the eye, ametropia is associated with distinct patterns of light sensitivity, regardless of glaucoma; (B) because myopes have retinal nerve fiber (RNF) bundles that lie closer to the fovea, there is an interaction effect between glaucoma severity and ametropia; and (C) because myopes have more nasalized CRVTs, they develop deeper central VF depression (Figure 1). Our study aims to help clinicians better identify and interpret glaucomatous VF loss patterns in myopic and hyperopic patients.

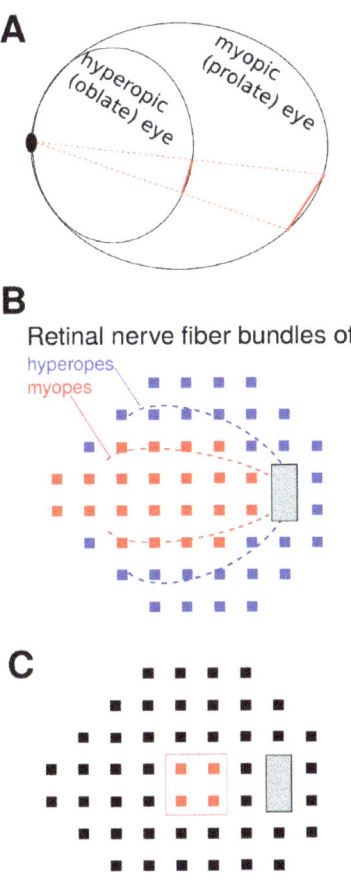

Figure 1. Schematic illustration of the three main hypotheses. (**A**) Ametropia is related to differences in eye length and shape, e.g., myopic eyes are longer, "curvier" (more prolate), and less regular. Therefore, we hypothesize relative differences of light sensitivity related to ametropia independent of glaucoma. (**B**) The two major retinal nerve fiber bundles, illustrated by dashed lines superimposed on the locations of a Humphrey 24-2 visual field (VF), are closer to the fovea for myopes (red lines) than for hyperopes (blue lines). Therefore, we hypothesize a center-periphery interaction effect between glaucoma severity and ametropia, schematically illustrated by the two different colors of the VF locations. (**C**) Myopia is correlated to a nasalization of the central retinal vessel trunk which, in turn, is related to glaucomatous central VF loss on the four central locations of the Humphrey 24-2 VF, illustrated in red. Therefore, we hypothesize deeper central VF depression for myopes, particularly for higher glaucoma severity.

2. Methods

The VFs used for this study were obtained through the Glaucoma Research Network, a multicenter consortium, which consists of Massachusetts Eye and Ear, Wilmer Eye Institute, New York Eye and Ear Infirmary, Wills Eye Hospital, and Bascom Palmer Eye Institute. The institutional review board of each participating institution approved this retrospective study. This study adheres to the Declaration of Helsinki and all federal and state laws.

2.1. Participants and Data

Our dataset consisted of SITA standard 24-2 VFs measured with the Humphrey Field Analyzer (HFA; Carl Zeiss Meditec, Dublin, CA, USA). The dataset used in this study consisted of all available VFs from the glaucoma services of Massachusetts Eye and Ear, Wilmer Eye Institute, New York Eye and Ear Infirmary, and Wills Eye Hospital, and the entire set of VF measurements from Bascom Palmer Eye Institute. The reliability criteria for VF selection were as follows: fixation losses $\leq$ 33%, false-negative rate $\leq$ 20%, and false-positive rate $\leq$ 20% [17,24–27]. If more than one measurement per eye fulfilled the reliability criteria, the most recent reliable VF was selected for each eye. VFs from the left eye were reflected along the vertical axis to match the orientation of the right eye, which is the standard orientation displayed in this paper. At testing time, the operator was required to enter the patient's distance refractive error into the HFA machine in order for the machine to determine the matching trial lens. These distance refractive error values were logged by the HFA and used in the present study. The HFA device automatically assigns a value of 0 to all participants wearing a contact lens; therefore, all eyes with a distance refractive error of 0 could not be distinguished whether they were naturally emmetropic, pseudophakic, and emmetropic due to successful cataract surgery, or corrected by contact lenses and thus were excluded from analysis. In our supplemental analyses, additional exclusion criteria were applied based on age, SE, and mean deviation (MD): patients younger than 18 years or older than 80 years, eyes with $-1.5\,D \leq SE \leq +1.0\,D$, and eyes with MD less than -18 dB were excluded.

2.2. Statistical Analyses

All statistical analyses were performed using the R platform [28]. For patients with minimal VF loss, defined as MD within ± 1 dB, mean PD and their standard deviations were plotted against SE for each VF location on the Humphrey 24-2. Linear regression slopes of PD and SE were calculated and plotted for patients with MD within ± 1 dB and for those with MD < -12 dB. Furthermore, PD values at each VF location were modeled by linear regression with SE, MD, and their interaction (SE $\times$ MD) as regressors, using the following equation: PD~SE + MD + (SE $\times$ MD). Finally, given our previous finding that CRVT nasalization was associated with VF loss in the central 4 VF locations [17], SE slopes were calculated for the 4 most central locations, as a function of the magnitude of MD. p values of the slopes were adjusted for multiple comparisons by the false discovery rate method [29]. A p value < 0.05 was considered statistically significant.

3. Results

A total of 120,019 VFs from 120,019 eyes of 70,495 patients met our inclusion criteria. Figure 2 summarizes the clinical and demographic information of the subjects.

In the analysis involving all eyes, MD had a weak but statistically significant correlation with SE (Pearson's r = 0.045, $p < 2.2 \times 10^{-16}$). Figure 3 shows the mean PD values at each of the 52 VF locations, grouped by bins of SE (bin centers: $-6, -4, -2, 0, 2, 4,$ and 6 Diopters (Ds), bin width: ± 1 D), for individuals with minimal VF loss (MD within ± 1 dB). The following general trend was observed: with increasing myopia (decreasing SE), PD values increased at the peripheral VF locations and decreased at the central VF locations; opposite effects were noted for hyperopia.

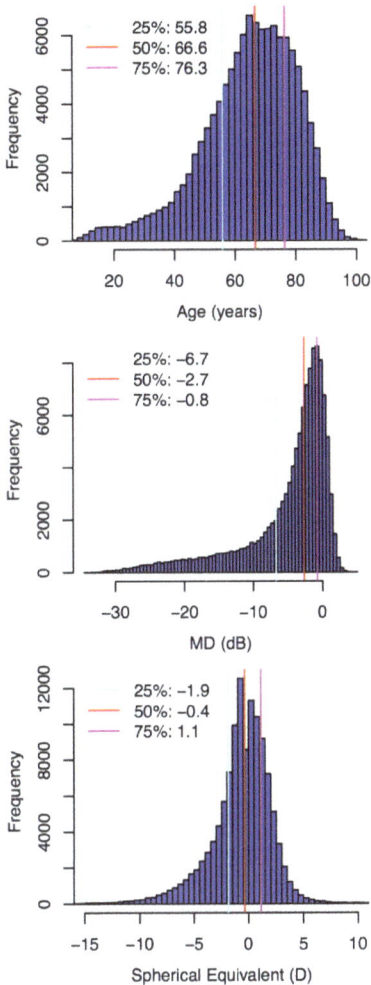

Figure 2. Demographic histograms of age, visual field mean deviation (MD), and spherical equivalent of refractive error (from top to bottom). Quartiles are denoted by vertical lines.

Given the generally monotonic pattern of correlation observed, linear regression of PD from SE was performed to quantify the relationship. The regression coefficients at each VF location are shown in Figure 4. For patients with minimal VF loss (MD within ±1 dB), positive coefficients were observed in the paracentral and temporal VFs, indicating that increased myopia was associated with decreased light sensitivity in these regions. Negative slopes were observed mostly in the Bjerrum and nasal step areas, indicating that increasing hyperopia was associated with lower light sensitivity in these regions (Figure 4A). These results were in line with the trend observed in Figure 3. The significant positive slopes ranged from 0.01 to 0.04, and significant negative slopes ranged from −0.01 to −0.11 ($p < 0.05$). This means that for individuals with at most mild glaucoma, high myopes (SE: −6 D) can have up to 0.48 dB lower and 1.3 dB higher PD values compared to high hyperopes (SE: +6 D) at individual VF locations.

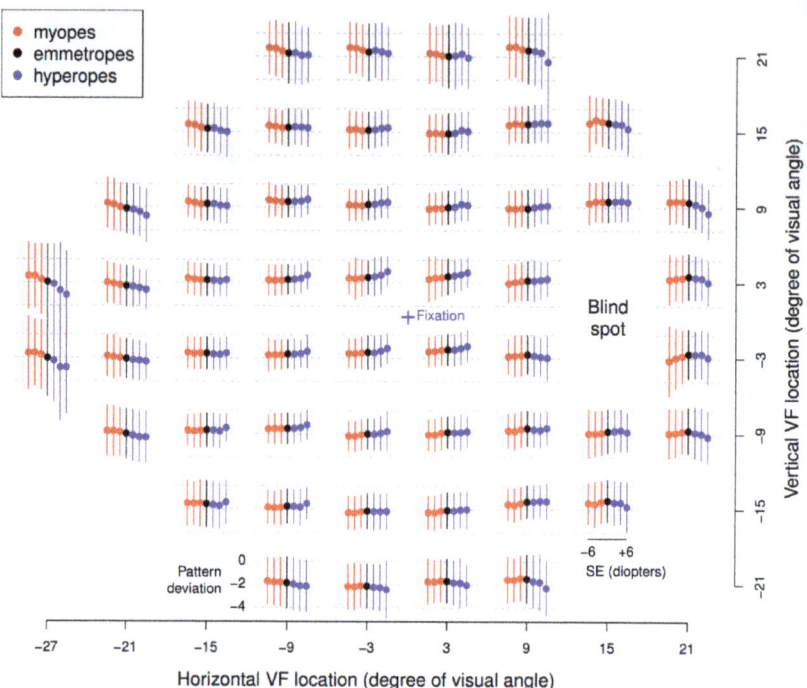

Figure 3. Mean pattern deviations (PD), illustrated by filled circles, and corresponding standard deviations (whiskers) grouped by bins of spherical equivalent (SE) of refractive error (bin centers: −6, −4, −2, 0, 2, 4, and 6 Diopters) for each visual field (VF) location for patients with VF mean deviations within ±1 dB. Each SE bin contains SEs within ±1 Diopter of the respective bin center. The location of fixation is denoted by the central blue cross. The two VF locations closest to the blind spot are omitted.

For patients with severe VF depression (MD < −12 dB), the pattern was slightly different: positive slopes were observed mostly in the paracentral VF, and negative slopes were observed in the Bjerrum and temporal regions (Figure 4B). This implies that increasing myopia was associated with VF depression in the paracentral region, and increasing hyperopia was associated with depression in Bjerrum and temporal regions. The magnitudes of the slopes were greater for severe VF loss compared to mild VF loss: the significant positive slopes ranged from 0.01 to 0.19, and significant negative slopes ranged from −0.02 to −0.23 ($p < 0.05$). This means that for severe glaucoma, high myopes (SE: −6 D) can have up to 2.3 dB lower and 2.8 dB higher PD values than high hyperopes (SE: +6 D) at individual VF locations.

To further explore the relationship between SE and PD, and to understand the role of VF loss severity on this correlation, linear regression was carried out with SE, MD, and their interaction term (SE × MD) as regressors. Figure 5A shows the "pure" SE effect on PD: when MD was not taken into account, myopes had a significantly lower light sensitivity in the paracentral and temporal VFs, but greater light sensitivity in the Bjerrum and nasal step regions. When the interactive effect of MD and SE was examined, myopic VF depression became localized to the paracentral and nasal step regions while hyperopic VF depression became more pronounced at the Bjerrum and temporal areas (Figure 5B). The significant positive interaction coefficients ranged from 0.002 to 0.012, and significant negative coefficients ranged from −0.002 to −0.01 ($p < 0.05$). The detailed regression coefficients for SE, MD, and SE × MD at each of the 52 VF locations are provided in Supplementary Materials Figure S1. As expected, the effect of MD alone on PD showed a highly significant correlation at every location.

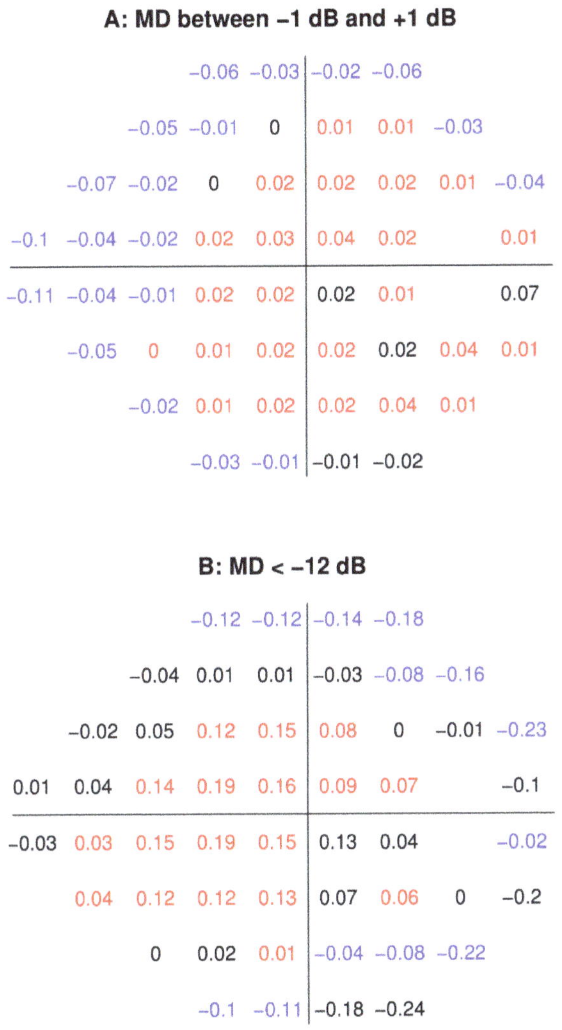

A: MD between −1 dB and +1 dB

			−0.06	−0.03	−0.02	−0.06	
		−0.05	−0.01	0	0.01	0.01	−0.03
	−0.07	−0.02	0	0.02	0.02	0.02	0.01	−0.04
−0.1	−0.04	−0.02	0.02	0.03	0.04	0.02		0.01
−0.11	−0.04	−0.01	0.02	0.02	0.02	0.01		0.07
	−0.05	0	0.01	0.02	0.02	0.02	0.04	0.01
		−0.02	0.01	0.02	0.02	0.04	0.01
			−0.03	−0.01	−0.01	−0.02	

B: MD < −12 dB

			−0.12	−0.12	−0.14	−0.18	
		−0.04	0.01	0.01	−0.03	−0.08	−0.16
	−0.02	0.05	0.12	0.15	0.08	0	−0.01	−0.23
0.01	0.04	0.14	0.19	0.16	0.09	0.07		−0.1
−0.03	0.03	0.15	0.19	0.15	0.13	0.04		−0.02
	0.04	0.12	0.12	0.13	0.07	0.06	0	−0.2
		0	0.02	0.01	−0.04	−0.08	−0.22
			−0.1	−0.11	−0.18	−0.24	

Figure 4. Spherical equivalent regression coefficients of pattern deviations at each visual field (VF) location for (**A**) patients with (at most) minor VF depression (mean deviation (MD) within ±1 dB) vs. (**B**) patients with severe VF depression (MD < −12 dB). Non-significant coefficients are colored in black, significant positive coefficients in red, and significant negative coefficients in blue. In short, at red/blue locations, myopes have more/less VF depression.

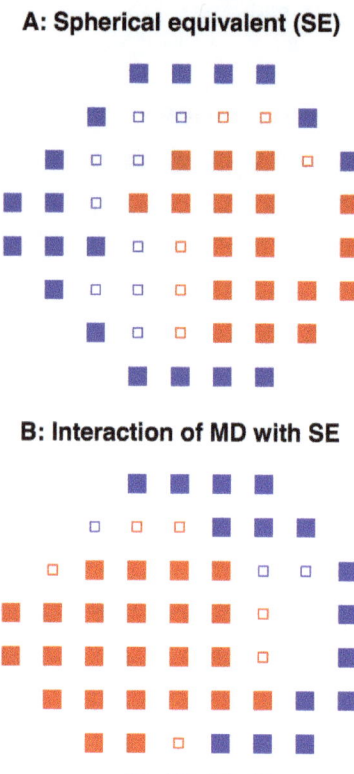

Figure 5. (**A**) Impact of spherical equivalent (SE) on visual field pattern deviations that are not explained by glaucoma severity (mean deviation, MD) and (**B**) interaction effects between glaucoma severity (MD) and SE. Significant locations are denoted by filled squares, non-significant locations by small, open squares. In label (**A**), red/blue locations denote positive/negative coefficients, i.e., locations where myopes have more/less VF depression regardless of glaucoma severity. In label (**B**), red/blue locations denote negative/positive coefficients of the interaction term (SE × MD). In short, at red/blue locations, increasing glaucoma severity is related to more/less VF depression in myopes.

Example VFs of myopic and hyperopic patients seen at Mass. Eye and Ear displaying these VF loss patterns are shown in Figure 6. With worsening glaucoma, myopic individuals tend to develop deeper paracentral VF defects, while hyperopic individuals tend to develop greater VF depression in the Bjerrum and temporal regions.

Finally, we examined the effect of SE on PD at the 4 most central VF locations (marked by the red squares in Figure 1C) as a function of VF loss severity. Myopia was significantly correlated with decreasing PD values at the central 4 locations ($p < 0.001$), and the correlation became stronger with decreasing MD (Table 1).

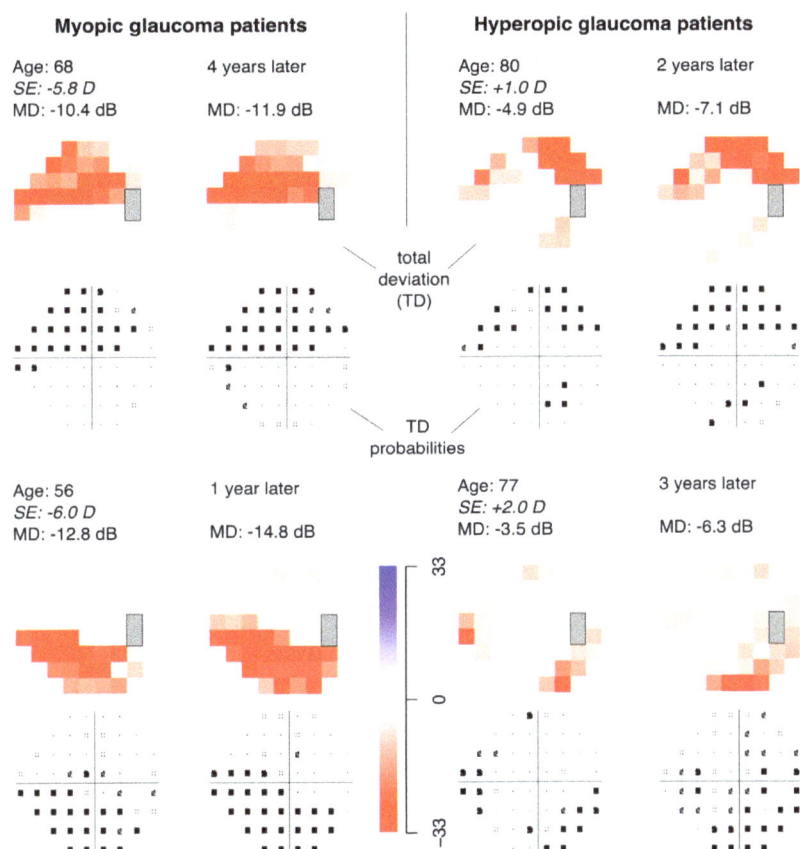

Figure 6. Example visual fields (VFs) of myopic and hyperopic patients with glaucoma, and the progression of VFs over time. Total deviation (TD) plots are shown for each patient: the color plots represent the numerical TD values (dB) and the grayscale plots represent the probability plots. In myopic patients (left panel), VF defects tend to be located in the paracentral and nasal step regions, whereas in hyperopic patients (right panel), VF defects tend to be located in the Bjerrum and temporal regions.

Table 1. Spherical equivalent regression coefficients of pattern deviations for the central four visual field (VF) locations on SITA 24-2 by VF loss severity. Each mean deviation (MD) bin contains MDs within ±3 dB of the respective bin center given in the first column. p values are adjusted for multiple comparisons.

MD Bin Center (dB)	SE Coefficient	p Value
0	0.03	6.82×10^{-46}
-6	0.05	3.22×10^{-14}
-12	0.06	0.000455
-18	0.12	7.04×10^{-5}
-24	0.20	5.92×10^{-6}

4. Discussion

In this study, we systematically investigated and quantified the effect of ametropia on retinal sensitivity at each VF location in the 24-2 pattern. While effects of myopia on specific VF defects have been reported [19–23], to our best knowledge, no prior work has examined this relationship in detail over the full range of ametropia and over the entire VF test locations. Additionally, we studied the interactive effect of ametropia and glaucoma severity on VF loss patterns. Our results show that while the effects of ametropia on individual PD values are small, there are distinct patterns of VF loss associated with myopia and hyperopia, and the relationship becomes stronger with increasing VF loss severity.

The Glaucoma Research Network dataset does not contain ophthalmic diagnoses, but given the origins of this large dataset, we may safely assume that VF loss occurring in these patients is mostly due to glaucoma. We first hypothesized that because of the structural variations in myopic and hyperopic eyes [8,9], there would be differences in light sensitivity depending on the degree of ametropia, regardless of the presence of VF loss. We demonstrate that in patients with minimal VF loss, patterns of light sensitivity differ among myopes and hyperopes, with myopes having relatively decreased sensitivity in the paracentral and temporal VF areas and hyperopes in the Bjerrum region and nasal step areas (Figure 4A). Notably, the different patterns in Figure 4A,B indicate a possibly independent effect of ametropia from that of nerve fiber anatomy associated with ametropia on VF loss. Therefore, we chose to statistically disentangle these two effects. Figure 5A shows the "pure SE effect", i.e., the effect without accounting for the variance explained by VF loss severity. As expected, a pattern similar to Figure 4A is seen, with myopes having decreased sensitivity in the paracentral, inferior Bjerrum, and temporal areas. These "pure SE effects" could originate from ocular anatomical parameters associated with (axial) ametropia, but could also result from lens related diseases (e.g., nuclear cataract) or even by trial lens related measurement artifacts. Without medical diagnoses, potentially confounding diseases could not be controlled for in the current study. In a previous work on high myopia, Ohno-Matsui et al. [23]. carefully controlled for diseases and excluded trial lens artifacts by applying soft contact lenses for perimetry. They studied 492 highly myopic eyes without known glaucoma: among the eyes with significant VF defects, temporal field defects were observed in 61.5% of the eyes with round discs, 75.0% of the eyes with vertically oval discs, and 68.2% of the eyes with obliquely oval discs. Consistent with their results, our study found the temporal field to be the dominant location of reduced sensitivity in myopia. While they focus only on extremely myopic patients, we examine the full range of ametropia and show that myopic and hyperopic individuals, regardless of VF loss severity, have distinct patterns of light sensitivity.

We also hypothesized that, given the anatomical differences in RNF bundle trajectories between myopic and hyperopic eyes, there would be an interaction effect of ametropia and glaucoma severity on VF patterns. As mentioned above, using linear modeling with the interaction term (SE × MD) as a regressor, we were able to disentangle the effect of SE from that of MD. Lens artifacts and diseases of the anterior segment such as cataracts are most likely additive to VF loss patterns but would not interact with glaucomatous VF loss severity. This means, the "pure SE effect" bundles all possibly artifactual lens effects and confounding diseases so that our SE × MD interaction results can likely be solely explained by retinal differences associated with ametropia, such as differences in nerve fiber anatomy. We demonstrate that with increasing severity of VF loss and degree of ametropia, myopes develop more profound paracentral and nasal step VF depressions, while hyperopes develop more depression in the Bjerrum and temporal VF points (Figures 4B and 5B). Furthermore, while myopia alone is associated with decreased sensitivity in the temporal sector and increased sensitivity in the nasal step sector, the pattern reverses when the interactive effect of ametropia and VF loss severity is examined. These distinct patterns indicate that different mechanisms are responsible for the effects of ametropia and glaucoma on VF loss.

We performed additional analyses after excluding subjects older than 80 years or younger than 18 years, as these patients might have a higher ratio of non-excluded pseudophakia (see Discussion) or not have age-matched controls, respectively. Similar effects on VF patterns were observed with or without the age exclusion criteria (Supplementary Materials Figure S2). Furthermore, we performed analyses after excluding eyes with

MD < −18 dB, because our dataset and others indicate that the pattern standard deviation and PD values begin to normalize at this degree of VF loss severity [30]. Again, similar effects were observed with this exclusion criterion (Supplementary Materials Figure S3), indicating that our results are not caused by potential non-linearities of the PD values. Finally, we re-analyzed the data after excluding eyes with lower absolute refractive error (−1.5 D ≤ SE ≤ +1.0 D) to exclude the vast majority of pseudophakics (see Discussion). Similar results were obtained with this exclusion criterion as well (Supplementary Materials Figure S4).

Given our findings, we further examined the effect of ametropia on light sensitivity at the 4 most central VF locations on the 24-2 plot representing macular function. This experimental design was inspired by our previous work [17] showing that CRVT nasalization was significantly correlated with VF depression only in the central sector (as defined by the annular scheme [17] and the Garway-Heath scheme [31]). In the current study, we demonstrate that myopia is significantly associated with VF loss in the central four locations and that the correlation becomes progressively stronger with increasing VF loss severity (Table 1). These results are consistent with our previous finding that myopes have more nasally located CRVTs [15], which in turn is associated with deeper central VF depression [16,17]. Although we cannot conclude any causal relationships, CRVT nasalization may explain the increased susceptibility of myopic eyes to central VF loss. We and others have speculated that CRVTs can act as stabilizing forces against glaucomatous deformation of the lamina cribrosa [17]. More nasally located CRVTs in myopic eyes can result in greater mechanical strain in the temporal area, making the macular region more susceptible to glaucomatous damage.

Our finding that myopic individuals are predisposed to central vision loss is consistent with previous studies showing an association between myopia and paracentral scotomas [19–22]. Mayama et al. focusing on the central 12 points on HFA 30-2 VFs of 313 glaucoma patients, reported that myopia is associated with damage in the lower cecocentral VF [19]. Myopia was also found to be a risk factor for VF progression in the upper paracentral subfield in 92 normal-tension glaucoma patients [20]. In a recent study, Dias et al. found myopia to be associated with the presence of parafoveal scotomas in 130 glaucomatous eyes with disc hemorrhage [21]. The current study agrees with these prior works and significantly expands upon them by analyzing a dataset of over 120,000 VFs pointwise, rather than focusing only on the presence of paracentral scotomas or a subset of VF locations. Using this systematic approach, we show that myopic VF depression not only affects the cecocentral and paracentral areas but also extends to the nasal step locations, forming an arcuate pattern that corresponds to the superior and inferior arcuate bundle trajectories. Our results support the recommendations from previous studies that myopic individuals, particularly those with high myopia, deserve closer monitoring for central field defects which are highly correlated with quality of life [32,33].

While our study does not provide direct mechanistic evidence, we briefly discuss potential physiologic explanations for the VF patterns observed. First, the effect of SE alone on VF light sensitivity is likely due to structural differences between myopic and hyperopic eyes. Myopia is associated with increased axial length, optic disc tilt, and torsion [8,9,12,15,34]. Furthermore, structural parameters such as optic disc torsion [35] and abrupt change in scleral curvature [23] have been associated with VF defects in myopic eyes. The stretching or bending of optic nerve fibers due to mechanical tension may explain the increased susceptibility of myopic eyes to develop VF loss at certain locations. On the other hand, the VF patterns seen from the interaction of ametropia and glaucoma suggest that differences in RNF anatomy are responsible for the effect. The major superotemporal and inferotemporal RNF bundles, i.e., the arcuate fibers, are particularly susceptible to damage and are preferentially lost in glaucoma [36,37]. These bundles lie closer to the fovea in myopic eyes, as shown as a schematic in Figure 1B [10–13]. The reciprocal patterns observed, in which myopic VF loss shifts centrally and nasally with worsening glaucoma and hyperopic VF loss occurs in the opposite direction, correspond well to the respective locations of the arcuate fiber trajectories in myopic and hyperopic eyes.

In the present study, ametropia was significantly correlated to VF loss severity, but the effect was weak ($r = 0.045$). This likely represents a clinically insignificant result, in line with our previous study of a smaller population ($n = 438$) showing no significant association between SE and MD [15]. Our recent studies have shown, however, that optic nerve related parameters associated with myopia have specific impacts on the abnormality patterns of RNFL thickness measured by optical coherence tomography (OCT) [13,38]. Consistent with these findings, the current study shows differences in the patterns of relative light sensitivity between myopes and hyperopes, resulting in an effect modification of glaucomatous VF loss. Indeed, the magnitude of ametropia's effect on individual PD values was small, and we would not expect ametropia alone to produce VF loss that mimics glaucoma. However, the overarching patterns of VF loss indicate that there are distinct zones of vulnerability in myopic and hyperopic eyes predisposing them to different patterns of VF loss. These patterns are exemplified in Figure 6 showing VF progression in myopic and hyperopic glaucoma patients.

There are several strengths of our study: first, we used a large sample size of over 120,000 eyes collected from multiple institutions to study the effect of ametropia on visual function. Second, we used a systematic and quantitative approach to examine the effect of the full spectrum of SE pointwise over the entire 24-2 VF, quantifying the effect of SE on PD values at each VF location. Finally, our study focuses on the interaction term (SE × MD) in the regression analysis, separating the effect of ametropia from that of VF loss severity. This specific study design addresses well-known challenges related to research on myopia and posterior eye diseases, as it filters out the various potential impacts of refractive error on the VF and allows to extract only those effects that are immediately relevant for glaucoma.

This study also has several limitations. First, because of the retrospective, cross-sectional nature of our study, we could establish associations between ametropia and VF patterns, but not causal relationships. Second, because axial length was not recorded by the HFA device, we used SE as an alternative. Third, in the absence of diagnostic information in our dataset, patients with lens related conditions could not be excluded from analysis. This is of particular relevance for cases of pseudophakia due to cataract surgery, which is a confounder when investigating impacts of ametropia on posterior eye diseases. We addressed this potential problem in two ways. First, as the prevalence of cataracts strongly increases with age, in a supplemental analysis we recalculated our results with subjects older than 80 years excluded. Second, in another supplemental analysis, we excluded all eyes with relatively mild refractive errors (-1.5 D $\leq$ SE $\leq +1.0$ D), which is a range into which the vast majority of eyes fall after cataract surgery [39]. For either of these two additional data analyses, the effects we found were similar to the original results and did not change any of our conclusions. Apart from pseudophakia, we would like to note again that our focus on the SE×MD interaction term would extract most lens related properties as those are likely additive to VF loss patterns but would not be expected to interact with glaucomatous VF loss severity. Fourth, this study was restricted to the 24-2 pattern test. The 10-2 VF test has higher sensitivity for central vision compared to the 24-2 [40] and may be better suited to examine the detailed pattern of central VF loss. Fifth, a linear association between SE and PD was observed at most, but not all, of the VF locations (Figure 3). Nonlinear regression may be used in future studies to better model the association. Finally, the current study focused on functional data (VFs) and not structural data (e.g., RNFL defects on OCT), so we could only speculate the anatomical basis of the observed VF patterns. Future work will focus on characterizing the structure-function relationship and the effect of ametropia on this relationship.

In conclusion, utilizing a large dataset of over 120,000 VFs, we characterized the effect of ametropia on the spatial pattern of VF loss as a function of glaucoma severity. We demonstrate that myopic and hyperopic individuals are predisposed to developing different patterns of VF loss. With worsening VF loss severity, individuals with myopia have increased depressions at the paracentral and nasal step regions; conversely, hyperopes have increased depressions in the Bjerrum and temporal regions. Clinicians should be aware of these effects from ametropia and take them into account when interpreting VF loss, particularly in patients with severe VF depression.

Supplementary Materials: The following are available online at https://www.mdpi.com/article/10.3390/jcm10132796/s1, Figure S1: Regression coefficients for each of the 52 visual field locations; Figure S2: Impact of spherical equivalent (SE) on visual field pattern deviations that is not explained by glaucoma severity (mean deviation, MD), excluding age larger than 80 years old; Figure S3: Impact of spherical equivalent (SE) on visual field pattern deviations that is not explained by glaucoma severity (mean deviation, MD), for MD less than −18 dB; Figure S4: Impact of spherical equivalent (SE) on visual field pattern deviations that is not explained by glaucoma severity (mean deviation, MD), excluding lower refractive error.

Author Contributions: E.Y.C. and T.E. designed the study. E.Y.C., R.C.S.W. and T.E. analyzed the data and wrote the paper. E.Y.C., R.C.S.W., T.T., L.R.P., L.Q.S., M.W., D.L., Q.J., H.W., N.B., M.V.B., S.Y., S.R.W., C.G.D.M., J.S.M., P.J.B., T.E. collected data from their associated institutions, discussed the results and commented on the manuscript. All authors have read and agreed to the published version of the manuscript.

Funding: This work was supported by NIH R21EY030142 (T.E., S.Y.), NIH R21EY030631 (T.E.), NIH R01EY030575 (T.E.), NIH R01EY015473 (L.R.P.), BrightFocus Foundation (M.W., T.E.), Lions Foundation (M.W., T.E.), Grimshaw-Gudewicz Foundation (M.W., T.E.), Research to Prevent Blindness (M.W., T.E.), NIH K99EY028631 (M.W.), Harvard Glaucoma Center of Excellence (M.W., T.E., L.Q.S.), the Eleanor and Miles Shore Fellowship (L.Q.S.), Departmental Grant from Research to Prevent Blindness (C.G.D.M.), NIH R01EY025253 (C.G.D.M.), the Alice Adler Fellowship (T.E.), and NIH NEI Core Grant P30EY003790 (E.Y.C., M.W., T.E., D.L., H.W., Q.J.).

Institutional Review Board Statement: The study was approved by the Mass. Eye and Ear Institutional Review Board (Protocol #: 2019P000936).

Informed Consent Statement: As only retrospective and fully de-identified data were used, the Mass. Eye and Ear Institutional Review Board waived the need for informed consent.

Data Availability Statement: The datasets and analysis programs are available from the corresponding author.

Conflicts of Interest: Tobias Elze: US patent PCT/US2014/052414. Tobias Elze and Mengyu Wang: US provisional patents 62/804,903, 62/909,386, 62/637,181. Nothing to report for any other author.

References

1. Ferreras, A.; Pablo, L.E.; Garway-Heath, D.F.; Fogagnolo, P.; García-Feijoo, J. Mapping standard automated perimetry to the peripapillary retinal nerve fiber layer in glaucoma. *Investig. Ophthalmol. Vis. Sci.* **2008**, *49*, 3018–3025. [CrossRef]
2. Advanced Glaucoma Intervention Study. 2. Visual field test scoring and reliability. *Ophthalmology* **1994**, *101*, 1445–1455. [CrossRef]
3. Jampel, H.D.; Singh, K.; Lin, S.C.; Chen, T.C.; Francis, B.A.; Hodapp, E.; Smith, S.D. Assessment of Visual Function in Glaucoma. *Ophthalmology* **2011**, *118*, 986–1002. [CrossRef]
4. Hood, D.C.; Kardon, R.H. A framework for comparing structural and functional measures of glaucomatous damage. *Prog. Retin. Eye Res.* **2007**, *26*, 688–710. [CrossRef]
5. Perkins, E.S.; Phelps, C.D. Open angle glaucoma, ocular hypertension, low-tension glaucoma, and refraction. *Arch. Ophthalmol.* **1982**, *100*, 1464–1467. [CrossRef]
6. Marcus, M.W.; de Vries, M.M.; Montolio, F.G.J.; Jansonius, N.M. Myopia as a Risk Factor for Open-Angle Glaucoma: A Systematic Review and Meta-Analysis. *Ophthalmology* **2011**, *118*, 1989–1994.e2. [CrossRef] [PubMed]
7. Shen, L.; Melles, R.B.; Metlapally, R.; Barcellos, L.; Schaefer, C.; Risch, N.; Herrinton, L.J.; Wildsoet, C.; Jorgenson, E. The Association of Refractive Error with Glaucoma in a Multiethnic Population. *Ophthalmology* **2016**, *123*, 92–101. [CrossRef] [PubMed]
8. Llorente, L.; Barbero, S.; Cano, D.; Dorronsoro, C.; Marcos, S. Myopic versus hyperopic eyes: Axial length, corneal shape and optical aberrations. *J. Vis.* **2004**, *4*, 288–298. [CrossRef] [PubMed]
9. Morgan, I.G.; Ohno-Matsui, K.; Saw, S.-M. Myopia. *Lancet* **2012**, *379*, 1739–1748. [CrossRef]
10. Kang, S.H.; Hong, S.W.; Im, S.K.; Lee, S.H.; Ahn, M.D. Effect of Myopia on the Thickness of the Retinal Nerve Fiber Layer Measured by Cirrus HD Optical Coherence Tomography. *Investig. Ophthalmol. Vis. Sci.* **2010**, *51*, 4075–4083. [CrossRef]

11. Hong, S.W.; Ahn, M.D.; Kang, S.H.; Im, S.K. Analysis of Peripapillary Retinal Nerve Fiber Distribution in Normal Young Adults. *Investig. Opthalmol. Vis. Sci.* **2010**, *51*, 3515–3523. [CrossRef] [PubMed]
12. Leung, C.K.-S.; Yu, M.; Weinreb, R.N.; Mak, H.K.; Lai, G.; Ye, C.; Lam, D.S.-C. Retinal Nerve Fiber Layer Imaging with Spectral-Domain Optical Coherence Tomography: Interpreting the RNFL Maps in Healthy Myopic Eyes. *Investig. Opthalmol. Vis. Sci.* **2012**, *53*, 7194–7200. [CrossRef]
13. Elze, T.; Baniasadi, N.; Jin, Q.; Wang, H. Ametropia, retinal anatomy, and OCT abnormality patterns in glaucoma. 1. Impacts of refractive error and interartery angle. *J. Biomed. Opt.* **2017**, *22*, 1. [CrossRef] [PubMed]
14. Vongphanit, J.; Mitchell, P.; Wang, J.J. Population prevalence of tilted optic disks and the relationship of this sign to refractive error. *Am. J. Ophthalmol.* **2002**, *133*, 679–685. [CrossRef]
15. Baniasadi, N.; Wang, M.; Wang, H.; Mahd, M.; Elze, T. Associations between Optic Nerve Head–Related Anatomical Parameters and Refractive Error over the Full Range of Glaucoma Severity. *Transl. Vis. Sci Technol.* **2017**, *6*, 9. [CrossRef]
16. Huang, H.; Jonas, J.B.; Dai, Y.; Hong, J.; Wang, M.; Chen, J.; Sun, X. Position of the central retinal vessel trunk and pattern of remaining visual field in advanced glaucoma. *Br. J. Ophthalmol.* **2013**, *97*, 96–100. [CrossRef]
17. Wang, M.; Wang, H.; Pasquale, L.R.; Baniasadi, N.; Shen, L.Q.; Bex, P.J.; Elze, T. Relationship Between Central Retinal Vessel Trunk Location and Visual Field Loss in Glaucoma. *Am. J. Ophthalmol.* **2017**, *176*, 53–60. [CrossRef] [PubMed]
18. Besombes, G.; Grunewald, F.; Ramdane, N.; Salleron, J.; Labalette, P.; Rouland, J.-F. Position of the central retinal vessel trunk and location of visual field and parapapillary nerve fibers damage in early to moderate glaucoma. *Investig. Ophthalmol. Vis. Sci.* **2014**, *55*, 950. [CrossRef]
19. Mayama, C.; Suzuki, Y.; Araie, M.; Ishida, K.; Akira, T.; Yamamoto, T.; Kitazawa, Y.; Funaki, S.; Shirakashi, M.; Abe, H.; et al. Myopia and advanced-stage open-angle glaucoma. *Ophthalmology* **2002**, *109*, 2072–2077. [CrossRef]
20. Sakata, R.; Aihara, M.; Murata, H.; Mayama, C.; Tomidokoro, A.; Iwase, A.; Araie, M. Contributing Factors for Progression of Visual Field Loss in Normal-tension Glaucoma Patients With Medical Treatment. *J. Glaucoma* **2013**, *22*, 250–254. [CrossRef]
21. Dias, D.T.; Almeida, I.; Sassaki, A.M.; Juncal, V.R.; Ushida, M.; Lopes, F.S.; Alhadeff, P.; Ritch, R.; Prata, T.S. Factors associated with the presence of parafoveal scotoma in glaucomatous eyes with optic disc hemorrhages. *Eye* **2018**, *32*, 1669–1674. [CrossRef] [PubMed]
22. Araie, M.; Arai, M.; Koseki, N.; Suzuki, Y. Influence of myopic refraction on visual field defects in normal tension and primary open angle glaucoma. *Jpn. J. Ophthalmol.* **1995**, *39*, 60–64. [PubMed]
23. Ohno-Matsui, K.; Shimada, N.; Yasuzumi, K.; Hayashi, K.; Yoshida, T.; Kojima, A.; Moriyama, M.; Tokoro, T. Long-term Development of Significant Visual Field Defects in Highly Myopic Eyes. *Am. J. Ophthalmol.* **2011**, *152*, 256–265.e1. [CrossRef] [PubMed]
24. Birt, C.M.; Shin, D.H.; Samudrala, V.; Hughes, B.A.; Kim, C.; Lee, D. Analysis of reliability indices from Humphrey visual field tests in an urban glaucoma population. *Ophthalmology* **1997**, *104*, 1126–1130. [CrossRef]
25. Newkirk, M.R.; Gardiner, S.K.; Demirel, S.; Johnson, C.A. Assessment of False Positives with the Humphrey Field Analyzer II Perimeter with the SITA Algorithm. *Investig. Opthalmol. Vis. Sci.* **2006**, *47*, 4632. [CrossRef]
26. Pasquale, L.R.; Kang, J.H.; Manson, J.E.; Willett, W.C.; Rosner, B.A.; Hankinson, S.E. Prospective Study of Type 2 Diabetes Mellitus and Risk of Primary Open-Angle Glaucoma in Women. *Ophthalmology* **2006**, *113*, 1081–1086. [CrossRef]
27. Pasquale, L.R.; Willett, W.C.; Rosner, B.A.; Kang, J.H. Anthropometric measures and their relation to incident primary open-angle glaucoma. *Ophthalmology* **2010**, *117*, 1521–1529. [CrossRef]
28. R Core Team. *R: A Language and Environment for Statistical Computing*; R Core Team: Vienna, Austria, 2014.
29. Benjamini, Y.; Hochberg, Y. Controlling the False Discovery Rate—A Practical and Powerful Approach to Multiple Testing. *J. R. Stat. Soc. Ser. B* **1995**, *57*, 289–300. [CrossRef]
30. Heo, D.W.; Kim, K.N.; Lee, M.W.; Lee, S.B.; Kim, C. Properties of pattern standard deviation in open-angle glaucoma patients with hemi-optic neuropathy and bi-optic neuropathy. *PLoS ONE* **2017**, *12*, e0171960. [CrossRef] [PubMed]
31. Garway-Heath, D.F.; Poinoosawmy, D.; Fitzke, F.W.; Hitchings, R.A. Mapping the visual field to the optic disc in normal tension glaucoma eyes. *Ophthalmology* **2000**, *107*, 1809–1815. [CrossRef]
32. Fujita, K.; Yasuda, N.; Oda, K.; Yuzawa, M. [Reading performance in patients with central visual field disturbance due to glaucoma]. *Nihon Ganka Gakkai Zasshi* **2006**, *110*, 914–918.
33. Coeckelbergh, T.R.M.; Brouwer, W.H.; Cornelissen, F.W.; Van Wolffelaar, P.; Kooijman, A.C. The effect of visual field defects on driving performance: A driving simulator study. *Arch. Ophthalmol.* **2002**, *120*, 1509–1516. [CrossRef] [PubMed]
34. Park, H.-Y.L.; Choi, S.I.; Choi, J.-A.; Park, C.K. Disc Torsion and Vertical Disc Tilt Are Related to Subfoveal Scleral Thickness in Open-Angle Glaucoma Patients With Myopia. *Investig. Opthalmol. Vis. Sci.* **2015**, *56*, 4927–4935. [CrossRef]
35. Lee, K.S.; Lee, J.R.; Kook, M.S. Optic disc torsion presenting as unilateral glaucomatous-appearing visual field defect in young myopic korean eyes. *Ophthalmology* **2014**, *121*, 1013–1019. [CrossRef]
36. Minckler, D.S. The organization of nerve fiber bundles in the primate optic nerve head. *Arch. Ophthalmol.* **1980**, *98*, 1630–1636. [CrossRef]
37. Hood, D.C.; Raza, A.S.; de Moraes, C.G.V.; Liebmann, J.M.; Ritch, R. Glaucomatous damage of the macula. *Prog. Retin. Eye Res.* **2013**, *32*, 1–21. [CrossRef] [PubMed]
38. Baniasadi, N.; Wang, M.; Wang, H.; Jin, Q.; Elze, T. Ametropia, retinal anatomy, and OCT abnormality patterns in glaucoma. 2. Impacts of optic nerve head parameters. *J. Biomed. Opt.* **2017**, *22*, 1–9. [CrossRef] [PubMed]

19. Lundström, M.; Dickman, M.; Henry, Y.; Manning, S.; Rosen, P.; Tassignon, M.-J.; Young, D.; Stenevi, U. Risk factors for refractive error after cataract surgery: Analysis of 282 811 cataract extractions reported to the European Registry of Quality Outcomes for cataract and refractive surgery. *J. Cataract Refract. Surg.* **2018**, *44*, 447–452. [CrossRef]
20. Hangai, M.; Ikeda, H.O.; Akagi, T.; Yoshimura, N. Paracentral scotoma in glaucoma detected by 10-2 but not by 24-2 perimetry. *Jpn. J. Ophthalmol.* **2014**, *58*, 188–196. [CrossRef] [PubMed]

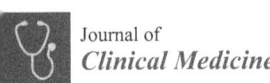

Article

Multifocal Femto-PresbyLASIK in Pseudophakic Eyes

Bojan Pajic [1,2,3,4,5,*], Horace Massa [3], Philipp B. Baenninger [6], Erika Eskina [7,8], Brigitte Pajic-Eggspuehler [1], Mirko Resan [5] and Zeljka Cvejic [2]

1. Eye Clinic Orasis, Swiss Eye Research Foundation, 5734 Reinach, Switzerland; brigitte.pajic@orasis.ch
2. Department of Physics, Faculty of Sciences, University of Novi Sad, Trg Dositeja Obradovica 4, 21000 Novi Sad, Serbia; zeljka.cvejic@df.uns.ac.rs
3. Department of Clinical Neurosciences, Division of Ophthalmology, Geneva University Hospitals, 1205 Geneva, Switzerland; horace.massa@hcuge.ch
4. Faculty of Medicine, University of Geneva, 1205 Geneva, Switzerland
5. Faculty of Medicine of the Military Medical Academy, University of Defense, 11000 Belgrade, Serbia; resan.mirko@gmail.com
6. Cantonal Hospital of Lucerne, Department of Ophthalmology, 6006 Lucerne, Switzerland; philipp.baenninger@luks.ch
7. Ophthalmological Department of Academy of Postgraduate Education FSBF FRCC of the FMBA of Russia, 125310 Moscow, Russia; erika.eskina@sfe.ru
8. Laser Surgery Clinic "SPHERE", 117628 Moscow, Russia
* Correspondence: bpajic@datacomm.ch; Tel.: +41-62-765-60-80

Citation: Pajic, B.; Massa, H.; Baenninger, P.B.; Eskina, E.; Pajic-Eggspuehler, B.; Resan, M.; Cvejic, Z. Multifocal Femto-PresbyLASIK in Pseudophakic Eyes. *J. Clin. Med.* **2021**, *10*, 2282. https://doi.org/10.3390/jcm10112282

Academic Editor: Kazuno Negishi

Received: 11 April 2021
Accepted: 21 May 2021
Published: 25 May 2021

Publisher's Note: MDPI stays neutral with regard to jurisdictional claims in published maps and institutional affiliations.

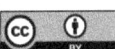

Copyright: © 2021 by the authors. Licensee MDPI, Basel, Switzerland. This article is an open access article distributed under the terms and conditions of the Creative Commons Attribution (CC BY) license (https://creativecommons.org/licenses/by/4.0/).

Abstract: Background: Presbyopia treatment in pseudophakic patients with a monofocal IOL is challenging. This study investigates the refractive results of femto-PresbyLASIK and analyzes presbyopia treatment in pseudophakic eyes. Methods: 14 patients with 28 pseudophakic eyes were treated with femto-PresbyLASIK. The dominant eye was targeted at a distance and the non-dominant eye at −0.5 D. The presbyopic algorithm creates a steepness in the cornea center by using an excimer laser that leads to corneal multifocality. Results: 6 months after surgery a refraction of −0.11 ± 0.13 D ($p = 0.001$), an uncorrected distance visual acuity of 0.05 ± 1.0 logMAR ($p < 0.001$) and an uncorrected near visual acuity of 0.15 ± 0.89 logMAR ($p = 0.001$) were achieved in the dominant eye. For the non-dominant eye, the refraction was −0.28 ± 0.22 D ($p = 0.002$), the uncorrected distance of visual acuity was 0.1 ± 1.49 logMAR, and the uncorrected near visual acuity was 0.11 ± 0.80 logMAR ($p < 0.001$). Spherical aberrations (Z400) were reduced by 0.21–0.3 μm in 32% of eyes, and by 0.31–0.4 μm in 26% of eyes. Conclusion: By steepening the central cornea while maintaining spherical aberrations within acceptable limits, PresbyLASIK created a corneal multifocality that safely improved near vision in both eyes. Thus, femto-PresbyLASIK can be used to treat presbyopia in pseudophakic eyes without performing intraocular surgery.

Keywords: presbyLASIK; excimer laser; multifocality; pseudophakic

1. Introduction

While patients are increasingly aware of the possibility that they do not need to wear spectacles after cataract surgery, if they have a simultaneous multifocal intraocular lens (IOL) placed, few patients are benefiting from this advanced technology. Indeed, the vast majority of patients are choosing a monofocal IOL. Limitations to the wider use of multifocal IOL might be their high cost, the careful patient selection that is required for good outcomes, or the patients' fear of side effects. Monofocal IOL placement after cataract surgery allows perfect vision, but only at one focal distance. This monovision can lead to patient dissatisfaction, and a desire to regain multifocality without corrective lenses. Unfortunately, solutions to restore multifocality remain scarce and poorly explored.

There are different ways to reach multifocality. The goal is to achieve the best possible visual outcome while maintaining a low level of optical disturbance. There are only 3 surgical options to treat presbyopia [1]. One option is to exchange the monofocal lens with a multifocal one, but this remains challenging, as treated eyes might be weakened by the first surgery. Thus, this does not have a high level of safety [2]. A second option would be the implantation of a multifocal add-on IOL [3], but this has several limitations. The power calculations of lenses are not as precise as with a laser. Deposits in the interface between the IOL in the bag and the add-on IOL might also disturb the vision. The rubbing of the add-on IOL against the iris tissues might induce ocular inflammation [4], or a pigment dispersion syndrome that risks elevated intraocular pressure and glaucoma. Lastly, this is an intraocular procedure that poses a certain amount of complication risk. The third option is to obtain multifocality at the corneal level. The concept of multifocal PresbyLASIK is an attractive correction method, because the surgical technique is based on the LASIK method. In contrast to a multifocal IOL implantation, minimal invasive surgery is necessary, because the eye does not need to be opened up. PresbyLASIK involves two steps. The first step is to correct ametropia for distance vision, and the second step is to make an addition for near vision. In multifocality, the central part of the cornea is most often adjusted for proximity, and the middle periphery is corrected for distance [5–10].

A conventional PresbyLASIK always represents a compromise between distance and near vision, since it creates unwanted aberrations, especially spherical aberrations in the central pupillary region. To minimize unwanted aberrations, today's PresbyLASIK treatment algorithms are wavefront-guided. Compared to the well-established treatment of presbyopia with a multifocal IOL, PresbyLASIK is a newer surgical technique, but it has the advantage of being less invasive than implanting an IOL, because the eye does not need to be opened up. On the other hand, the use of PresbyLASIK is much more demanding. Patient selection and the interpretation of objective preoperative topographic and wavefront analyses are challenging. In particular, decisions based on the Zernike polynomial analysis of the cornea have a high influence on the surgical result.

It is not sufficient to use the general LASIK criteria for PresbyLASIK application. The lack of encouraging treatment results of PresbyLASIK to date is likely because the indication for surgery was on LASIK criteria, and corresponding refraction and other parameters from the wavefront analysis were not taken into account [11]. Moreover, even if wavefront analysis is done perfectly, it must be adapted to pupillary diameter in the mesopic condition [12].

The PresbyLASIK, in particular the Supracor algorithm, was already successfully used with presbyopic phakic eyes [11,13,14]. Therefore, in this retrospective study, we assessed refractive outcomes after PresbyLASIK in pseudophakic patients.

2. Materials and Methods

We included 14 patients with 28 pseudophakic eyes in this retrospective case series. The same surgeon performed all surgical procedures. The study was approved by the Ethics Committee in Novi Sad (34–08.18). This study was conducted in accordance with the Protocol, the Declaration of Helsinki, and all applicable regulatory requirements.

In the following Table 1, all significant preoperative PresbyLASIK data were listed of all 14 patients, such as mean age, UDVA, CDVA, UNVA, CNVA for the dominant and non-dominant eye, as well as the refraction preoperative levels for the dominant and non-dominant eyes. The mean period between cataract surgery and presbyopia was 8.93 ± 3.82 (range 6–16) months (Table 1).

Table 1. Details regarding preoperative data prior to PresbyLASIK, inclusive preoperative refraction, visual acuity in logMAR, and time elapsed since cataract surgery in months.

	Mean + SD	Range
Age	55.9 ± 13.1 Years	(Range 37–74)
UDVA before: Dominant eye	0.42 ± 1.13	0.3–0.5
CDVA before: Dominant eye	0.10 ± 0.87	0.0–0.2
UNVA before: Dominant eye	0.45 ± 1.0	0.7–0.3
CNVA before: Dominant eye	0.19 ± 0.81	0.3–0.1
UDVA before: Non-dominant eye	0.33 ± 0.83	0.5–0.2
CDVA before: Non-dominant eye	0.11 ± 0.85	0.2–0.0
UNVA before: Non-dominant eye	0.53 ± 1.2	0.7–0.4
CNVA before: Non-dominant eye	0.20 ± 0.83	0.3–0.1
Preoperative refraction: dominant eye	−1.14 ± 0.73 sph −0.96 ± 0.77 cyl −1.62 ± 1.03 sph aquiv	−2.0−−0.25 −2.0−0 −3.0−−0.5
Preoperative refraction: non-dominant eye	−0.59 ± 0.81 sph −1.23 ± 0.67 cyl −1.23 ± 1.03 sph aquiv	−1.75−±0.25 −2.0−−0.25 −2.63–0.13
Time elapsed since the cataract surgery (months)	8.93 ± 3.82	6–16

Inclusion criteria were a dissatisfaction with myopic refraction obtained with a monofocal IOL with manifest refraction spherical equivalent (MRSE) between −0.5 and −4.0 diopters (D), astigmatism of 2.50 D or less, mean keratometry between 41.00 and 46.00 D, a central corneal thickness of 540 µm or more, a mesopic pupil diameter between 4 and 6 mm, and a kappa angle of less than 6°. Exclusion criteria were the presence of ocular surface disease, clinically significant corneal opacity, posterior segment ocular pathologies, and abnormal corneal topography. All pseudophakic patients received the same IOL (Nidek NS 60YG, Nidek CO. LTD., Gamagori, Japan) during the cataract surgery.

All patients had a complete ophthalmologic examination prior to surgery, including manifest refraction, cycloplegic refraction, slit lamp microscopy of the anterior ocular segment, dilated fundoscopy and intraocular pressure measurement. The preoperative examination also included corneal topography with the Orbscan II system (Technolas Perfect Vision GmbH, Munich, Germany) and Pentacam (Oculus optical devices, Wetzlar, Germany). Wavefront aberrometry measurements were performed preoperatively with the Zywave II aberrometer (Technolas Perfect Vision GmbH) with undilated pupils and pupillometry. Eye dominance was determined by means of a "hole test". The measurement was carried out under scotopic conditions. The aberration analysis was carried out in a 6-mm zone.

Uncorrected near (UNVA) and distance (UDVA) visual acuity, and corrected near (CNVA) and distance (CDVA) visual acuity, were assessed using Snellen visual charts for distance vision and the Jaeger Scale for near vision, and then converted into a logarithm of the minimum angle of resolution (logMAR) notation. In all examinations, the eyes were not dilated. The examinations were performed at baseline, then postoperatively at 1 week, 1 month, 3 months and 6 months. Bilateral LASIK multifocal aspheric corneal ablation treatment was performed at least 6 months after cataract surgery.

The procedures were completed using the Supracor PresbyLASIK algorithm with a Teneo 317 excimer laser (Technolas Perfect Vision GmbH, Munich, Germany). The dominant eye of the patient was planned as plano for distance, while the non-dominant eye was slightly aimed at myopia of −0.5 D. However, we simulated the desired postoperative outcome before surgery using a contact lens. In the 14 patients included in the study, the distance setting was considered comfortable for the dominant eye. The LASIK incision was performed using a femtosecond laser (Ziemer Ophthalmic Systems, LDV, Port, Switzerland) with a target flap thickness of 110 μm. The hinge was set superior in each case, with a flap diameter of 9.5 mm.

Our presbyLASIK protocol included a treatment algorithm with 2 phases. In the first phase, the dominant eye is treated for emmetropia and the non-dominant eye to aim for −0.5 diopters myopia with the excimer laser. The Munnerlyn formula [15] was used to determine the feasibility of the ablative process. In a second phase, but in the same treatment, a central steepness is achieved by ablation in a 3–6 mm zone and, in principle, is an addition for near vision. A multifocality is created in the cornea, which seamlessly represents a correction for near, intermediate and distance vision (Figure 1). Multifocality was created in both treated eyes during PresbyLASIK. To counteract the spherical aberration induced by this multifocal treatment, the laser applied additional wavefront-guided correction.

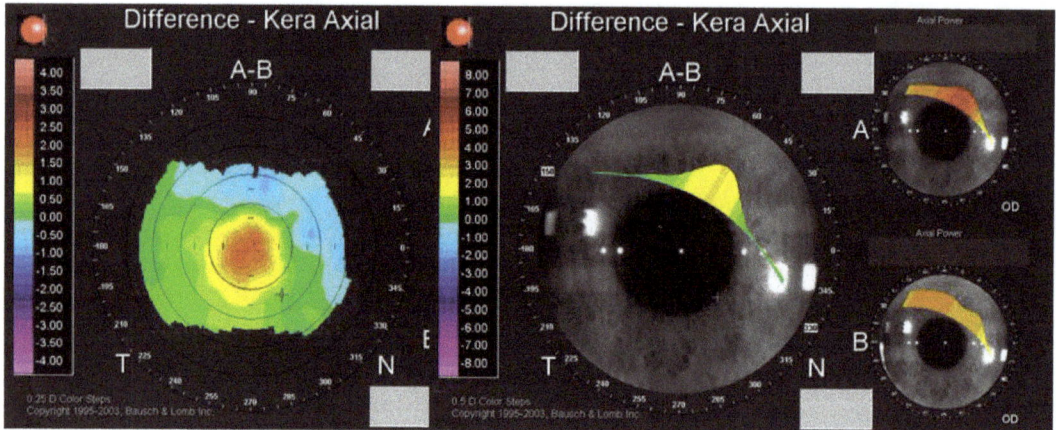

Figure 1. Topographical imaging showing a central steepness of the cornea created using the Supracor PresbyLASIK algorithm.

This wavefront-guided correction reduces higher-order aberrations (HOA), as shown by the point spread function (PSF). It can be qualitatively appreciated in a patient example of how the PSF was significantly reduced after wavefront-guided presbyLASIK (Figure 2). The focus was mainly on the correction of spherical aberration.

The postoperative topical regime was Tobradex (Alcon Laboratories, Inc., Fort Worth, TX, USA) 3 times daily for seven days, and topical hyaluronic acid 0.15% 3 times daily for a month.

Statistical analysis was performed using the IBM SPSS Statistics version 22.0 (IBM Corp., Armonk, NY, USA). The Kolmogorov–Smirnov and Shapiro–Wilk tests were used to test the data sets for normal distribution. If $p > 0.05$, the data set was considered normally distributed. If the data sets were parametric, they were calculated using the Pearson normality test, an unpaired t-test and ANOVA test. For the non-parametric data sets, the Friedmann test was used for further analysis. Significance was considered to be when $p < 0.05$.

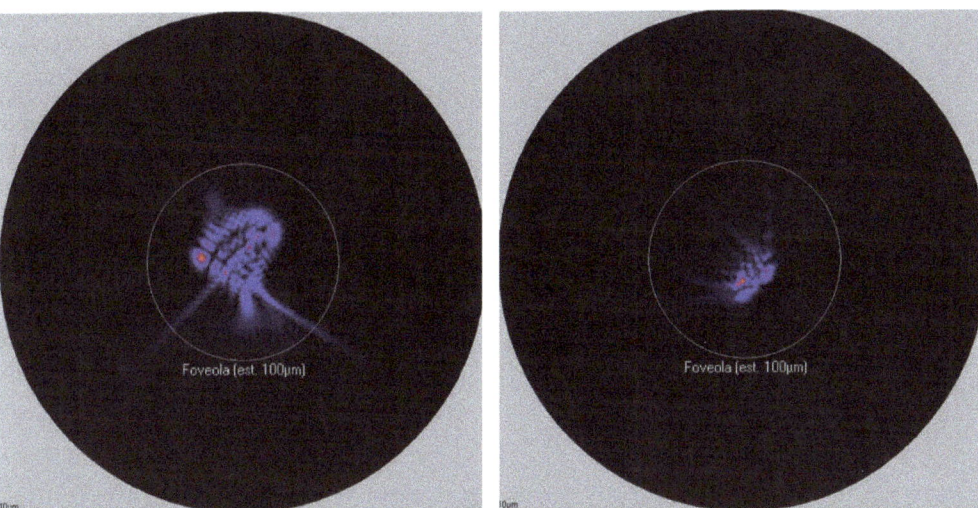

Figure 2. Reduction of PSF after wavefront-guided presbyLASIK.

3. Results

A total of 28 eyes in 14 patients were treated, of which 9 (64%) were female and 5 (36%) were male. The mean age was 56 ± 13 years. Mean preoperative MRSE was −1.43 ± 1.03 D (range: −0.50 to −3.0 D), mean sphere −0.87 ± 0.81 D (range: −2.00 to 0.25 D) and mean cylinder −1.13 ± 0.73 D (range: 0.00 to −2.00 D). The mean preoperative monocular CDVA was 0.1 ± 0.85 logMAR (Snellen) and the CNVA, 0.19 ± 0.82 logMAR (Jaeger 5).

3.1. Dominant Eye

3.1.1. Refraction

The mean preoperative refraction in the dominant eye was −1.63 ± 1.03 D. Distance adjustment was aimed for emmetropia. The mean postoperative refraction was −0.04 ± 0.29 D, 0.01 ± 0.28 D and −0.11 ± 0.13 D after 1, 3 and 6 months, respectively (Figure 3). Refraction significantly improved from preoperative testing to 1-month postoperative testing ($p = 0.001$), without further significant changes at later times ($p = 0.37$) and ($p = 0.42$).

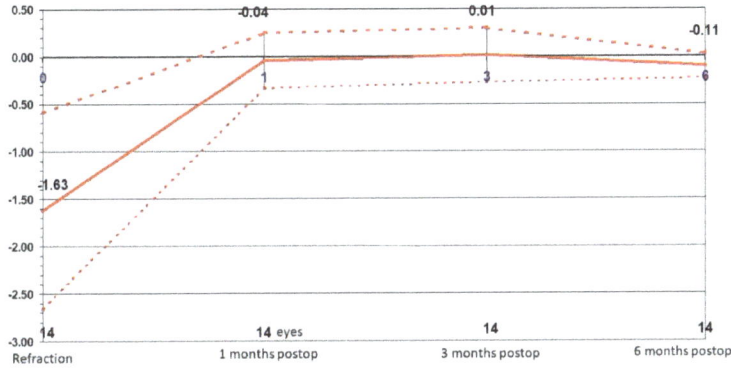

Figure 3. Stability: Change in refraction over time in the dominant eye.

3.1.2. Distance Vision

At the 1-week postoperative test, 93% of eyes had a UDVA better than 0.2 logMAR, while the remainder had better than 0.3 logMAR. At 1 month after surgery, 50% of eyes had a UDVA of 0.1 logMAR, 36% had a UDVA of 0.2 logMAR, and the remainder (14%) had a UDVA of 0.3 logMAR. These same percentages persisted at 3 months, postoperatively (50%, UDVA of 0.1 logMAR; 36%, 0.2 logMAR; 14%, 0.3 logMAR. At 6 months, postoperatively, 57% of eyes had UDVA of 0.0 logMAR and the remainder of eyes (43%) had a 0.1 logMAR (Figure 4). Preoperative UDVA was 0.42 ± 1.15 logMAR and increased to 0.14 ± 1.05 logMAR, 0.21 ± 1.10 logMAR, 0.07 ± 1.05 and 0.05 ± 1.00 logMAR 1 week, 1 month, 3 and 6 months postoperatively, respectively. Compared to the preoperative value, the increase to each postoperative value was significant ($p < 0.001$). Visual acuity significantly increased between the first postoperative week and the third postoperative month ($p = 0.014$) and from the first postoperative month to the third postoperative month ($p = 0.017$).

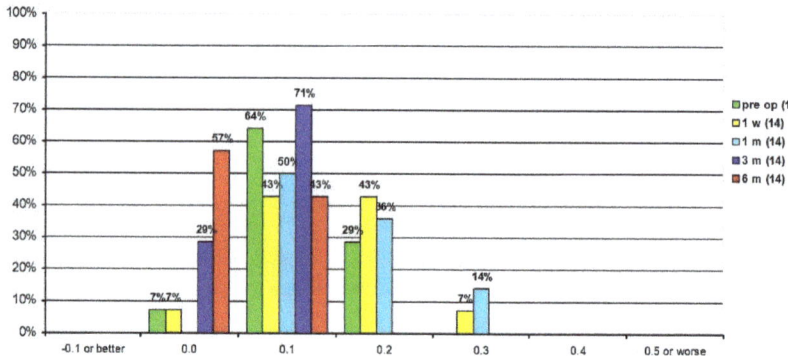

Figure 4. Uncorrected distance visual acuity percentage distribution.

The mean CDVA was 0.10 ± 0.89 logMAR preoperatively. CDVA fluctuated from 0.12 ± 0.83 logMAR at 1 week postoperatively, 0.14 ± 1.05 logMAR at 1 month postoperatively, 0.05 ± 1.0 logMAR at 3 months postoperatively, to 0.03 ± 1.05 logMAR at 6 months postoperatively. CDVA increased significantly from preoperative values to those obtained at 3 months ($p = 0.027$) and 6 months ($p = 0.003$), postoperatively. There was also a significant increase in CDVA from the first postoperative week to the third postoperative month ($p = 0.003$), and the sixth postoperative month ($p < 0.001$). CDVA also significantly increased from the first postoperative month to the third postoperative month ($p < 0.001$) and to the sixth postoperative month ($p < 0.001$). There was no significant change in CDVA after the third postoperative month.

CDVA was also assessed in terms of safety. At 1 week postoperatively, CDVA was unchanged in 71% of eyes, while 29% lost 1 line of CDVA. At 1 month postoperatively, CDVA was unchanged in 71% of eyes, but 14% lost 1 or 2 lines of CDVA, respectively. At 3 months postoperatively, CDVA was unchanged in 50% of eyes, while the other half gained 1 line. By 6 months, 21% of eyes had unchanged CDVA and 79% gained 1 line (Figure 5).

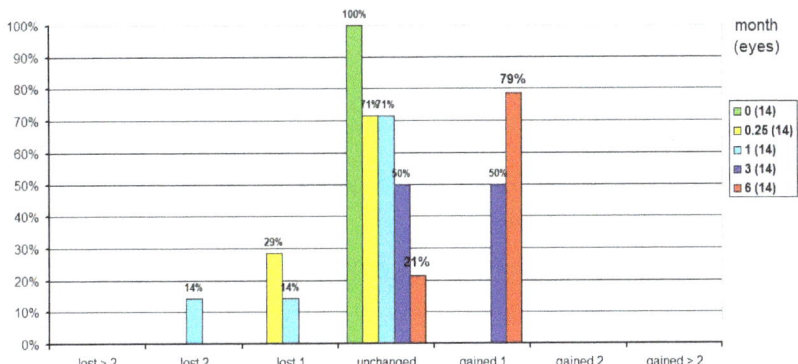

Figure 5. Safety: Changes in corrected distance visual acuity over time compared to preoperative values.

The cumulative CDVA at 1 week postoperatively was 0.3 logMAR or better in all eyes, 0.2 logMAR or better in 93%, 0.1 logMAR or better in 50%, and 0 logMAR or better in 7% of eyes. At 1 month postoperatively, CDVA was 0.3 logMAR or better in all eyes, 0.2 logMAR or better in 86% and 0.1 logMAR or better in 50%. At 3 months postoperatively, CDVA was already 0.1 logMAR or better in all eyes, and 29% had CDVA of 0 logMAR or better. At 6 months postoperatively, all eyes had a 0.1 logMAR or better and 57% had a CDVA of 0 logMAR or better (Figure 6).

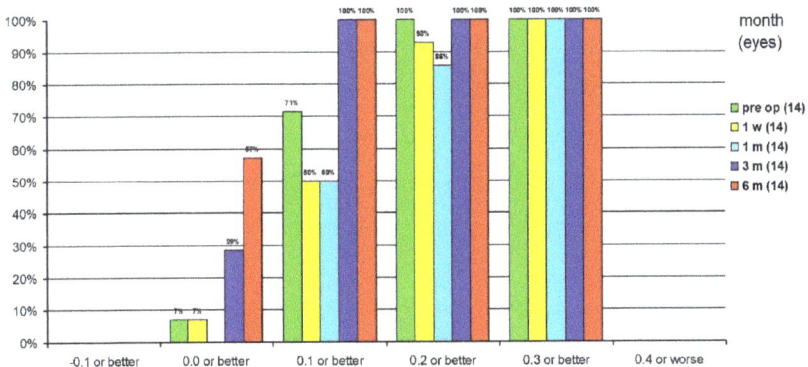

Figure 6. Cumulative corrected distance visual acuity.

The cumulative UDVA at 1 week postoperatively was 0.3 logMAR or better in all eyes, 0.2 logMAR or better in 93% of eyes, and 0.1 logMAR or better in 50% of eyes. One month postoperatively, UDVA was 0.3 logMAR or better in all eyes, 0.2 logMAR or better in 93% of eyes and 0.1 logMAR or better in 7% of eyes. Three months postoperatively, UDVA was already 0.2 logMAR or better in all eyes, 93% of eyes had UDVA of 0.1 logMAR or better and 21% of eyes had UDVA of 0 logMAR. At 6 months postoperatively, all eyes had a 0.1 logMAR or better and 57% of eyes had a UDVA of 0 logMAR or better (Figure 7).

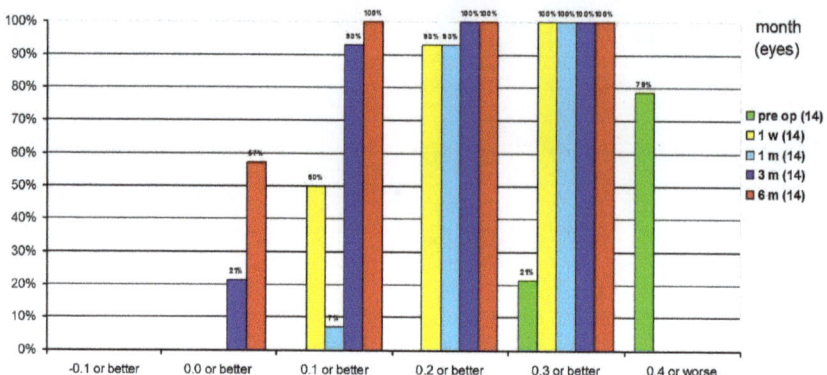

Figure 7. Cumulative uncorrected distance visual acuity.

3.1.3. Near Vision

The mean preoperative UNVA was 0.46 ± 1.0 logMAR. At 1 week postoperatively UNVA increased to 0.13 ± 0.77 logMAR, 1 month postoperatively to 0.09 ± 0.89 logMAR, 3 months postoperatively to 0.14 ± 0.89 logMAR and 6 months postoperatively to 0.15 ± 0.89 logMAR. The difference in UNVA was significant at each time point compared to preoperative values ($p < 0.001$).

The CNVA was 0.19 ± 0.80 logMAR preoperative. One week postoperatively, there was a slight visual improvement to 0.10 ± 0.89 logMAR, 1 month postoperatively to 0.08 ± 1.04 logMAR, 3 months postoperatively 0.10 ± 1.0 logMAR and 6 months postoperatively to 0.10 ± 0.96 logMAR. Visual acuity only increased significantly between the preoperative values and 1 month postoperatively ($p = 0.007$). Otherwise, there was no other significant improvement compared to preoperative values ($p > 0.05$).

3.2. Non-Dominant Eye

3.2.1. Refraction

The refraction target value was set at -0.5 D. The mean preoperative refraction was -1.23 ± 1.03 D, -0.29 ± 0.35 D at 1 month postoperatively, -0.26 ± 0.32 D at 3 months postoperatively and -0.28 ± 0.22 D at 6 months postoperatively. Refraction significantly changed at 1 month ($p = 0.001$), 3 months ($p = 0.004$) and 6 months ($p = 0.002$), compared to preoperative values (Figure 8).

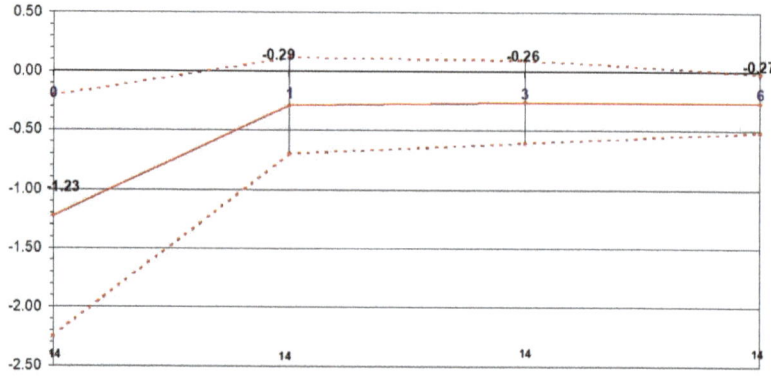

Figure 8. Stability: Change in refraction over time in the non-dominant eye.

3.2.2. Distance Vision

At 1 week postoperatively, 7% of eyes had an uncorrected distance visual acuity (UDVA) of 0 logMAR, 21% of 0.1 logMAR, 50% of 0.2 logMAR and 21% of 0.3 logMAR, respectively. By 1 month after surgery, 14% of eyes had a UDVA of 0.1 logMAR and 86% had a UDVA of 0.2 logMAR. At 3 months postoperatively, 71% of eyes had a UDVA of 0.1 logMAR and 29% of 0.2 logMAR. Six months postoperatively, 14% had a UDVA of 0 logMAR and 86% of 0.1 logMAR (Figure 9). The mean UDVA was 0.33 ± 0.82 logMAR preoperatively, and increased to 0.17 ± 0.85 logMAR, 0.19 ± 1.30 logMAR, 0.12 ± 1.15 logMAR and 0.1 ± 1.40 logMAR at 1-week, 1-, 3- and 6-month postoperative examinations, respectively. Compared to preoperative values, there was a significant improvement in UDVA after 3 and 6 months postoperatively ($p < 0.001$). Between the first postoperative week and the third and sixth postoperative month, there was a significant improvement in UDVA ($p = 0.031$ and $p = 0.004$). Between the first and third postoperative months, there was an improvement in UDVA ($p = 0.01$). All other parameters were not significant.

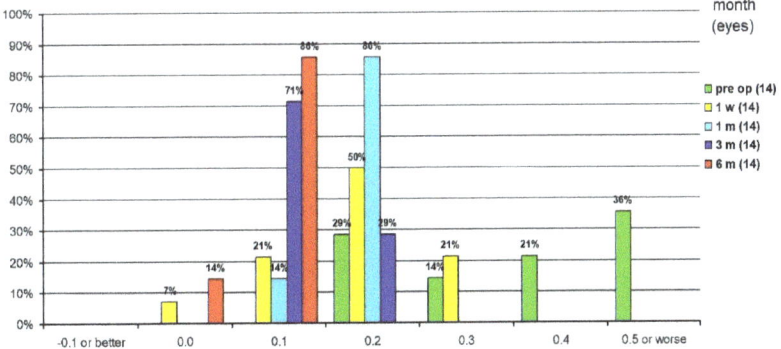

Figure 9. Distribution of uncorrected distance visual acuity.

The mean CDVA was 0.11 ± 0.85 logMAR preoperatively, 0.13 ± 0.77 logMAR, 0.12 ± 1.10 logMAR, 0.08 ± 1.05 logMAR and 0.05 ± 1.0 logMAR at 1-week, 1-, 3- and 6-month postoperative examinations, respectively. A significant increase in CDVA was observed between preoperative tests and 6 months postoperatively ($p = 0.02$). From the first postoperative week to the third postoperative month ($p = 0.01$), and to the sixth postoperative month ($p < 0.001$), there was a significant increase in CDVA. Compared to the first postoperative month, CDVA significantly increased at the third postoperative month ($p = 0.036$), and at the sixth postoperative month ($p = 0.002$). All other tested parameters to CDVA did not vary significantly with time.

CDVA was assessed in terms of safety. At 1 week postoperatively, 43% of eyes were unchanged, 43% lost 1 line of CDVA, and 7% 2 lines. At 1 month postoperatively, 64% of eyes were unchanged. While 7% of eyes gained 1 line of CDVA, 29% lost 1 line of CDVA. At 3 months postoperatively, 64% of eyes were unchanged and 36% gained 1 line of CDVA. By 6 months, 50% of eyes were unchanged, 36% gained 1 line and 7% gained 2 lines of CDVA (Figure 10).

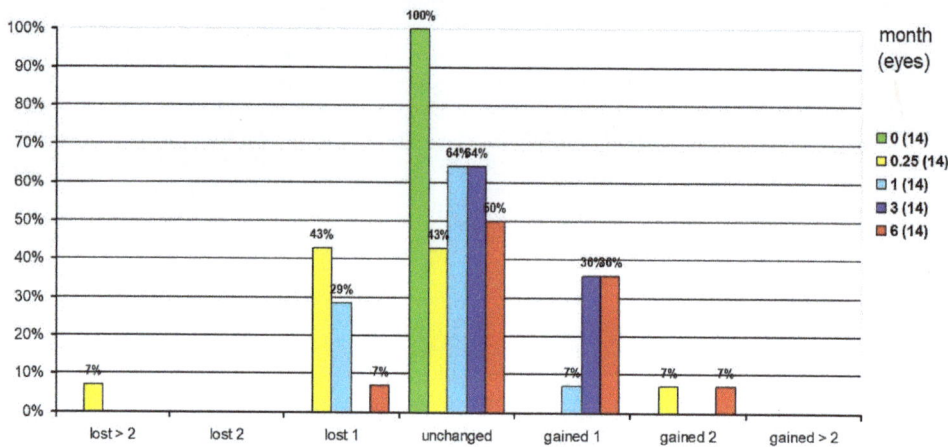

Figure 10. Safety: Changes of corrected distance visual acuity in percentage.

The cumulative CDVA at 1 week postoperatively was 0.4 logMAR or worse in 7% of eyes, 0.3 logMAR or better in 93%, 0.2 logMAR or better in 86%, 0.1 logMAR or better in 29% and 0 logMAR or better in 29%. At 1 month postoperatively, CDVA was 0.2 logMAR or better in all eyes and 0.1 logMAR or better in 64%. At 3 months postoperatively, CDVA was already 0.1 logMAR or better in all eyes, and 21% had CDVA of 0 logMAR or better. At 6 months postoperatively, all eyes had a 0.1 logMAR or better and 29% had a CDVA of 0 logMAR or better (Figure 11).

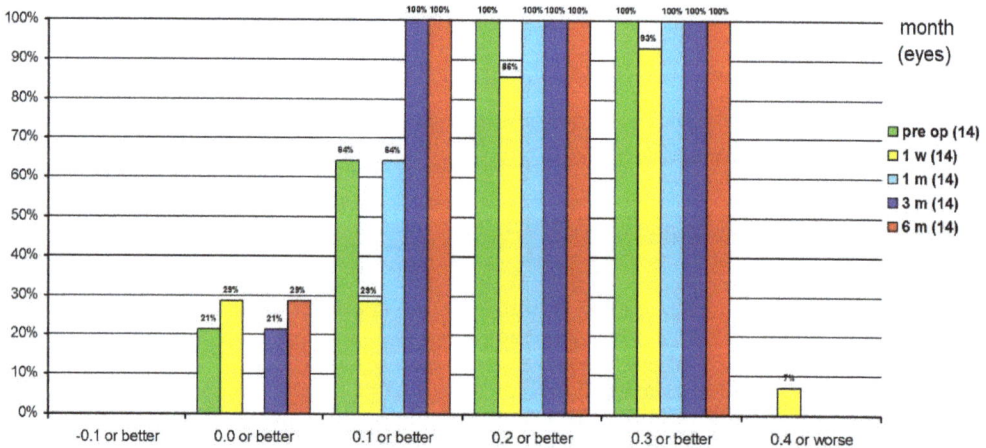

Figure 11. Cumulative corrected distance visual acuity in percentage.

The cumulative UDVA at 1 week postoperatively was 0.3 logMAR or better in all eyes, 0.2 logMAR or better in 79% of eyes, 0.1 logMAR or better in 29%, and 0 logMAR or better in 7%. One month postoperatively, UDVA was 0.2 logMAR or better in all eyes, and 0.1 logMAR or better in 14% of eyes. Three months postoperatively, UDVA was already 0.2 logMAR or better in all eyes, and 71% of eyes had a UDVA of 0.1 logMAR or better. At 6 months postoperatively, all eyes had a 0.1 logMAR or better and 14% had a UDVA of 0 logMAR or better (Figure 12).

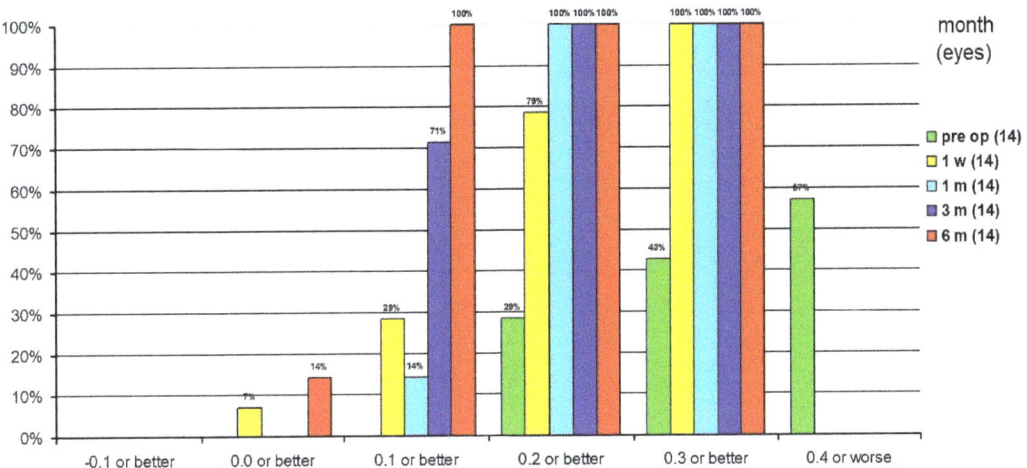

Figure 12. Cumulative uncorrected distance visual acuity.

3.2.3. Near Vision

The mean UNVA was 0.54 ± 1.22 logMAR preoperatively. Postoperative examinations at 1 week, then at 1, 3, and 6 months, revealed that near vision increased to 0.10 ± 0.82 logMAR, 0.09 ± 0.89 logMAR, 0.1 ± 0.77 logMAR and 0.11 ± 0.80 logMAR, respectively. Compared to the preoperative values, postoperative visual acuity increased significantly at each time point ($p < 0.001$).

The mean preoperative CNVA was 0.19 ± 0.82 logMAR. It increased to 0.08 ± 1.05 logMAR 1 week post-operatively and remained stable at each time point until at least 6 months, the last time they were tested. Postoperative CNVA values were significantly better than preoperative values ($p = 0.02$).

3.3. Higher-Order Aberrations

The RMS of higher-order aberrations (RMS-HOA) (at 6 mm diameter) increases in mean by 0.07 ± 0.1 μm from preoperatively to 6 months postoperative values ($p = 0.04$), which is significant. Customized treatment decreased the spherical aberration (Z400) decrease in mean by 0.36 ± 0.12 μm ($p < 0.001$). Quatrefoil aberrations (Z440) decreased significantly at 6 months ($p < 0.001$), compared to the preoperative values in mean, by 0.29 ± 0.11 μm ($p < 0.001$). The total coma RMS did not significantly increase in mean, changing by 0.03 ± 0.07 μm ($p = 0.35$). The total trefoil RMS did not significantly decrease, changing by 0.02 ± 0.05 μm ($p = 0.28$).

4. Discussion

In our study, postoperative UDVA and UNVA were better than preoperative values for all our patients. All patients in the study could be considered as spectacles-free for driving or for reading in standard conditions.

Most ophthalmologists consider that having a residual accommodation is an advantage for near visual acuity [16], and for some, it might be considered a necessary capacity for good outcomes. Herein, it could be demonstrated that even without any residual accommodation—all of our patients were pseudophakic—it is possible to obtain a monocular UNVA of almost 0.1 logMAR and 0.15 logMAR with PresbyLASIK in non-dominant and dominant eyes, respectively. Indeed, the target refraction values of the dominant eye (set to plano) were achieved, as confirmed by the visual acuity of 0.1 logMAR or more at 6 months postoperatively. As expected, UNVA was slightly lower, averaging 0.14 logMAR at 6 months after surgery. In the non-dominant eye (set to -0.5 D), the target refraction value of −0.5 D was not perfectly reached; we found a slight overcorrection with a mean postoperative refraction value of −0.27 D at 6 months postoperatively. This led to a rather high uncorrected distance vision of at least 0.1 logMAR. The uncorrected near vision was 0.11 logMAR due to the slight overcorrection, which was only slightly better than in the dominant eye. Satisfaction was high among all patients, because the patients were very well informed and knew what to expect. However, it must be taken into account that the situation could be somewhat different with a larger group of patients. In any case, patient information is eminently important, especially for PresbyLASIK.

Conventional femto-PresbyLASIK is always a compromise between distance and near correction, as it creates unwanted aberrations in the pupillary region, especially spherical aberrations. If not taken into account, spherical aberrations might lead to an unsatisfactory quality of vision. With the wavefront-guided treatment, however, spherical aberrations could decrease, giving improved visual outcomes. In our study, we attempted to account for the most clinically relevant aberrations, namely, spherical aberrations (Z400). The approach allowed us to significantly decrease Z400 aberrations, even in a multifocal treatment, which usually frequently induces spherical aberrations. The Z300 (i.e., coma and trefoil) aberrations are not usually affected during multifocal treatment, as long as it is centered on the corneal apex. Therefore, we excluded patients with a kappa angle over 6°. Wavefront-guided treatments are also apparently effective in correcting the aberration induced not only by the cornea but also by the intraocular lens [17].

Similar studies have been made recently to determine the feasibility of presbyopia correction using LASIK technologies. A recent study used an aspheric ablation profile to increase spherical aberrations and enhance near vision associated with a micro-monovision [18]. However, as expected, increasing spherical aberration was associated with a decrease in far vision (UDVA of 0.08 logMAR at 6 months), with a micro-monovision that was not well tolerated in 4% of patients.

If we compare our pseudophakic population to phakic patients having undergone a wavefront-guided presbyLASIK treatment, we obtain quite similar results in terms of UDVA and UNVA. In another study, a UDVA and a UNVA of 0.22 logMAR and 0.30 logMAR, respectively, and a 0.1 logMAR Snellen equivalent in the non-dominant eye, were achieved [19].

Compared to the treatment of presbyopia with multifocal IOLs, which is considered to be already established, wavefront-guided PresbyLASIK is a newer surgical technique, with the advantage that it is less invasive than implanting an IOL, because the treatment is applied on the eye surface. On the other hand, the application of wavefront-guided PresbyLASIK is much more demanding regarding the indication and interpretation of the objective preoperative topographic and wavefront analyses, which have a high influence on the surgical result. Wavefront-guided femto-PresbyLASIK significantly alters the biomechanical and optical properties of the cornea, which have a major influence on the surgical outcome. It is not sufficient to apply the general LASIK criteria for the indication of wavefront-guided femto-PresbyLASIK. This is probably also the reason for the not universally encouraging treatment results, because the surgical indication was made on the basis of the LASIK criteria, and the corresponding refraction and other parameters from the wavefront analysis were not taken into account. In this sense, it can be assumed that not only the suitable patients received wavefront-guided femto-PresbyLASIK treatment [11].

Our study has a few limitations. First, there is a need for an adequately sized randomized trial, since our study was a retrospective analysis with a limited number of participants. However, it must be emphasized that all patients included in this study were in a pseudophakic state, and only later requested enhancement after cataract surgery had been performed. Indeed, an alternative would have been to perform a LASIK treatment with a so-called monovision LASIK (i.e., one eye for distance and the other for near vision). In this technique, the patient selection is less crucial [20], but the non-dominant eye has a drastic decrease in far vision, and stereoscopic vision is impacted [21]. Therefore, up to 15% of patients who undergo monovision LASIK may be dissatisfied [22]. Second, we could not compare our patient population to patients who had multifocal lens implantation. Therefore, extrapolating our results to this population of patients is not possible.

The industry and researchers should focus on more accurate or innovative wavefront-guided PresbyLASIK protocols, especially addressing the needs of pseudophakic patients, as this problem affects a large number of people in their early sixties, and could substantially improve the quality of life for these patients. Even if our results are very encouraging, there is still some room for progress. It is conceivable that an entire eye-adapted treatment protocol could be developed for each patient, based on the spherical aberration of the cornea and the IOL.

Clinicians should be aware of more precise refractive outcomes after LASIK in patients with a monofocal IOL than a multifocal IOL [23]. If the patient is not carefully selected, the surgical outcome may be worse with a multifocal IOL due to the larger optical aberrations and reduced targeting accuracy compared to LASIK. Indeed, using a laser to adapt the size of the optic and transition zone might offer a more customized treatment profile [24].

Finally, clinicians should also manage patient expectations and anxiety. In our study, UDVA fluctuated a lot during the first six months. This is a natural phenomenon caused by corneal remodeling. Initially, the multifocal treatment plan leads to light myopization, and UDVA decreases. Then the corneal epithelium compensates for the irregular corneal shape induced by laser treatment by flattening the surface, which is associated with an emmetropic shift and a slight decrease in near visual acuity. Near-vision decrease was very low, at 6 months in the dominant eye, and insignificant in the non-dominant eye.

5. Conclusions

Steepening the central cornea with wavefront-guided PresbyLASIK creates a corneal multifocality, which improved near vision in both eyes. The procedure was safe, as postoperative spherical aberration was within acceptable limits. Wavefront-guided femto-PresbyLASIK offers the possibility of treating presbyopia in pseudophakic eyes without having to perform intraocular surgery.

Author Contributions: B.P. developed the study design, acquired clinical data, performed statistical calculations, and substantially contributed to writing the paper. H.M. developed the methodology and contributed substantially to writing the manuscript. P.B.B. substantially contributed by advising on the paper's contents. E.E. performed substantial data curation and contributed to the study design. B.P.-E. collected the study data and advised on the paper's contents. M.R. performed data analysis and substantially contributed the study design. Z.C. contributed substantially to the methodology and statistical calculations and substantially contributed to writing the paper. All authors have read and agreed to the published version of the manuscript.

Funding: This research received no external funding.

Institutional Review Board Statement: The study was conducted according to the guidelines of the Declaration of Helsinki and approved by the Ethics Committee of Eye Center Vidar Orasis Swiss (protocol code 2018-34).

Informed Consent Statement: Informed consent was obtained from all subjects involved in the study.

Data Availability Statement: The data presented in this study are available on request from the authors; the datasets, in particular, are archived in the clinics treated. The data are not publicly available as they contain information that could compromise the privacy of the participants.

Conflicts of Interest: The authors declare no conflict of interest.

References

1. Fernández-Buenaga, R.; Alió, J.L.; Ardoy, A.L.P.; Quesada, A.L.; Cortés, L.P.; Barraquer, R.I. Resolving Refractive Error After Cataract Surgery: IOL Exchange, Piggyback Lens, or LASIK. *J. Refract. Surg.* **2013**, *29*, 676–683. [CrossRef]
2. El Awady, H.E.; Ghanem, A.A. Secondary piggyback implantation versus IOL exchange for symptomatic pseudophakic residual ametropia. *Graefe's Arch. Clin Exp. Ophthalmol.* **2013**, *251*, 1861–1866. [CrossRef]
3. Donoso, R.; Rodríguez, A. Piggyback implantation using the AMO Array multifocal intraocular lens. *J. Cataract. Refract. Surg.* **2001**, *27*, 1506–1510. [CrossRef]

4. Singh, H.; Modabber, M.; Safran, S.G.; Ahmed, I.I.K. Laser iridotomy to treat uveitis-glaucoma-hyphema syndrome secondary to reverse pupillary block in sulcus-placed intraocular lenses: Case series. *J. Cataract. Refract. Surg.* **2015**, *41*, 2215–2223. [CrossRef]
5. Alarcón, A.; Anera, R.G.; Villa, C.; del Barco, L.J.; Gutierrez, R. Visual quality after monovision correction by laser in situ keratomileusis in presbyopic patients. *J. Cataract. Refract. Surg.* **2011**, *37*, 1629–1635. [CrossRef]
6. Uthoff, D.; Pölzl, M.; Hepper, D.; Holland, D. A new method of cornea modulation with excimer laser for simultaneous correction of presbyopia and ametropia. *Graefe's Arch. Clin. Exp. Ophthalmol.* **2012**, *250*, 1649–1661. [CrossRef]
7. Baudu, P.; Penin, F.; Mosquera, S.A. Uncorrected binocular performance after biaspheric ablation profile for presbyopic corneal treatment using AMARIS with the PresbyMAX module. *Am. J. Ophthalmol.* **2013**, *155*, 636–647.e1. [CrossRef] [PubMed]
8. Jackson, W.B.; Tuan, K.-M.A.; Mintsioulis, G. Aspheric Wavefront-Guided LASIK to Treat Hyperopic Presbyopia: 12-Month Results with the VISX Platform. *J. Refract. Surg.* **2011**, *27*, 519–529. [CrossRef]
9. Jung, S.W.; Kim, M.J.; Park, S.H.; Joo, C.K. Multifocal Corneal Ablation for Hyperopic Presbyopes. *J. Refract. Surg.* **2008**, *24*, 903–910. [CrossRef]
10. Luger, M.H.; Ewering, T.; Arba-Mosquera, S. One-year experience in presbyopia correction with biaspheric multifocal central presbyopia laser in situ keratomileusis. *Cornea* **2013**, *32*, 644–652. [CrossRef]
11. Pajic, B.; Massa, H.; Eskina, E.N. Presbyopiekorrektur mittels Laserchirurgie. *Klin. Mon. Augenheilkd.* **2017**, *234*, e29–e42. [CrossRef]
12. Tabernero, J.; Atchison, D.A.; Markwell, E.L. Aberrations and Pupil Location under Corneal Topography and Hartmann-Shack Illumination Conditions. *Investig. Opthalmol. Vis. Sci.* **2009**, *50*, 1964–1970. [CrossRef] [PubMed]
13. Pajic, B.; Pajic-Eggspuehler, B.; Mueller, J.; Cvejic, Z.; Studer, H. A Novel Laser Refractive Surgical Treatment for Presbyopia: Optics-Based Customization for Improved Clinical Outcome. *Sensors* **2017**, *17*, 1367. [CrossRef] [PubMed]
14. Pajic, B.; Cvejic, Z.; Massa, H.; Pajic-Eggspuehler, B.; Resan, M.; Studer, H. Laser Vision Correction for Regular Myopia and Supracor Presbyopia: A Comparison Study. *Appl. Sci.* **2020**, *10*, 873. [CrossRef]
15. Munnerlyn, C.R.; Koons, S.J.; Marshall, J. Photorefractive keratectomy: A technique for laser refractive surgery. *J. Cataract. Refract. Surg.* **1988**, *14*, 46–52. [CrossRef]
16. Liu, F.; Zhang, T.; Liu, Q. One year results of presbyLASIK using hybrid bi-aspheric micro-monovision ablation profile in correction of presbyopia and myopic astigmatism. *Int. J. Ophthalmol.* **2020**, *13*, 271–277. [CrossRef]
17. Seiler, T.G.; Wegner, A.; Senfft, T.; Seiler, T. Dissatisfaction After Trifocal IOL Implantation and Its Improvement by Selective Wavefront-Guided LASIK. *J. Refract. Surg.* **2019**, *35*, 346–352. [CrossRef]
18. Elmohamady, M.N.; Abdelghaffar, W.; Bayoumy, A.S.M.; Gad, E.A. Correction of pseudophakic presbyopia using Lasik with aspheric ablation profiles and a micro-monovision protocol. *Int. Ophthalmol.* **2021**, *41*, 79–86. [CrossRef]
19. Kohnen, T.; Böhm, M.; Herzog, M.; Hemkeppler, E.; Petermann, K.; Lwowski, C. Near visual acuity and patient-reported outcomes in presbyopic patients after bilateral multifocal aspheric laser in situ keratomileusis excimer laser surgery. *J. Cataract. Refract. Surg.* **2020**, *46*, 944–952. [CrossRef]
20. Reilly, C.D.; Lee, W.B.; Alvarenga, L.; Caspar, J.; Garcia-Ferrer, F.; Mannis, M.J. Surgical monovision and monovision reversal in LASIK. *Cornea* **2006**, *25*, 136–138. [CrossRef] [PubMed]
21. Smith, C.E.; Allison, R.S.; Wilkinson, F.; Wilcox, L.M. Monovision: Consequences for depth perception from large disparities. *Exp. Eye Res.* **2019**, *183*, 62–67. [CrossRef] [PubMed]
22. Peng, M.Y.; Hannan, S.; Teenan, D.; Schallhorn, S.J.; Schallhorn, J.M. Monovision LASIK in emmetropic presbyopic patients. *Clin. Ophthalmol.* **2018**, *12*, 1665–1671. [CrossRef] [PubMed]
23. Piñero, D.P.; Espinosa, M.J.A.; Alió, J.L. LASIK Outcomes Following Multifocal and Monofocal Intraocular Lens Implantation. *J. Refract. Surg.* **2010**, *26*, 569–577. [CrossRef] [PubMed]
24. Reinstein, D.Z.; Archer, T.J.; Carp, G.I.; Stuart, A.J.; Rowe, E.L.; Nesbit, A.; Moore, T. Incidence and Outcomes of optical zone enlargement and recentration after previous myopic LASIK by topography-guided custom ablation. *J. Refract. Surg.* **2018**, *34*, 121–130. [CrossRef]

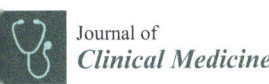

Article

Quality of Life in Presbyopes with Low and High Myopia Using Single-Vision and Progressive-Lens Correction

Adeline Yang [1,*,†], Si Ying Lim [2,†], Yee Ling Wong [1], Anna Yeo [3], Narayanan Rajeev [2] and Björn Drobe [1]

1. Essilor R&D AMERA, Essilor International, Singapore 339346, Singapore; yeeling.wong@essilor.com.sg (Y.L.W.); drobeb@essilor.com (B.D.)
2. School of Chemical & Life Sciences, Singapore Polytechnic, Singapore 139651, Singapore; siying100@hotmail.com (S.Y.L.); Narayanan_RAJEEV@sp.edu.sg (N.R.)
3. Education & Professional Services, Essilor AMERA, Singapore 339338, Singapore; anna.yeo@essilor.com.sg
* Correspondence: adeline.yang@essilor.com.sg; Tel.: +65-91814194
† Both authors contributed equally to this work.

Abstract: This study evaluates the impact of the severity of myopia and the type of visual correction in presbyopia on vision-related quality of life (QOL), using the refractive status and vision profile (RSVP) questionnaire. A total of 149 subjects aged 41–75 years with myopic presbyopia were recruited: 108 had low myopia and 41 had high myopia. The RSVP questionnaire was administered. Rasch analysis was performed on five subscales: perception, expectation, functionality, symptoms, and problems with glasses. Highly myopic subjects had a significantly lower mean QOL score (51.65), compared to low myopes (65.24) ($p < 0.001$). They also had a significantly lower functionality score with glasses (49.38), compared to low myopes (57.00) ($p = 0.018$), and they had a worse functionality score without glasses (29.12), compared to low myopes (36.24) ($p = 0.045$). Those who wore progressive addition lenses (PAL) in the high-myope group ($n = 25$) scored significantly better, compared to those who wore single-vision distance (SVD) lenses ($n = 14$), with perception scores of 61.19 and 46.94, respectively ($p = 0.029$). Highly myopic presbyopes had worse overall QOL and functionality, both with and without glasses, compared to presbyopes with low myopia. High-myopic PAL users had a better perception outcome than SVD lens wearers. Low-myopic PAL wearers had a better QOL than SVD wearers.

Keywords: myopia; quality of life; RSVP questionnaire; presbyopia

1. Introduction

Presbyopia is a global problem affecting 1.8 billion people worldwide [1], of which at least 826 million were not adequately corrected as of 2015 [2]. The number of presbyopes is set to increase to 2.1 billion by 2030, against a backdrop of an ageing global population where the median age could reach 40 years by 2050 [3]. While the impact of presbyopia can be minimised easily by using visual correction such as spectacles, contact lenses, or refractive surgery, up to 34% of presbyopes in developed countries do not have adequate correction [4]. This is compounded by the projected rise in myopia's prevalence and severity globally, which will have a further impact on the quality of life (QOL) for presbyopes [3].

In people with both presbyopia and myopia, adequate correction for near and far vision is crucial for daily activities. The negative impact of presbyopia on both visual functions and QOL has been demonstrated with the use of questionnaires [5,6]. Similarly, the detrimental impact of myopia on vision-related outcomes has been shown in previous studies [7–9]. However, there is a lack of studies that look at the collective impact of myopia and presbyopia on QOL, the correction habits of presbyopic patients, and the impact of the combination of corrections utilised on their QOL. The refractive status and vision profile (RSVP) questionnaire and visual analogue scale (VAS) are methods that are well established, validated, and can be used to capture outcomes that cannot be measured through objective clinical assessments, enabling better management of the clinical practice and research evaluation of new treatments [10–15].

Therefore, this study aims to evaluate the QOL of presbyopes with low and high myopia and to determine how different optical corrections, namely progressive addition lenses (PAL) and single-vision distance (SVD) lenses, affect the QOL outcomes of presbyopes with various myopia severity.

2. Materials and Methods

2.1. Study Population

A total of 149 people aged 41 to 75 years, who had both myopia and presbyopia, participated in this study in the period between August 2016 and March 2018. Presbyopia was defined as the need for reading glasses, near addition, or, in some cases, removing the distance correction. Myopia was defined as spherical equivalent (SE) of ≤ -0.50 diopters (D). All participants were myopic, with no more than 2.00 D of astigmatism in either eye; with anisometropia of less than 1.50 D; and with no history of any eye diseases (such as cataracts, glaucoma, age-related macular degeneration, or other eye complications) or surgeries.

The study adhered to the tenets of the Declaration of Helsinki, and ethics approval was obtained from the Singapore Polytechnic Ethics Review Committee. All tests were administered at the Singapore Polytechnic Optometry Centre after obtaining written informed consent from all participants.

2.2. Examinations

Only participants with distance visual acuity of at least 0.3 LogMAR (measured using the Early Treatment Diabetic Retinopathy Study (ETDRS) chart), near visual acuity of at least N5 (using the N-point near chart), and at least 1.9 log contrast sensitivity (using the Pelli-Robson Contrast Sensitivity chart with habitual correction) were included in the study. Study participants did not undergo any refraction assessment; thus, their distant spectacle power was used as the refractive error. Spectacle power was measured with an automated focimeter (Topcon, CL.100; Topcon Corporation, Tokyo, Japan).

2.3. Questionnaires

A detailed questionnaire was used to collect demographic (age, gender, occupation), ocular, and general medical history from the participants for the purpose of screening. In total, 182 were screened before 149 were recruited. The questionnaire was administered by research staff and completed by the participants themselves.

The original RSVP questionnaire consists of 42 questions. Four questions were omitted, as they were contact lens-related and did not apply to our study objective. There were 38 questions on the different types of vision-dependent activities to assess the level of difficulty in performing daily activities (Table 1). The items used a five-point rating scale. The 38 items were divided into the following five subscales: perception (5 items), expectation (5 items), functionality (14 items), and visual symptoms (13 items).

The current state of health (1 item) was measured using the VAS. This is a measure of perception that ranges across a continuum of values. VAS is a horizontal line, 100 mm in length, anchored by a word descriptor at the end—in this case, the "worst imaginable health state" at zero, and the "best imaginable health state" at 100.

Table 1. Summary of the refractive status and vision profile (RSVP) questionnaire.

Questions	Scale
Perception	
(1) I worry about my vision. (2) My vision holds me back. (3) I am frustrated with my vision. (4) My vision makes me less self-sufficient. (5) Because of my vision, there are things I am afraid to do.	(1) Never (2) Rarely (3) Sometimes (4) Often (5) Always
Expectation	
(1) I am frustrated to use glasses to get the best possible vision. (2) I could accept less than perfect vision if I didn't need glasses any more. (3) As long as I could see well enough to drive without wearing glasses, I wouldn't mind having a vision that was less than perfect. (4) I am only satisfied with my life if I have very sharp vision without glasses. (5) I think my vision will be worse in the future.	(1) Strongly disagree (2) Disagree (3) Neither agree nor disagree (4) Agree (5) Strongly agree
Functionality (With and without correction)	
(1) Watching TV or movies (2) Working or outdoor activities (3) Taking care of or playing with children (4) Seeing your alarm clock (5) Seeing clearly when you wake up (6) Seeing a clock on the wall (7) Doing your job (8) Doing sports/recreation (9) Swimming (10) Your social life (11) Reading and near work (12) Driving at night (13) Driving in the rain (14) Driving when there is a glare from oncoming headlights	(1) Not applicable (2) No difficulty at all (3) A little difficulty (4) Moderate difficulty (5) Severe difficulty (6) So much difficulty that I did not do the activity with this type of correction
Visual Symptoms (With and without correction)	
(1) Your eyes feeling irritated (2) Drafts (from heating or air-conditioning) blowing into your eyes (3) Eyes being sensitive to light (4) Pain in your eyes (5) Changes in your vision during the day (6) Your vision is cloudy or foggy (7) Glare (reflections off shiny surfaces, snow) (8) Things looking different out of one eye versus the other (9) Seeing a halo around lights (10) Seeing in dim light (11) Your depth perception (12) Things appearing distorted (13) Judging distance when going up or down steps (stairs, curbs)	
The current state of health Your own health state today	0 (worst imaginable health state) to 100 (best imaginable health state) using a visual analogue scale

2.4. Statistical Analysis

A Rasch analysis was used to transform the data, and, for further analysis, we used the Andrich rating scale model, with Winsteps software, version 3.68; (Winsteps, Chicago, IL, USA) [16,17]. The transformed scores were scaled from 0 to 100, with a higher score indicating better satisfaction and better QOL. Rasch analysis uses the raw score from the questionnaire and expresses the respondent's outcome on a linear scale, which accounts for the unequal difficulties across all test items. The Rasch analysis was done for the overall QOL and the five subscales of perception, expectation, functionality, symptoms, and problems with glasses.

A chi-square test was used to test for differences in the proportion of participants between groups, and an analysis of variance (ANOVA) was used for the difference in the mean QOL between the groups, using statistical software Statistica, version 13.2 (TIBCO Software Inc., Palo Alto, CA, USA). Values of $p < 0.05$ were taken to be statistically significant differences.

3. Results

Of the 149 participants with both myopia and presbyopia, 108 (72.5%) were presbyopic with low myopia (SE $\leq$ −0.50 D to SE > −5.00 D), and 41 (27.5%) were presbyopic with high myopia (SE $\leq$ −5.00 D), with a mean age (±SD) of 52.1 ± 6.9 years. Moreover, 89 (59.7%) of the participants were females, and 60 (40.3%) were males. There was a significant difference in the distribution of gender, especially in the highly myopic group ($p = 0.04$). This difference in gender distribution did not have any effect on the QOL score (F (1, 145) = 0.30; $p = 0.49$), even with the additional effect among the myope group (F (1, 145) = 0.79; $p = 0.32$). Of the 41 with high myopia, most (85%) had an SE in the range of −5.00 D to −9.00 D. The power of the study was 99.4%, with an effect size of 0.83.

Eighty (53.7%) wore PALs, 61 (40.9%) wore SVD lenses, one (0.7%) wore single-vision near lenses, four (2.7%) wore bifocals, and the remaining three (2%) did not wear glasses. Among those with high myopia, 14 (35.9%) were SVD wearers, and 25 (64.1%) were PAL wearers. Among those with low myopia, 47 (46.1%) were SVD wearers, and 55 (53.9%) were PAL wearers. There were more females in the low-myopic group than in the high-myopic group ($p = 0.04$), and the distance-corrected habitual visual acuity was significantly better in the low-myopic group (−0.09 ± 0.09 logMAR) compared to the high-myopic group (−0.04 ± 0.09 logMAR) ($p = 0.003$) (Table 2).

Table 2. Baseline characteristics of presbyopic participants with low myopia and high myopia (n = 149). Mean ± standard deviation. PAL, progression addition lens; SVD, single-vision distance lens; VAS, visual analogue scale. * Statistically significant with p-value of <0.05.

	Low Myopia (n = 108)	High Myopia (n = 41)	p-Value
Mean age (years)	51.8 ± 6.6	52.8 ± 7.7	0.43
Gender, n (%)			
Female	70 (64.8%)	19 (46.3%)	0.04 *
Male	38 (35.2%)	22 (53.7%)	
Mean spherical equivalent, diopters	−3.1 ± 1.7	−5.6 ± 2.4	<0.001 *
Type of glasses, n (%)			
PAL	55 (50.9%)	25 (61.0%)	0.40
SVD	47 (43.5%)	14 (34.1%)	0.50
Others	6 (5.6%)	2 (4.9%)	-
Mean distance visual acuity, LogMAR	−0.09 ± 0.09	−0.04 ± 0.09	0.003 *
Mean near visual acuity, LogMAR	0.25 ± 0.20	0.25 ± 0.14	0.57
Mean log contrast sensitivity	1.94 ± 0.02	1.94 ± 0.03	0.22
Current health (VAS)	77.48 ± 1.50	73.07 ± 2.42	0.12

The health-state score was significantly correlated with the QOL score, but the correlation was weak, $r^2 = 0.10$ ($p < 0.05$). The health-state score was similar between the two myopic groups ($p = 0.43$), and between the PAL- and SVD-lens wearers ($p = 0.81$).

High myopes had a significantly lower overall QOL (51.7) than low myopes (65.2) ($p < 0.001$; Figure 1). High myopes also had significantly poorer functionality with glasses, with a score of 29.1, compared with those of presbyopes with low myopia, with a score of 36.2 ($p = 0.01$). Similarly, presbyopes with high myopia had poorer functionality without glasses (49.4) than low myopes (57.0; $p = 0.04$).

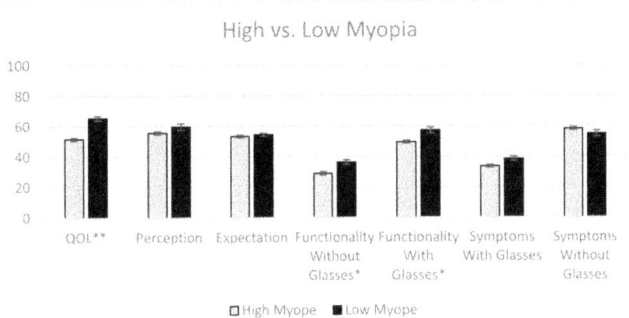

Figure 1. The quality of life (QOL) scores of presbyopes with low myopia versus high myopia, with error bars representing standard error. * Statistically significant, with a p-value of <0.05; ** statistically significant, with a p-value of <0.001.

With glasses, a greater proportion of high myopes had difficulty driving at night (low myopes 27.5% vs. high myopes 54.2%) (X^2 (1, $n = 93$) = 5.6; $p = 0.02$) and driving in the rain (11.3% low myopes vs. 36.7% high myopes; X^2 (1, $n = 92$) = 8.3; $p = 0.004$). High myopes also had more issues swimming with correction (19.4% low myopes vs. 36.7% high myopes; X^2 (1, $n = 92$) = 4.5; $p = 0.03$). Without glasses, high myopes had greater difficulty reading and doing near work (42% low myopes vs. 83.9% high myopes; X^2 (1, $n = 131$) = 16.6; $p < 0.001$). They were also less able to see clearly when they woke up (42.3% vs. 88.2%; X^2 (1, $n = 131$) = 21.4; $p < 0.001$) or see the alarm clock (40.4% vs. 80.0%; X^2 (1, $n = 129$) = 16.0; $p < 0.001$).

For presbyopes with low myopia, the group using PAL had significantly better overall QOL than SVD lens users ($p = 0.04$; Figure 2), although there was no significant difference between SVD lens and PAL wearers in all the other subscales, such as perception, expectation, functionality, and symptoms.

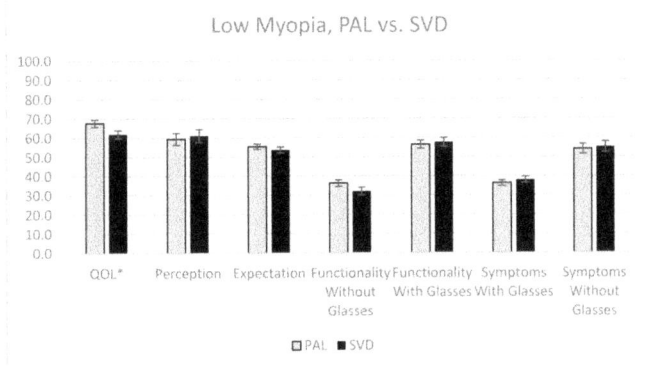

Figure 2. The QOL scores of presbyopes with low myopia who wore PAL and SVD lenses for all five subscales, with error bars representing standard error. * Statistically significant, with p-value of <0.05.

In the group of presbyopes with high myopia, those who wore PAL had significantly better perception (61.2) than those who wore SVD lenses (46.9; $p = 0.03$). High myopes wearing SVD lenses stated that they were more often afraid to do things because of their vision (SVD 57.1% vs. PAL 28%; X^2 (1, n = 39) = 4.3; p = 0.04), and were more frustrated with their glasses (71.4% vs. 32.0%; X^2 (1, n = 39) = 5.6; p = 0.02). No other significant differences were found for the other subscales, for presbyopes with high myopia wearing PAL and SVD lenses (Figure 3).

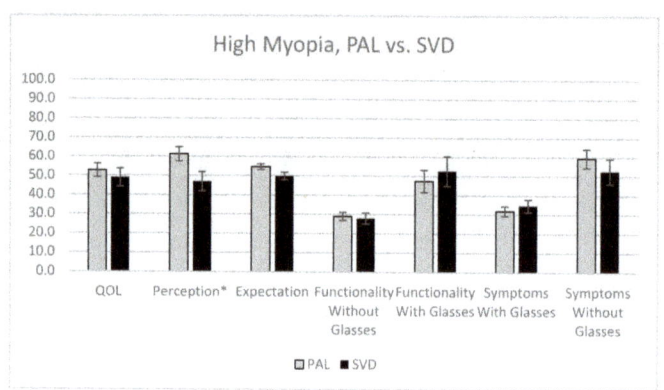

Figure 3. The QOL scores of highly myopic presbyopes who wore PAL and SVD lenses for all five subscales, with error bars representing standard error. * Statistically significant, with p-value of <0.05.

4. Discussion

4.1. Significant Findings

Presbyopes with high myopia had poorer overall QOL compared to those with low myopia. Similarly, high myopes had worse functionality scores compared to low myopes. Compared to SVD users, PAL users, on average, had better overall QOL scores for both myopic groups. PAL users also had better perception scores for high myopes. The difference in gender distribution did not have a significant effect on the QOL score.

The highly myopic group had significantly poorer visual acuity, with a difference of 0.05 logMAR, which equates to 2–3 letters from the visual acuity chart. This slight decrease in visual acuity may not be considered clinically significant by clinicians. However, it may have a tangible effect, contributing to poorer QOL and functionality outcomes with glasses. Therefore, this study's outcome from the QOL reflected the tangible effects of reduced vision felt by the participants, which were often dismissed as insignificant by clinicians.

Reduced best-corrected visual acuity with spectacle lenses in high myopia has been found in previous studies [9,18–25]. In addition, there was a higher proportion of high myopes who experienced severe trouble with driving at night and in the rain [26]. Besides visual acuity affecting the corrected vision of high myopes, the night vision threshold [26], higher-order aberration [20,21], and larger pupil size may also contribute to poorer vision under dim lighting, as experienced when driving at night and in the rain. Further physiological stretching from axial elongation due to myopia also reduces the function and resolution of photoreceptors [22,26]. Some studies also found reduced contrast sensitivity at high spatial frequencies in fully corrected high myopes, which may contribute to reduced functionality with glasses [27]. However, we did not find any differences in contrast sensitivity between low and high myopic groups, as found by Collins et al. [19]. Further investigation is required to measure contrast sensitivity at different spatial frequencies in order to elucidate the underlying cause of reduced functionality with glasses.

It was expected that the difference in the refractive error between high- and low-myopic groups (−5.52 ± 2.4 D compared to −3.1 ± 1.7 D; p < 0.001) would have a significant impact on the unaided visual acuity of high-myopic groups, even though it was not measured. With significantly poorer vision without glasses, a higher proportion of high-myopic presbyopes would have issues seeing both far and near, as they are severely under-corrected for both distances. This would result in a poorer outcome in functionality without glasses for the high-myopic group. The poorer outcome in QOL regarding uncorrected vision was also reflected in other studies [18,28,29]. Our study shows that a larger proportion of high myopes had difficulty reading and doing near work, as well as waking up with clear vision and looking at an alarm clock without glasses. All the affected activities, as mentioned above, were near-distance activities, as also reported in other studies [18,29]. The lack of distance activities reported without glasses was due to the inability to carry them out without glasses. No high myopes drove without glasses.

This study found that highly myopic PAL wearers had a better score for perception subscales compared to SVD lens wearers. In the perception subscale, highly myopic SVD lens wearers were more "afraid to do things due to their vision" and were also more "frustrated with their glasses." SVD lenses only correct distance vision and not near vision; hence, highly myopic SVD lens wearers will have poor near and intermediate vision, with or without glasses. To overcome blurred vision due to working distance, they may need to remove and put on SVD glasses more frequently, adding to the frustration. Compared with SVD wearers, low-myopic PAL wearers also had a significantly better overall QOL, with no other difference in the other subscales. Despite the lack of a significant difference in each subscale, the significant differences in the overall QOL may be due to the additive effect of multiple components. Other studies have found that near vision is affected while using SVD lenses for presbyopes, while having better outcomes using PAL [30–33]. Poorer near and intermediate vision with SVD lenses may significantly affect QOL outcomes in low myopes; they may also significantly affect the perception subscale for high myopes. Moreover, Pesudovs et al., 2006 found that PAL wearers have reduced sensitivity to light, eye pain, and redness compared to SVD lens wearers, while doing near work, for early presbyopes [33]. As such, the visual comfort from PAL could be another factor in this outcome.

4.2. Strengths and Limitations of the Study

This is the first study that explores the correction habits of presbyopes and the impact of the severity of myopia on QOL. This study was able to measure the subjective differences between the severity of myopia and the types of visual correction, which was otherwise not significantly different from clinical measures. However, the recruitment rate of patients with high myopia (27.5%) was much lower compared with those having low myopia (72.5%). This, however, is a reflection of myopia's prevalence in the population [3]. Refraction and axial length measurements were not conducted to directly link the causal effect of refractive error and elongation of the eye to the QOL outcome. Unaided visual acuity and contrast sensitivity with spatial frequencies need to be measured to directly understand the contribution of these factors to some of the subscales, such as functionality with and without glasses. More details such as the lens design of PAL should be included in order to further understand whether it has an impact on QOL. Though the RSVP questionnaire has been shown to be deficient in several psychometric properties with underutilised response scales, it was chosen not only because it was validated but also because it includes measures for quality of vision and life [11–15,34–36].

4.3. Suggestions for Future Work

From this study, the QOL assessment recorded outcomes that could not be measured through typical clinical tests or may be deemed clinically insignificant. Hence, such questionnaires should be administered during dispensing to achieve higher success rates. Work should be done to understand which are the important and contributing subscales for each eye condition and interventions, in order to apply the right questionnaire for each condition. A systematic review could be done on all types of vision correction used for presbyopia, such as PAL, SVD, contact lenses, and intraocular lenses, in order to understand their impact on QOL.

5. Conclusions

This study was able to measure significant subjective feedback from the RSVP questionnaire that was not found clinically (visual acuity). It was found that a significantly higher proportion of highly myopic presbyopes reported lower vision-related QOL across both the QOL and functionality subscales. Despite having similar best-corrected vision, PAL wearers had better QOL outcomes than SVD lens wearers with low myopia. Moreover, PAL wearers with high myopia had better perception than SVD wearers with high myopia. Therefore, wearing PAL could be a better option to improve the QOL in myopic presbyopes of various myopia levels.

Author Contributions: Conceptualisation, B.D., A.Y. (Anna Yeo) and N.R.; methodology, A.Y. (Anna Yeo), N.R., S.Y.L. and A.Y. (Adeline Yang); formal analysis, Y.L.W., S.Y.L. and A.Y. (Adeline Yang); investigation, N.R. and S.Y.L.; resources, A.Y. (Anna Yeo) and B.D.; writing—original draft preparation, S.Y.L. and A.Y. (Adeline Yang); writing—review and editing, B.D., Y.L.W., A.Y. (Anna Yeo) and N.R.; supervision, A.Y. (Adeline Yang), A.Y. (Anna Yeo) and N.R.; project administration, A.Y. (Adeline Yang), A.Y. (Anna Yeo) and N.R.; funding acquisition, B.D. and A.Y. (Anna Yeo). All authors have read and agreed to the published version of the manuscript.

Funding: This research was done in collaboration with Essilor International. Students and staff were not paid by this collaboration, and participants were remunerated SGD 20 each for taking part in this study.

Institutional Review Board Statement: IRB approval No.: 201604-01. The study was conducted according to the guidelines of the Declaration of Helsinki and approved by the Institutional Review Board (or Ethics Committee) of Singapore Polytechnic (Protocol code: 201604-01 and Date of approval: 25-07-2016).

Informed Consent Statement: Informed consent was obtained from all subjects involved in the study.

Data Availability Statement: Please contact corresponding author for data.

Acknowledgments: To Charmaine, Eunice, Gao Jun, Gao Ming, Huda, Joseph, Kelly, Lynn, Rui Qi, Yi Xin, Zhan Foong, and Zhixun for their assistance in collecting the data.

Conflicts of Interest: Adeline Yang, Yee Ling Wong, Anna Yeo, and Björn Drobe are employees of Essilor International.

Abbreviations

Quality of life (QOL), spherical equivalent (SE), diopters (D), refractive status and vision profile (RSVP), progressive addition lenses (PAL), single vision distance (SVD) lenses, visual analogue scales (VAS).

References

1. World Population Prospects—Population Division. United Nations. 2020. Available online: https://population.un.org/wpp/ (accessed on 15 January 2020).
2. Holden, B.A.; Fricke, T.R.; Ho, S.M.; Wong, R.; Schlenther, G.; Cronje, S.; Burnett, A.; Papas, E.; Naidoo, K.S.; Frick, K.D. Global vision impairment due to uncorrected presbyopia. *Arch. Ophthalmol.* **2008**, *126*, 1731–1739. [CrossRef] [PubMed]
3. Holden, B.; Fricke, T. Global Prevalence of myopia and high myopia and temporal trends from 2000 through 2050. *Ophthalmology* **2016**, *123*, 1036–1042. [CrossRef] [PubMed]
4. Fricke, T.R.; Tahhan, N.; Resnikoff, S.; Papas, E.; Burnett, A.; Ho, S.M.; Naduvilath, T.; Naidoo, K.S. Global prevalence of presbyopia and vision impairment from uncorrected presbyopia: Systematic review, meta-analysis, and modelling. *Ophthalmology* **2018**, *125*, 1492–1499. [CrossRef] [PubMed]
5. Lu, Q.; Congdon, N. Quality of life and near vision impairment due to functional presbyopia among rural Chinese adults. *Investig. Opthal. Vis. Sci.* **2011**, *52*, 4118–4123. [CrossRef]
6. Muhammad, N.; Alhassan, M. Visual function and vision-related quality of life in a presbyopic adult population of Northwestern Nigeria. *Niger Med. J.* **2015**, *56*, 317–322. [CrossRef]
7. McDonnell, P.J.; Lee, P.; Spritzer, K.; Lindblad, A.S.; Hays, R.D. Associations of presbyopia with vision-targeted health-related quality of life. *Arch. Ophthalmol.* **2003**, *121*, 1577–1581. [CrossRef]

8. Kumaran, S.; Balasubramaniam, S. Refractive error and vision-related quality of life in South Indian children. *Optom. Vis. Sci.* **2015**, *92*, 272–278. [CrossRef]
9. Rose, K.; Harper, R.; Tromans, C.; Waterman, C.; Goldberg, D.; Haggerty, C.; Tullo, A. Quality of life in myopia. *Br. J. Ophthalmol.* **2000**, *84*, 1031–1034. [CrossRef]
10. Black, N. Patient reported outcome measures could help transform healthcare. *Br. Med. J.* **2013**, *346*, f167. [CrossRef]
11. Elliott, D.; Pesudovs, K. Vision-related quality of life. *Optom. Vis. Sci.* **2007**, *84*, 656–658. [CrossRef]
12. Vitale, S. The Refractive Status and Vision Profile A Questionnaire to Measure Vision-Related Quality of Life in Persons with Refractive Error. *Ophthalmology* **2000**, *107*, 1529–1539. [CrossRef]
13. Nichols, J.J. Reliability and Validity of Refractive Error–Specific Quality-of-Life Instruments. *Arch. Ophthalmol.* **2003**, *121*, 1289. [CrossRef]
14. Khadka, J.; McAlinden, C.; Pesudovs, K. Quality Assessment of Ophthalmic Questionnaires. *Optom. Vis. Sci.* **2013**, *90*, 720–744. [CrossRef]
15. Wu, X.Y.; Ohinmaa, A.; Johnson, J.A.; Veugelers, P.J. Assessment of Children's Own Health Status Using Visual Analogue Scale and Descriptive System of the EQ-5D-Y: Linkage between Two Systems. *Qual. Life Res.* **2013**, *23*, 393–402. [CrossRef]
16. Andrich, D. A rating formulation for ordered response categories. *Psychometrika* **1978**, *43*, 561–573. [CrossRef]
17. Linacre, J.M. *Winsteps Rasch Measurement Computer Program*; Winsteps: Chicago, IL, USA, 2006.
18. Lamoureux, E.L.; Wang, J.; Aung, T.; Saw, S.M.; Wong, T.Y. Myopia and quality of life: The Singapore Malay Eye Study (SiMES). *Investig. Ophthalmol. Vis. Sci.* **2008**, *49*, 4469.
19. Collins, J.W.; Carney, L.G. Visual performance in high myopia. *Curr. Eye Res.* **1990**, *9*, 217–223. [CrossRef]
20. Cheng, X.U.; Bradley, A.; Hong, X.; Thibos, L.N. Relationship between refractive error and monochromatic aberrations of the eye. *Optom. Vis. Sci.* **2003**, *80*, 43–49. [CrossRef]
21. Paquin, M.P.; Hamam, H.; Simonet, P. Objective measurement of optical aberrations in myopic eyes. *Optom. Vis. Sci.* **2002**, *79*, 285–291. [CrossRef]
22. Atchison, D.A.; Pritchard, N.; Schmid, K.L. Peripheral refraction along the horizontal and vertical visual fields in myopia. *Vis. Res.* **2006**, *46*, 1450–1458. [CrossRef]
23. Chen, P.C.; Woung, L.C.; Yang, C.F. Modulation transfer function and critical flicker frequency in high-myopia patients. *J. Formos Med. Assoc.* **2000**, *99*, 45–48. [PubMed]
24. Kawabata, H.; Adachi-Usami, E. Multifocal electroretinogram in myopia. *Investig. Ophthalmol. Vis. Sci.* **1997**, *38*, 2844–2851.
25. Westall, C.A.; Dhaliwal, H.S.; Panton, C.M.; Sigesmun, D.; Levin, A.V.; Nischal, K.K.; Héon, E. Values of electroretinogram responses according to axial length. *Doc Ophthalmol.* **2001**, *102*, 115–130. [CrossRef] [PubMed]
26. Mashige, K. Night vision and glare vision thresholds and recovery time in myopic and hyperopic eyes. *Afr. Vis. Eye Health* **2010**, *69*, a136. [CrossRef]
27. Jaworski, A.; Gentle, A.; Zele, A.J.; Vingrys, A.J.; McBrien, N.A. Altered visual sensitivity in axial high myopia: A local postreceptoral phenomenon? *Investig. Ophthalmol. Vis. Sci.* **2006**, *47*, 3695–3702. [CrossRef]
28. Kandel, H.; Khadka, J.; Goggin, M.; Pesudovs, K. Impact of refractive error on quality of life: A qualitative study. *Clin. Exp. Ophthalmol.* **2017**, *45*, 677–688. [CrossRef]
29. Smith, T.S.; Katz, J.; Khatry, S.; Le Clerk, S.; Patel, I.; Hyon, B.; Tielsch, J. The impact of uncorrected presbyopia on performance in tasks of daily living and vision-related quality of life in rural Nepal. *Investig. Ophthalmol. Vis. Sci.* **2009**, *50*, 3966.
30. Sivardeen, A.; McAlinden, C.; Wolffsohn, J.S. Presbyopic correction use and its impact on quality of vision symptoms. *J. Optom.* **2020**, *13*, 29–34. [CrossRef]
31. Chu, B.S.; Wood, J.M.; Collins, M.J. Effect of presbyopic vision corrections on perceptions of driving difficulty. *Eye Contact Lens* **2009**, *35*, 133–143. [CrossRef]
32. Chu, B.S.; Wood, J.M.; Collins, M.J. The effect of presbyopic vision corrections on nighttime driving performance. *Investig. Ophthalmol. Vis. Sci.* **2010**, *51*, 4861–4866. [CrossRef]
33. Pesudovs, K.; Garamendi, E.; Elliott, D.B. The contact lens impact on quality of life (CLIQ) questionnaire: Development and validation. *Investig. Ophthalmol. Vis. Sci.* **2006**, *47*, 2789–2796. [CrossRef]
34. Kandel, H.; Khadka, J.; Lundström, M.; Goggin, M.; Pesudovs, K. Questionnaires for Measuring Refractive Surgery Outcomes. *J. Refract Surg.* **2017**, *33*, 416–424. [CrossRef]
35. Kandel, H.; Khadka, J.; Goggin, M.; Pesudovs, K. Patient-reported Outcomes for Assessment of Quality of Life in Refractive Error: A Systematic Review. *Optom. Vis. Sci. Off. Publ. Am. Acad. Optom.* **2017**, *94*, 1102–1119. [CrossRef]
36. Garamendi, E.; Pesudovs, K.; Stevens, M.J.; Elliott, D.B. The Refractive Status and Vision Profile: Evaluation of psychometric properties and comparison of Rasch and summated Likert-scaling. *Vis. Res.* **2006**, *46*, 1375–1383. [CrossRef]

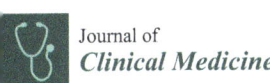

Article

Factors Influencing Contrast Sensitivity Function in Eyes with Mild Cataract

Kazutaka Kamiya [1,*], Fusako Fujimura [1], Takushi Kawamorita [1], Wakako Ando [2], Yoshihiko Iida [2] and Nobuyuki Shoji [2]

[1] Visual Physiology, School of Allied Health Sciences, Kitasato University, Kanagawa 2520373, Japan; f-fujimu@kitasato-u.ac.jp (F.F.); kawa2008@kitasato-u.ac.jp (T.K.)
[2] Department of Ophthalmology, School of Medicine, Kitasato University, Kanagawa 2520374, Japan; wakako@kitasato-u.ac.jp (W.A.); sparkle.i.4415@gmail.com (Y.I.); nshoji@kitasato-u.ac.jp (N.S.)
* Correspondence: kamiyak-tky@umin.ac.jp; Tel.: +81-42-778-8464; Fax: +81-42-778-2357

Abstract: This study was aimed to evaluate the relationship between the area under the log contrast sensitivity function (AULCSF) and several optical factors in eyes suffering mild cataract. We enrolled 71 eyes of 71 patients (mean age, 71.4 ± 10.7 (standard deviation) years) with cataract formation who were under surgical consultation. We determined the area under the log contrast sensitivity function (AULCSF) using a contrast sensitivity unit (VCTS-6500, Vistech). We utilized single and multiple regression analyses to investigate the relevant factors in such eyes. The mean AULSCF was 1.06 ± 0.16 (0.62 to 1.38). Explanatory variables relevant to the AULCSF were, in order of influence, logMAR best spectacle-corrected visual acuity (BSCVA) ($p < 0.001$, partial regression coefficient B = −0.372), and log(s) ($p = 0.023$, B = −0.032) (adjusted R^2 = 0.402). We found no significant association with other variables such as age, gender, uncorrected visual acuity, nuclear sclerosis grade, or ocular HOAs. Eyes with better BSCVA and lower log(s) are more susceptible to show higher AULCSF, even in mild cataract subjects. It is indicated that both visual acuity and intraocular forward scattering play a role in the CS function in such eyes.

Keywords: contrast sensitivity; cataract; AULCSF; visual acuity; intraocular scattering; higher-order aberrations

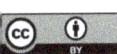

1. Introduction

Cataract still remains a major cause of visual impairment worldwide [1]. The prevalence rate of cataract increases with age, according to population-based studies on lens opacities [2,3]. Cataract has a greater impact on the quality of life of older adults, including increased difficulties in daily activities, compared with other common age-related conditions [4,5]. Cataract importantly increases scattered light, when light passes through the eye media, generating a veil of straylight over the retina that degrades vision, a phenomenon called straylight. This veiling luminance over the retina affects the retinal image quality, diminishing contrast and increasing the sensitivity to glare. Actually, it has been demonstrated that the amount of scattered light was objectively assessed by the double-pass instrument, as an objective scatter index (OSI) in cataract patients [6], and that this index can be used for cataract classification [7]. The comparison compensation method has been successfully applied in order to subjectively assess intraocular straylight by the logarithmic straylight value (log(s)) [8–10]. It has been shown that visual acuity and straylight are rather independent aspects of the overall quality of vision in cataract patients [11]. Cataracts have been reported to notably influence driving performance in older subjects, and that the OSI has high predictive power when it comes to simulated driving performance in older drivers [12]. Likewise, straylight has been shown to be the best parameter for predicting simulated driving performance in older drivers [13]. It has also been known that visual functions apart from visual acuity may be more associated with visual complaints that impact the quality of life.

Since conventional visual acuity testing may not be suitable for the assessment of detailed visual quality [14], contrast sensitivity (CS) testing will be clinically helpful for this evaluation, especially in eyes with mild cataract. Adamsons et al. stated that preoperative measurement of contrast sensitivity can help determine who with early cataract with mild impairment in visual acuity is most likely to report subjective improvement in vision [15]. Superstein et al. showed that spatial contrast sensitivity testing provided an objective assessment of patients who had good visual acuity yet also had functional complaints [16], and that should be considered as adjuncts to visual acuity testing in evaluating certain cataract patients [17]. The deterioration in CS function is caused not only by cataract formation itself, but also by the aging process and its consequent effect on visual processing and on the retina. We previously reported that intraocular forward scattering plays a more vital role in CS function than higher-order aberrations (HOAs) in myopic subjects [18]. However, the effect of light scatter and HOAs on CS function has not been fully elucidated in eyes having mild cataract. It may provide basic insights on understanding detailed visual performance in mild cataract patients. The goal of the current study is twofold; to quantitatively determine CS function in eyes with mild cataract, and to assess the background factors affecting CS function using single and multiple regression analyses in such eyes.

2. Materials and Methods

2.1. Study Population

We registered with the University Hospital Medical Information Network Clinical Trial Registry (000034854). Seventy-one eyes of 71 consecutive subjects (mean age ± standard deviation; 71.4 ± 10.7 years, 34 men and 37 women), who completed optical examinations for cataract surgery consultation, and who had no other ocular diseases, except for mild cataract, were enrolled in the current study. Only subjects in whom we could reproducibly quantify all optical parameters using the straylight meter, as well as the Hartmann–Shack aberrometry, were defined as mild cataract in this study. We randomly selected only one eye per subject for statistical analysis, when a bilateral cataract occurred. This retrospective study was approved by the Institutional Review Board at Kitasato University Hospital (B16-67), and followed the tenets of the Declaration of Helsinki. Our Institutional Review Board waived the requirement for informed consent for this retrospective review.

2.2. Assessment of Contrast Sensitivity Function

We measured the CS function using a contrast sensitivity unit (VCTS-6500, Vistech) under photopic conditions (500 lux). We conducted this test with the best spectacle correction at a distance of 2.5 m. We determined the area under the log contrast sensitivity function (AULCSF) by the CS data, as described previously [19]. Briefly, we plotted the log of CS as a function of log spatial frequency and fitted third-order polynomials to the data. We integrated the fitted function between the fixed limits of log spatial frequencies of 0.18 (corresponding to 1.5 cycles/degree) to 1.26 (corresponding to 18 cycles/degree), and determined the obtained value as the AULCSF.

2.3. Assessment of Visual Acuity, Nuclear Sclerosis and Cataract Type

We performed visual acuity measurement using a Snellen chart at 5 m, with and without spectacle correction. Two cataract specialists assessed the grade of nuclear sclerosis of the crystalline lens according to the Emery-Little classification, and the cataract type was divided into three subgroups (nuclear sclerosis, cortical, and posterior subcapsular cataract subgroups), based on slit-lamp biomicroscopy after mydriasis. We defined as cases those subjects who presented with an advanced form of 1 of the 3 types of cataract, regardless of the concomitant presence of the remaining 2 types of cataract. In addition, we investigated the relationship of the AULCSF with the logarithm of the minimal angle of resolution (logMAR) of best spectacle-corrected visual acuity (BSCVA) and log(s) in early cataract eyes with logMAR BSCVA of 0.05 or better.

2.4. Assessment of Intraocular Forward Scattering and Higher-Order Aberrations

We measured the retinal straylight, as a measure of subjective forward scattering, using the C-Quant straylight meter (Oculus Optikgeräte, GmbH, Wetzlar, Germany). Briefly, a test field that consists of a dark circle divided into two semicircles and is surrounded by a ring-shaped flickering light. A counter-phase compensation light is presented in one of the semicircles, reducing the flicker perception on that side. The subjects are instructed to select which semicircle is flickering more intensely. We repeated this process 3 times with different levels of compensation light, resulting in a logarithmic straylight value (log(s)) [8–10]. We used the measurement only when the estimated standard deviation was <0.08 and the quality factor for psychometric sampling was >1.00 [9].

We determined ocular HOAs for a 4-mm pupil after mydriasis using the Hartmann-Shack aberrometry (KR-1W, Topcon, Tokyo, Japan). We separately calculated the root mean square of the 3rd- and 4th-order coefficients.

2.5. Statistical Analysis

We used commercially-available statistical software (Bellcurve for Excel, Social Survey Research Information Co., Ltd., Tokyo, Japan) for statistical analyses. We conducted stepwise multiple regression analysis to assess the relationship of the CS function with several parameters. We utilized the AULCSF as the dependent variable, and age, gender, logMAR of uncorrected visual acuity (UCVA) and BSCVA, nuclear sclerosis grade, log(s), ocular 3rd-order aberrations, and ocular 4th-order aberrations as the explanatory variables. We also conducted Spearman's rank correlation test to evaluate the relationships between the AULCSF and other variables. We applied a one-way analysis of variance for the analysis of the AULCSF among the 3 cataract subgroups. We described the results as mean ± standard deviation, and deemed a p-value < 0.05 statistically significant.

3. Results

Table 1 shows the patient demographics in the present study. The mean AULSCF was 1.06 ± 0.16 (range, 0.62 to 1.38). The AULCSF was 1.07 ± 0.11, 1.08 ± 0.16, and 1.01 ± 0.20, in the nuclear sclerosis, cortical, and posterior subcapsular cataract subgroups. We found no significant differences in the AULCSF among the three subgroups (analysis of variance, $p = 0.391$). Table 2 summarizes the results of multiple regression analysis. The relevant explanatory variables were logMAR BSCVA ($p < 0.001$, partial regression coefficient B = −0.372) and log(s) ($p = 0.023$, B = −0.032) (adjusted $R^2 = 0.402$). The equation was described as follows: AULCSF = (−0.372 × logMAR BSCVA) + (−0.032 × log(s)) + 1.385. There were no significant associations with other explanatory variables such as age, gender, UCVA, nuclear sclerosis grade, ocular 3rd-order HOAs, or ocular 4th-order HOAs. The standardized partial regression coefficient was determined in order to investigate the level of each variable's influence. The most relevant variable was logMAR BSCVA, followed by the log(s). Table 2 shows similar results by single regression analysis. Figures 1 and 2 show significant associations between the AULCSF and logMAR BSCVA ($r = −0.640$, $p < 0.001$), and those between the AULCSF and the log(s) ($r = −0.427$, $p < 0.001$), respectively. With better BSCVA, lower log(s), or both, the AULSCF became significantly higher in eyes having mild cataract. On the other hand, we found no significant correlations of the AULCSF with ocular 3rd-order aberrations ($r = −0.144$, $p = 0.264$), or 4th-order aberrations ($r = −0.167$, $p = 0.194$). For subgroup analysis in 26 early cataract eyes with logMAR BSCVA of 0.05 or better, we also found significant correlations between the AULCSF and logMAR BSCVA ($r = −0.388$, $p = 0.049$), and those between the AULCSF and the log(s) ($r = −0.405$, $p = 0.040$), but no significant correlations between the AULCSF and 3rd-order aberrations ($r = −0.249$, $p = 0.220$), or those between the AULCSF and 4th-order aberrations ($r = −0.128$, $p = 0.532$).

Table 1. Demographic and visual functional data of the study population.

Patient Demographics and Visual Function	
Age (years)	71.4 ± 10.7 years (95% CI, 50.5 to 92.3 years)
Gender (Male:Female)	34:37
LogMAR UCVA	0.67 ± 0.49 (95% CI, −0.29 to 1.62)
LogMAR BSCVA	0.16 ± 0.19 (95% CI, −0.22 to 0.54)
Sphere (D)	−1.10 ± 4.18 D (95% CI, −9.28 to 7.09 D)
Cylinder (D)	1.05 ± 0.90 D (95% CI, −0.71 to 2.80 D)
Grade of nuclear sclerosis	2.08 ± 0.19 (95% CI, 1.16 to 3.02)
Log(s)	1.93 ± 1.08 (95% CI, −0.18 to 4.05)
Ocular 3rd-order aberrations (μm)	0.21 ± 0.12 μm (95% CI, −0.03 to 0.45 μm)
Ocular 4th-order aberrations (μm)	0.13 ± 0.06 μm (95% CI, 0.01 to 0.25 μm)
AULCSF	1.06 ± 0.16 (95% CI, 0.75 to 1.37)

CI = confidence interval, logMAR = logarithm of the minimal angle of resolution, UCVA = uncorrected visual acuity, BSCVA = best spectacle-corrected visual acuity, D = diopter, AULSCF = area under the log contrast sensitivity function.

Table 2. Results of correlation analysis and stepwise multiple regression analysis to select variables relevant to the area under the log contrast sensitivity function (AULCSF) in eyes with mild cataract.

Variables	Spearman Correlation Coefficient	p-Value	Partial Regression Coefficient	Standardized Partial Regression Coefficient	p-Value
Log(s)	−0.427	<0.001	−0.032	−0.241	0.023
LogMAR BSCVA	−0.640	<0.001	−0.372	−0.467	<0.001
Age (years)	−0.149	0.213	not included		-
Gender (male = 0, female = 1)	0.096	0.428	not included		-
LogMAR UCVA	−0.150	0.211	not included		-
Grade of nuclear sclerosis	−0.128	0.287	not included		-
Ocular 3rd-order aberrations (μm)	−0.144	0.264	not included		-
Ocular 4th-order aberrations (μm)	−0.167	0.194	not included		-
			1.385	Constant	

LogMAR = logarithm of the minimal angle of resolution, BSCVA = best spectacle-corrected visual acuity, UCVA = uncorrected visual acuity.

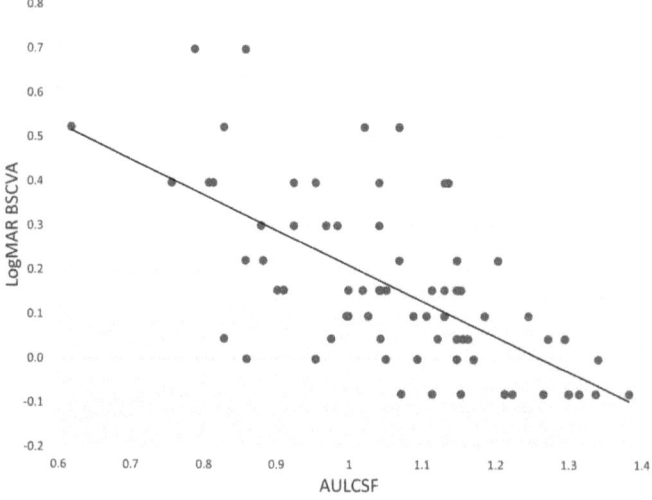

Figure 1. A scatterplot between the AULSCF and logMAR best spectacle-corrected visual acuity (Spearman correlation coefficient r = −0.640, $p < 0.001$).

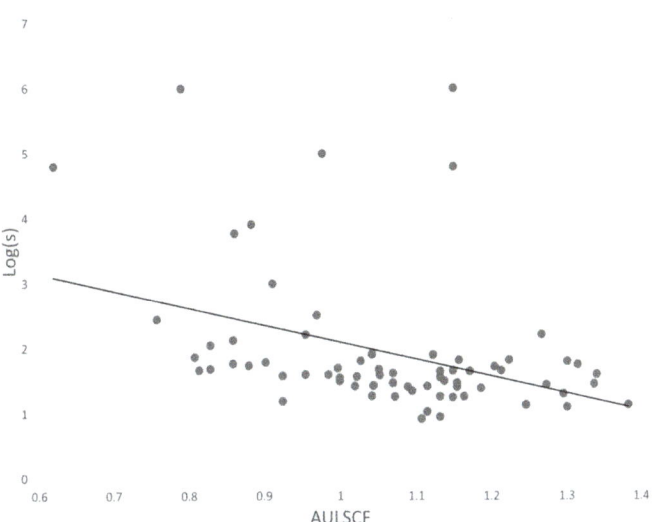

Figure 2. A scatterplot between the AULSCF and log(s) (Spearman correlation coefficient r = −0.427, p < 0.001).

4. Discussion

In the current study, our findings showed that both BSCVA and log(s) were significantly correlated with the CS function in eyes with mild cataract, although some of the variance has remained unanswered, as confirmed by the moderate R^2 value (0.402). Since CS can be affected by multiple factors, such as retina and brain processing [20,21], it is reasonable that the CS function cannot be totally clarified by the optics. To the best of our knowledge, this is the first study to determine the detailed clinical factors affecting the CS function by single and multiple regression analyses in mild cataract subjects.

With regard to visual acuity and CS function for cataract, Adamsons et al. described that the CS scores were lower for patients having mild lens opacities than for patients having clear lenses at high spatial frequencies, suggesting that decreased visual function for patients with early cataracts whose visual acuity is only minimally impaired [22]. Fujikado et al. reported that the AULCSF was moderately associated with the HOAs as well as with intraocular scattering in eyes having cataract [23]. Shandiz et al. found a significant loss of CS at all frequencies with increasing cataract severity, indicating that the AULCSF may provide additional information compared with standard visual acuity tests in patients with early cataracts [24]. Visual acuity encompasses a narrow central visual angle (0.02 degrees), whereas CS encompasses an angle of approximately 0.30 degrees. It is understandable that BSCVA was significantly associated with the AULSCF in the present study. It is suggested that BSCVA is one of the most relevant factors influencing the CS function for clinical use, even in eyes having mild cataract.

With regard to log(s) and CS function for cataract, van den Berg et al. and van der Meulen et al. demonstrated that visual acuity was not strongly correlated with straylight, indicating that each measurement shows different aspects of quality of vision [11,25]. Palomo-Álvarez et al. stated that the mean straylight (1.38 ± 0.24) in the cataract group was significantly worse than that (1.17 ± 0.11) in the control group [26]. Their findings of log(s) in cataract patients were slightly lower than our findings, presumably because of the differences in patient age (67.96 ± 7.11 years vs. 71.4 ± 10.7 years), cataract type, and cataract grade. Paz Filgueira et al. showed that straylight meter measurements demonstrate the loss of CS resulting from nuclear and posterior subcapsular opacities [27]. Martínez-Roda et al. found significant associations of the grading according to the lens opacities classification system III [28] with log(s) and OSI, although they were slightly stronger with

OSI for all cataract types [29]. These previous and our current findings indicate that the increase in intraocular forward scattering caused by the changes in the transparency of the crystalline lens, contributes to the loss of CS function.

With regard to HOAs and CS function for cataract, we found no significant associations of the AULCSF with ocular 3rd-order or 4th-order aberrations in mild cataract population in the current study. Kuroda et al. mentioned that both light scattering and optical aberration of the lens leads to the loss of CS in mild cataract [30]. Fujikado et al. also found a significant correlation between the AULCSF and HOAs in cataract population [23]. The differences in the sample size, the methodology of the measurements, the distribution of patient age, cataract severity, and other background factors, may explain this discrepancy between the previous and current findings.

We have several limitations to this study. Firstly, it was performed in a retrospective fashion, and there was no control group without cataract. Considering that straylight was subjectively assessed using the compensation comparison method, a randomized, controlled study with a control group may provide further information for confirming our findings. Secondly, we only included mild cataract subjects in whom we could reliably quantify all optical metrics with these devices. Accordingly, the study population might be biased, since severe cases that were not measurable for these metrics, including dense and mature cataracts, were excluded from the present study. Thirdly, we evaluated the CS function only under photopic conditions. Although the CS function under mesopic and scotopic conditions is likely to be somewhat related to that under photopic conditions, a further study under such conditions would be ideal to confirm our findings. Fourthly, our optical findings might be influenced by other functions, such as cognitive function or motor function in these older patients, especially in the case of the C-Quant testing, although we confirmed that all participants had no history of cognitive or motor impairment.

5. Conclusions

In summary, our findings demonstrated that eyes with better BSCVA and eyes with lower log(s) showed higher AULCSF in eyes having mild cataract, although the most variance remained unclear. Based on our results, both visual acuity and intraocular forward scattering play some role in predicting the CS function in mild cataract subjects. Further research in a large cohort of cataract patients with various stages will be necessary to confirm the authenticity of these results.

Author Contributions: Conceptualization, K.K., T.K., and N.S.; data curation, F.F., W.A. and Y.I.; investigation, F.F., T.K., and W.A.; methodology, K.K.; supervision, N.S.; visualization, K.K.; writing—review and editing, K.K. All authors have read and agreed to the published version of the manuscript.

Funding: This research received no external funding.

Institutional Review Board Statement: The study was conducted according to the guidelines of the Declaration of Helsinki, and approved by the Institutional Review Board at Kitasato University Hospital (B16-67).

Informed Consent Statement: Our Institutional Review Board waived the requirement for informed consent for this retrospective review.

Data Availability Statement: The data that support the findings of this study are available from the corresponding author, K.K., upon reasonable request.

Conflicts of Interest: The authors declare no conflict of interest.

Abbreviations

CS: contrast sensitivity; HOAs: higher-order aberrations; AULCSF: area under the log contrast sensitivity function; logMAR: logarithm of the minimal angle of resolution; log(s): logarithmic straylight; UCVA: uncorrected visual acuity; BSCVA: best spectacle-corrected visual acuity.

References

1. Khairallah, M.; Kahloun, R.; Bourne, R.; Limburg, H.; Flaxman, S.R.; Jonas, J.B.; Keeffe, J.; Leasher, J.; Naidoo, K.; Pesudovs, K.; et al. Number of people blind or visually impaired by cataract worldwide and in world regions, 1990 to 2010. *Investig. Ophthalmol. Vis. Sci.* **2015**, *56*, 6762–6769. [CrossRef]
2. Klein, B.E.K.; Klein, R.; Linton, K.L.P. Prevalence of age-related lens opacities in a population: The Beaver Dam Eye Study. *Ophthalmology* **1992**, *99*, 546–552. [CrossRef]
3. Mitchell, P.; Cumming, R.G.; Attebo, K.; Panchapakesan, J. Prevalence of cataract in Australia: The Blue Mountains eye study. *Ophthalmology* **1997**, *104*, 581–588. [CrossRef]
4. Steinberg, E.P.; Tielsch, J.M.; Schein, O.D.; Javitt, J.C.; Sharkey, P.; Cassard, S.D.; Legro, M.W.; Diener-West, M.; Bass, E.B.; Damiano, A.M.; et al. The VF-14. An index of functional impairment in patients with cataract. *Arch. Ophthalmol.* **1994**, *112*, 630–638. [CrossRef] [PubMed]
5. Cahill, M.T.; Banks, A.D.; Stinnett, S.S.; Toth, C.A. Vision-related quality of life in patients with bilateral severe age-related macular degeneration. *Ophthalmology* **2005**, *112*, 152–158. [CrossRef]
6. Artal, P.; Benito, A.; Pérez, G.M.; Alcón, E.; De Casas, A.; Pujol, J.; Marín, J.M. An objective scatter index based on double-pass retinal images of a point source to classify cataracts. *PLoS ONE* **2011**, *6*, e16823. [CrossRef] [PubMed]
7. Vilaseca, M.; Romero, M.J.; Arjona, M.; Luque, S.O.; Ondategui, J.C.; Salvador, A.; Güell, J.L.; Artal, P.; Pujol, J. Grading nuclear, cortical and posterior subcapsular cataracts using an objective scatter index measured with a double-pass system. *Br. J. Ophthalmol.* **2012**, *96*, 1204–1210. [CrossRef] [PubMed]
8. Franssen, L.; Coppens, J.E.; van den Berg, T.J. Compensation comparison method for assessment of retinal straylight. *Invest. Ophthalmol. Vis. Sci.* **2006**, *47*, 768–776. [CrossRef]
9. Coppens, J.E.; Franssen, L.; van den Berg, T.J. Reliability of the compensation comparison method for measuring retinal stray light studied using Monte-Carlo simulations. *J. Biomed. Opt.* **2006**, *11*, 054010. [CrossRef]
10. Van Den Berg, T.J.; Van Rijn, L.J.; Michael, R.; Heine, C.; Coeckelbergh, T.; Nischler, C.; Wilhelm, H.; Grabner, G.; Emesz, M.; Barraquer, R.I.; et al. Straylight effects with aging and lens extraction. *Am. J. Ophthalmol.* **2007**, *144*, 358–363. [CrossRef]
11. van den Berg, T.J.T.P. The (lack of) relation between straylight and visual acuity. Two domains of the point-spread-function. *Ophthalmic Physiol. Opt.* **2017**, *37*, 333–341. [CrossRef]
12. Ortiz-Peregrina, S.; Ortiz, C.; Salas, C.; Casares-López, M.; Soler, M.; Anera, R.G. Intraocular scattering as a predictor of driving performance in older adults with cataracts. *PLoS ONE* **2020**, *15*, e0227892. [CrossRef] [PubMed]
13. Ortiz-Peregrina, S.; Ortiz, C.; Casares-López, M.; Castro-Torres, J.J.; Jiménez Del Barco, L.; Anera, R.G. Impact of age-related vision changes on driving. *Int. J. Environ. Res. Public Health* **2020**, *17*, 7416. [CrossRef] [PubMed]
14. Jindra, L.F.; Zemon, V. Contrast sensitivity testing: A more complete assessment of vision. *J. Cataract Refract. Surg.* **1989**, *15*, 141–148. [CrossRef]
15. Adamsons, I.A.; Vitale, S.; Stark, W.J.; Rubin, G.S. The association of postoperative subjective visual function with acuity, glare, and contrast sensitivity in patients with early cataract. *Arch. Ophthalmol.* **1996**, *114*, 529–536. [CrossRef] [PubMed]
16. Superstein, R.; Boyaner, D.; Overbury, O.; Collin, C. Glare disability and contrast sensitivity before and after cataract surgery. *J. Cataract Refract. Surg.* **1997**, *23*, 248–253. [CrossRef]
17. Superstein, R.; Boyaner, D.; Overbury, O. Functional complaints, visual acuity, spatial contrast sensitivity, and glare disability in preoperative and postoperative cataract patients. *J. Cataract Refract. Surg.* **1999**, *25*, 575–581. [CrossRef]
18. Kamiya, K.; Shimizu, K.; Iijima, A.; Kobashi, H. Factors influencing contrast sensitivity function in myopic eyes. *PLoS ONE* **2014**, *9*, e113562.
19. Applegate, R.A.; Howland, H.C.; Sharp, R.P.; Cottingham, A.J.; Yee, R.W. Corneal aberrations and visual performance after radial keratotomy. *J. Refract. Surg.* **1998**, *14*, 397–407. [CrossRef]
20. Snyder, A.W.; Srinivasan, M.V. Human psychophysics: Functional interpretation for contrast sensitivity versus spatial frequency curve. *Biol. Cybern.* **1979**, *32*, 9–17. [CrossRef] [PubMed]
21. Virsu, V.; Rovamo, J. Visual resolution, contrast sensitivity, and the cortical magnification factor. *Exp. Brain Res.* **1979**, *37*, 475–494. [CrossRef] [PubMed]
22. Adamsons, I.; Rubin, G.S.; Vitale, S.; Taylor, H.R.; Stark, W.J. The effect of early cataracts on glare and contrast sensitivity. A pilot study. *Arch. Ophthalmol.* **1992**, *110*, 1081–1086. [CrossRef] [PubMed]
23. Fujikado, T.; Kuroda, T.; Maeda, N.; Ninomiya, S.; Goto, H.; Tano, Y.; Oshika, T.; Hirohara, Y.; Mihashi, T. Light scattering and optical aberrations as objective parameters to predict visual deterioration in eyes with cataracts. *J. Cataract Refract. Surg.* **2004**, *30*, 1198–1208. [CrossRef]
24. Shandiz, J.H.; Derakhshan, A.; Daneshyar, A.; Azimi, A.; Moghaddam, H.O.; Yekta, A.A.; Yazdi, S.H.; Esmaily, H. Effect of cataract type and severity on visual acuity and contrast sensitivity. *J. Ophthalmic Vis. Res.* **2011**, *6*, 26–31.
25. van der Meulen, I.J.; Gjertsen, J.; Kruijt, B.; Witmer, J.P.; Rulo, A.; Schlingemann, R.O.; van den Berg, T.J. Straylight measurements as an indication for cataract surgery. *J. Cataract Refract. Surg.* **2012**, *38*, 840–848. [CrossRef]
26. Palomo-Álvarez, C.; Puell, M.C. Capacity of straylight and disk halo size to diagnose cataract. *J. Cataract Refract. Surg.* **2015**, *41*, 2069–2074. [CrossRef]
27. Paz Filgueira, C.; Sánchez, R.F.; Issolio, L.A.; Colombo, E.M. Straylight and visual quality on early nuclear and posterior subcapsular cataracts. *Curr. Eye Res.* **2016**, *41*, 1209–1215. [CrossRef]

28. Chylack, L.T., Jr.; Wolfe, J.K.; Singer, D.M.; Leske, M.C.; Bullimore, M.A.; Bailey, I.L.; Friend, J.; McCarthy, D.; Wu, S.Y. The lens opacities classification system III. The longitudinal study of cataract study group. *Arch. Ophthalmol.* **1993**, *111*, 831–836. [CrossRef] [PubMed]
29. Martínez-Roda, J.A.; Vilaseca, M.; Ondategui, J.C.; Almudí, L.; Asaad, M.; Mateos-Pena, L.; Arjona, M.; Pujol, J. Double-pass technique and compensation-comparison method in eyes with cataract. *J. Cataract Refract. Surg.* **2016**, *42*, 1461–1469. [CrossRef]
30. Kuroda, T.; Fujikado, T.; Maeda, N.; Oshika, T.; Hirohara, Y.; Mihashi, T. Wavefront analysis in eyes with nuclear or cortical cataract. *Am. J. Ophthalmol.* **2002**, *134*, 1–9. [CrossRef]

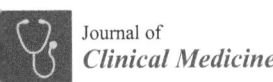

Article

Axial Length and Prevalence of Myopia among Schoolchildren in the Equatorial Region of Brazil

Erisa Yotsukura [1,2,†], Hidemasa Torii [1,2,†], Hiroko Ozawa [1,†], Richard Yudi Hida [1,3,4], Tetsuro Shiraishi [5], Ivan Corso Teixeira [6], Yessa Vervloet Bertollo Lamego Rautha [3], Caio Felipe Moraes do Nascimento [6], Kiwako Mori [1,2], Miki Uchino [1], Toshihide Kurihara [1,2,*], Kazuno Negishi [1,*] and Kazuo Tsubota [1,7,*]

1. Department of Ophthalmology, Keio University School of Medicine, 35 Shinanomachi, Shinjuku-ku, Tokyo 160-8582, Japan; erisa.tsutsui@gmail.com (E.Y.); hidemasatorii@yahoo.co.jp (H.T.); hiroko1011@gmail.com (H.O.); ryhida@gmail.com (R.Y.H.); morikiwako@gmail.com (K.M.); uchinomiki@yahoo.co.jp (M.U.)
2. Laboratory of Photobiology, Keio University School of Medicine, 35 Shinanomachi, Shinjuku-ku, Tokyo 160-8582, Japan
3. Department of Ophthalmology, Universidade de Sao Paulo, Av. Dr. Enéas Carvalho de Aguiar, 255-Cerqueira César, São Paulo SP 05402-000, Brazil; yessa.rautha@yahoo.com.br
4. Department of Ophthalmology, Universidade Federal de Sao Paulo, R. Botucatu, 822-Vila Clementino, São Paulo SP 04039-032, Brazil
5. Department of Obstetrics and Gynecology, Keio University School of Medicine, 35 Shinanomachi, Shinjuku-ku, Tokyo 160-8582, Japan; shiraishi15.5@gmail.com
6. Department of Ophthalmology, Santa Casa de Sao Paulo, Rua Dr. Cesario Mota Junior, 112-Vila Buarque, São Paulo SP 01221-010, Brazil; ivancorso@gmail.com (I.C.T.); caiofmn@gmail.com (C.F.M.d.N.)
7. Tsubota Laboratory, Inc., 304 Toshin Shinanomachi-Ekimae Bldg., 34 Shinanomachi Shinjuku-ku, Tokyo 160-0016, Japan
* Correspondence: kurihara@z8.keio.jp (T.K.); kazunonegishi@keio.jp (K.N.); tsubota@z3.keio.jp (K.T.); Tel.: +81-3-5363-3204 (T.K.); +81-3-3353-1211 (K.N.); +81-3-3353-1211 (K.T.)
† These authors contributed equally to the work and request triple first authorship.

Abstract: The prevalence of myopia is increasing globally, and the outdoor light environment is considered as a possible factor that can retard myopia. The aim of this study was to evaluate the prevalence of myopia and the light environment in Aracati, equatorial Brazil. We surveyed 421 children (421 right eyes; mean age, 10.6 years) and performed ocular examinations that included non-cycloplegic refraction and axial length (AL). Multiple regression analyses were performed to identify factors affecting myopia such as time spent outdoors and in near work. We measured illuminance and violet light irradiance in Aracati. The mean spherical equivalent (SE) and AL were −0.44 ± 1.38 diopters (D) and 22.98 ± 0.87 mm, respectively. The prevalence of myopia (SE ≤ −0.75 D) and high myopia (SE ≤ −6.0 D/AL ≥ 26.0 mm) was 20.4 and 1.4/0.48%, respectively. Multiple regression analyses showed that myopia was not associated with lifestyle factors. The average illuminance in Aracati was about 100,000 lux from morning to evening. The current results reflect the ALs and the prevalence of myopia among Brazilian schoolchildren. There is a possibility that the light environment in addition to other confounding factors including racial differences affects the ALs and refractive errors.

Keywords: myopia; refractive error; axial length; school children; light environment; violet light; illuminance

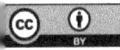

1. Introduction

Myopia, a common refractive error, mainly results from continuous increases in axial length (AL) [1]. The etiology of myopia is thought to be an interaction of genetic and environmental factors. However, the precise mechanism remains unclear. The prevalence of myopia has recently increased worldwide, especially in east Asia [2]. Currently, China has a high prevalence of myopia, while the prevalence rates have ranged from 20 to 80% for the previous 60 years; in other parts of the world such as the United States and Europe, the prevalence rates have doubled during the past 50 years [3]. We also recently reported that the prevalence of myopia among elementary school and junior high school children in Tokyo was 76.5 and 94.9%, respectively [4]. These rapid worldwide increases in myopia during a relatively short period must have resulted from changes in environmental factors and not genetic factors.

Outdoor activity is a factor that can suppress myopia onset [5–9] and progression [9] as reported by several studies including a meta-analysis. Spending more than 2 h daily outdoors is preferable [6,7,9]. The mechanism of the effects of outdoor activity remains unknown, but a possible reason is that outdoor activity can suppress myopia not only because of light illuminance [10,11] but also because of the short wavelength light, including violet light (360–400 nm wavelength) [12–14], that is abundant outdoors [12]. We reported that violet light might suppress myopia progression not only in chicks but also in children with mild myopia and adults with high myopia [12,13]. Based on those results, we hypothesized that the prevalence of myopia is lower in equatorial areas of Brazil, which have higher amounts of sunlight than other areas.

Numerous environmental factors have been associated with myopia progression in schoolchildren [15–19]; however, few studies have evaluated AL in schoolchildren using these factors, and those studies were mostly conducted in Asia [4,20]. To date, no reports have been published about AL and its associated factors in equatorial regions where the sunlight is intense, although a couple of studies have reported refractive data without AL among Brazilian schoolchildren [21–23]. Thus, using a questionnaire, we also evaluated the association between AL and environmental factors. We clarified the prevalence of myopia among schoolchildren in the equatorial region of Brazil by measuring refractive errors and ALs, and we investigated the light environment including the light illuminance and the violet light irradiance in Brazil.

2. Materials and Methods

2.1. Study Design and Participants

This cross-sectional study included 421 right eyes of 421 Brazilian schoolchildren (age range, 5–19 years; average age, 10.6 ± 2.9 (standard deviation) years; participation rate, 74.3%) who underwent a medical check-up that included the measurement of height and weight in the Professor Antonio Monteiro School in Pedregal, Aracati City, Ceará, Brazil, in August 2017. Aracati City is in the equatorial area of Brazil. We explained the study to the parents of the students. The students provided informed assent, and the parents provided written informed consent. All students who agreed to participate in this study underwent a medical examination. The inclusion criteria were children who could undergo an eye examination and had no previous ocular disease. The exclusion criteria were the presence of active ocular inflammation or systemic disease. In the questionnaire, we asked about a past history of systemic disease, and we evaluated active ocular inflammation during an ophthalmic medical examination. The Keio University School of Medicine Ethics Committee, and the Institutional Review Board and Ethics Committee of Penha Eye Institute approved this study. All the procedures involving human subjects were conducted in accordance with the tenets of the Declaration of Helsinki.

2.2. Measures

All participants underwent eye examinations that included measurement of refractive errors and AL. We also recorded the height, weight, and body mass index (BMI) of the participants.

The refractive errors were measured in a non-cycloplegic state using an autorefractometer (VISUREF100, Carl Zeiss Meditec AG, Jena, Germany). We used the automatic fogging system to reduce the effects of accommodation when we measured the refraction. The ALs were measured by partial coherence interferometry biometry (IOLMaster® 500, Carl Zeiss Meditec AG, Jena, Germany). Four trained ophthalmologists performed all the examinations, and the data were recorded. The device measured the AL five times and averaged the data. The spherical equivalent (SE) was defined as the spherical power plus half of the negative cylinder power. Myopia was defined as an SE of -0.75 diopters (D) or worse, and high myopia, as an SE ≤ -6.0 D or an AL ≥ 26.0 mm. Because the SE (Pearson correlation coefficient = 0.689, $p < 0.001$) and the AL (Pearson correlation coefficient = 0.959, $p < 0.001$) for the right and left eyes were similar for this study, only the results for the right eye are presented. All participants with any ocular disease were immediately treated and sent for further follow-up in Fortaleza City, Ceará, Brazil.

Illuminance was measured using the LX-1108 (MOTHERTOOL CO., Ltd., Ueda, Japan), and violet light irradiance was measured using VL-M-A1 (NEW OPTO, Ltd., Kawasaki, Japan). These data were collected outside in Aracati, Brazil (at 37° west longitude, 4° south latitude). All data were collected on sunny days at approximately 7:00, 10:00, 13:00, and 16:00 local time on 19 August 2017.

2.3. Questionnaire

A questionnaire in Portuguese was administered before the visit. If the participants were too young to complete the questionnaire by themselves, Brazilian staff members interviewed them and completed the questionnaire with the help of their parents. Information on sociodemographic factors were collected, including age, sex, and family economic status. Using a questionnaire, we asked their parents about the average time of activity during one recent month. The children's near work was assessed by asking (1) how many hours the child spent daily reading or studying for school assignments and for pleasure, using a computer, watching television, and playing with electronics, and (2) the distance when the child was reading. The children's outdoor activity was measured by asking how long they spent in the sun daily while outdoors. The family economic status was assessed by asking for the entire family monthly income: less than BRL 1000, BRL 1000 to 3000, BRL 3000 to 5000, more than BRL 5000, or unknown. BRL 1 was equivalent to USD 0.18 on 19 August 2020. Parental myopia was assessed by asking the following question: "Is the child's parent myopic?". The response categories were "one parent", "both parents", "neither", and "unknown". Since some responded that the time spent sleeping was only 120 min/day during one recent month, we considered that the answers indicating that the children spent less than 300 min a day as unrealistic ($n = 8$) and treated them as if they were not a response.

2.4. Statistical Analysis

To evaluate the factors affecting the SE and AL, we performed multiple regression analyses (stepwise variable selection for regression). The Pearson correlation coefficient was used to assess simple correlations between the SE, AL, and several variables, such as age, sex (males = 0, females = 1), BMI, time spent outdoors, time spent in near work, family economic status, and parental myopia. Multiple regression analyses were performed, in which significant variables ($p < 0.20$) with simple correlations were compared. We confirmed that there was no multicollinearity. All p values were 2-sided. $p < 0.05$ was considered to be statistically significant. All statistical analyses were performed using the SPSS version 24.0 software (IBM, Chicago, IL, USA).

3. Results

3.1. Study Population

Table 1 shows the characteristics of the current study population and results of the questionnaire. The mean SE was -0.44 ± 1.38 D, and the mean AL was 22.98 ± 0.87 mm for all the participants. The average time spent outdoors was 155.9 ± 104.3 min/day, and the average time spent doing near work was 516.4 ± 248.3 min/day. Figure 1 shows the distribution of the subjects by age. The distributions of the SE and AL are shown in Figures 2 and 3, respectively.

Table 1. Characteristics of the current study population and results of the questionnaire.

	Number of Cases	Mean ± Standard Deviation (Range)
Age (years)		10.6 ± 2.9 (5.0–19.0)
Number of students	421	
Males	212	
Females	209	
Height (cm)	417	144.5 ± 15.6 (110.0–179.0)
Weight (kg)	416	40.4 ± 13.9 (16.7–91.2)
BMI (kg/m^2)	416	18.8 ± 3.6 (12.1–31.9)
SE (D)	421	−0.44 ± 1.38 (−12.63–7.25)
AL (mm)	416	22.98 ± 0.87 (20.16–26.90)
Time spent outdoors (min/day)	123	155.9 ± 104.3 (9.3–540.0)
Time spent in near work (min/day)	121	516.4 ± 248.3 (60.0–1096.5)
Time spent sleeping (min/day)	113	507.8 ± 100.7 (300.0–875.0)
Family economic status		
Less than BRL 1000	42	
BRL 1000 to 3000	19	
BRL 3000 to 5000	5	
More than BRL 5000	5	
Unknown	171	
Number of parents with myopia		
0	158	
1	38	
2	6	
Unknown	219	

Abbreviations: SE, spherical equivalent; AL, axial length; BMI, body mass index; D, diopter. BRL 1 was equivalent to USD 0.18 on 19 August 2020.

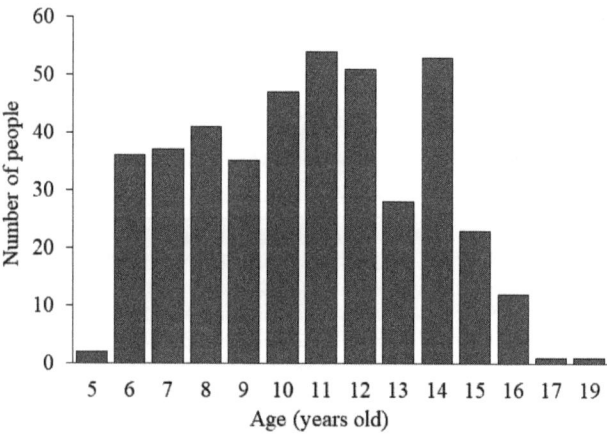

Figure 1. The distribution of subjects at each age: The ages of the participants in this study were mainly distributed from 6 to 16 years. The average age was 10.6 years.

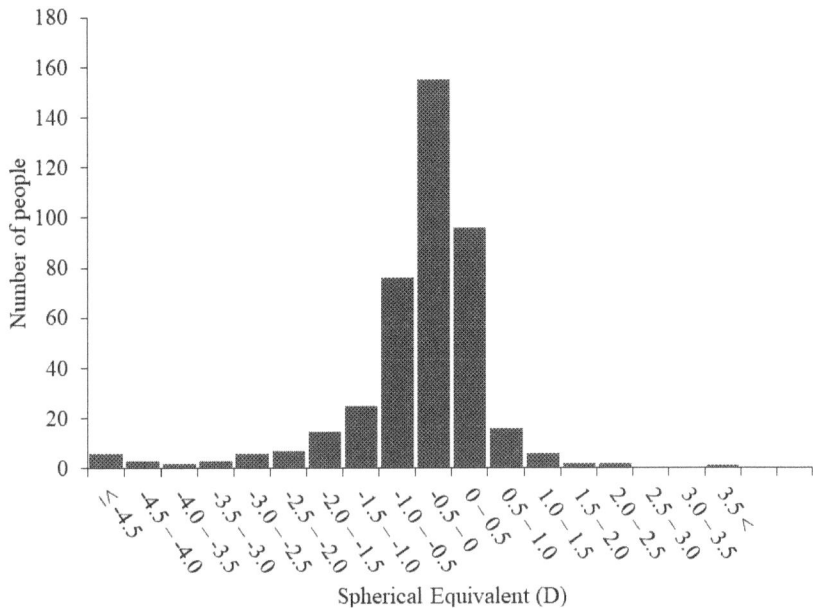

Figure 2. The distribution of SE. The participants in this study were primarily emmetropic (average, −0.44 diopters). Abbreviations: SE, spherical equivalent; D, diopters.

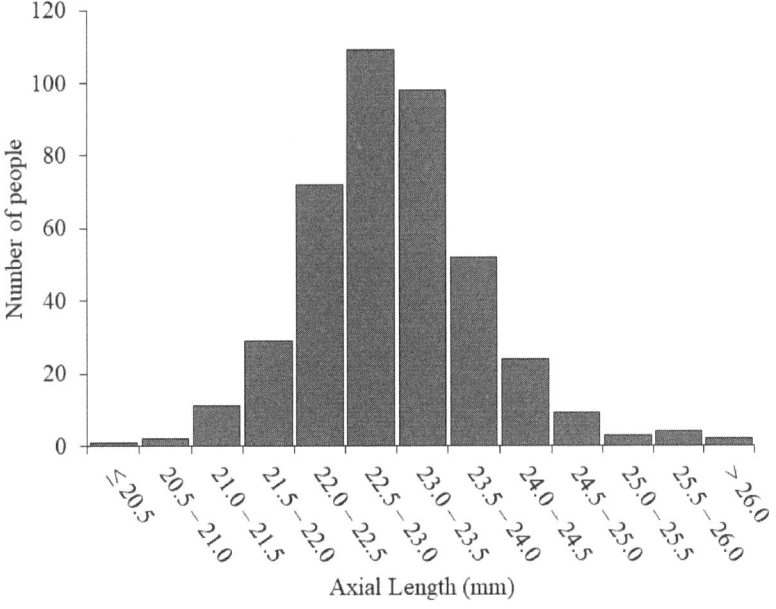

Figure 3. The distribution of the axial lengths (ALs). The ALs of the participants in this study were primarily in the 21.0 to 24.5 mm range (average, 22.98 mm).

The prevalence of myopia (SE ≤ -0.75 D) was 20.4%, and the prevalence of high myopia (SE ≤ -6.0 D) was 1.4% among all the students. Based on the AL, the prevalence of high myopia (AL ≥ 26.0 mm) was 0.48% among all the students.

3.2. Illuminance and Violet Light Irradiance

The illuminance and violet light (360–400 nm) irradiance values in Aracati and Tokyo are shown in Figure S1 (The illuminance and violet light irradiance in Tokyo and Aracati). The illuminance (lux) at 7:00, 10:00, 13:00, and 16:00 local time in Aracati/Tokyo was 92,000/76,000, 103,000/93,300, 107,500/106,000, and 80,000/54,000, respectively (Figure S1A). The violet light irradiance ($\mu W/cm^2$) at 7:00, 10:00, 13:00, and 16:00 local time in Aracati/Tokyo was 1650/1120, 2300/2000, 2320/1950, and 1030/468, respectively (Figure S1B).

3.3. Factors Affecting SE and AL According to Simple Correlation and Multiple Regression Analyses

Table 2 shows the results of simple correlation and multiple regression analyses between the SE and the variables. The results indicate that myopia is associated with older age (coefficient = -0.170; $p < 0.001$). Based on the results of the multiple regression analyses between the AL and the variables, the AL was associated with older age ($p < 0.001$), male sex ($p < 0.001$), and higher BMI ($p = 0.01$) (Table 3). Lifestyle factors were included ($n = 114$), and less sleep time was associated with a longer AL according to simple correlation (coefficient = -0.184; $p = 0.025$). The results of multiple regression analysis show that the AL was significantly associated with older age and male sex (coefficient = 0.119 and -0.405, respectively; $p = 0.001$ and 0.002, respectively).

Table 2. Results of simple correlation and multiple regression analysis between SE and variables ($n = 416$).

Variable	Univariate Analysis		Multivariate Analysis		
	Correlation Coefficient	p Value	Coefficient	Standard Error	p Value
Age (years)	−0.170	<0.001 *	−0.082	0.023	<0.001 *
Sex (males = 0, females = 1)	−0.041	0.201	N/A	N/A	≥0.05
BMI	−0.075	0.062	N/A	N/A	≥0.05

* Significant correlation according to the Pearson correlation test; Abbreviations: SE, spherical equivalent; BMI body mass index; N/A, not applicable.

Table 3. Results of simple correlation and multiple regression analysis between AL and variables ($n = 414$).

Variable	Univariate Analysis		Multivariate Analysis		
	Correlation Coefficient	p Value	Coefficient	Standard Error	p Value
Age (years)	0.326	<0.001 *	0.079	0.015	<0.001 *
Sex (males = 0, females = 1)	−0.267	<0.001 *	−0.438	0.078	<0.001 *
BMI	0.248	<0.001 *	0.031	0.012	0.01 *

* Significant correlation according to the Pearson correlation test; Abbreviations: AL, axial length; BMI, body mass index.

4. Discussion

The current results show that the mean refractive error among the Brazilian schoolchildren was -0.44 ± 1.38 D, the myopia prevalence in Aracati was 20.4%, and the prevalence of high myopia was 1.4%. In the current study, the mean AL was 22.98 ± 0.87 mm, and based on the AL, the prevalence of high myopia (AL ≥ 26.0 mm) was 0.48%. These results show a possibility that children in an equatorial area of Brazil might have shorter ALs than those in other studies [4,24–26] (Figure 4). A search of PubMed was undertaken for articles including the search terms "axial length", "children", and "myopia", and we chose the references in which the age was same as in our study (7 and 12 years old) and the studies that included more than 300 participants. In the current study, the mean ALs of the schoolchildren aged 7 and 12 years were 22.63 and 23.29 mm, respectively, which were the shortest among these studies [4,24–26] (Figure 4A,B). Possible reasons why the mean ALs of the schoolchildren aged 7 and 12 years in the current study were the shortest among these studies [4,24–26] are race and extended time of outdoor activity. Unfortunately, we could not obtain accurate information about the participants' races. The mechanism of outdoor activity's effect remains unknown, but a possible reason is the strong light environment including light illuminance [10,11] and the short wavelength of the light [12–14] that is abundant outdoors. We measured them only during 1 day, but there were no such published data, and we used them as Supplementary Data.

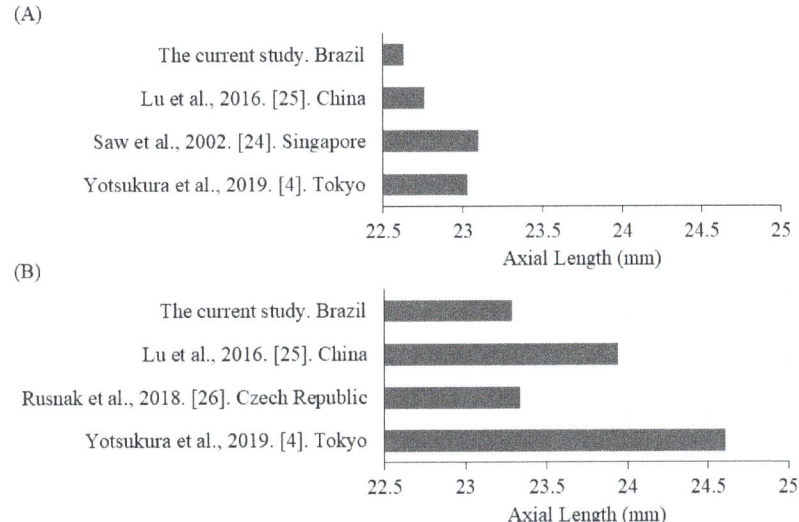

Figure 4. Comparison of the axial lengths (ALs) of (**A**) 7 and (**B**) 12 year-old schoolchildren in the current study with those from previous studies. Compared with some previous studies, the ALs of both the 7 and 12 year-old schoolchildren in the current study were the shortest.

We also compared our data with a previous study from Brazil to eliminate the racial differences. According to a previous study [27], which reported the ALs among Brazilian schoolchildren in Campinas (at 46° west longitude, 23° south latitude), the mean ALs were 22.5, 23.0, and 23.2 mm among the children aged 6, 10, and 14 years, respectively. In the current study, the mean ALs were 22.5, 23.0, and 23.0 mm (almost plateaued) among the children aged 6, 10, and 14 years, respectively. The mean ALs were the same for those aged 6 and 10 years, though we focused on the ALs of those aged 14 years. In Campinas, the mean AL for those aged 14 years was 23.2 mm; on the other hand, it was 23.0 mm in Aracati. The results indicate that the AL might plateau in Aracati at around 10 years because the mean ALs were same for those aged 10 and 14 years. These results show that the mean ALs of the adolescent children in Aracati plateaued and were shorter than those in Campinas. These results indicate that the ALs of children near the equatorial region where the sun light is intense in the same country might be short without factors such as the time spent outdoors and genetic backgrounds.

Several studies have suggested that increased time spent in near work is a possible risk factor for myopia [18,28–32]. Indeed, the time spent doing near work has been increasing recently among students [33,34]. When we evaluated the time spent doing near work in Aracati, the mean time was 516.4 min/day. By contrast, the time spent doing near work in Tokyo was 274.0 min/day [4]. However, in our previous study, which reported the prevalence of myopia among schoolchildren in Tokyo, we asked parents about the average time of activity excluding school time; therefore, it is possible that the time spent doing near work is almost the same in Aracati and Tokyo.

Outdoor activity is a well-known factor that suppresses myopia onset [7,35–40], and some clinical studies [41–43] have reported that outdoor activity may suppress myopia progression. In the current study, the mean time spent outdoors among Brazilian children was 155.9 min/day. However, the mean time spent outdoors among Japanese elementary school children was 78.3 min/day [4], which was about half of that in Aracati. Some studies have reported that spending more than 2 h daily outdoors can suppress myopia [6,7]. According to the results of the current study, the low prevalence of myopia in Aracati may be associated with the extended amount of time engaged in outdoor activities despite the long periods spent doing near work. However, the time spent engaged in outdoor activities was not significantly associated with myopia in the current study. We consider this because the mean time spent outdoors among children in Aracati was over 2 h daily (155.9 min daily). The effect of decreasing the risk of incident myopia almost plateaued under that condition, i.e., over 2 h daily of outdoor activity, according to a systematic review of the effects of outdoor activity against myopia [8]. For that reason, the time spent outdoors was not significantly associated with myopia in the current study.

The outdoor light environment, including the illuminance and wavelength, is now attracting attention in attempts to retard myopia [14]. High illuminance levels have been effective against myopia in some animal experiments [11,44,45]. Furthermore, we recently found that 360 to 400 nm violet light, which is abundant in sunlight, suppressed myopia progression in both chicks and humans [12], i.e., not only in children with mild myopia but also in adults with high myopia [13]. Therefore, we measured the illuminance and violet light irradiance in the current study. Although we did not compare the illuminance and irradiance of violet light globally and annually, a website titled "World Weather Online" [46] shows the ultraviolet index (UVI), which was developed by the World Health Organization and is a measure of UV radiation levels. The calculated annual average UVI in 2017 was 6.75 in Aracati, 6.92 in Singapore, and 4.25 in Tokyo [46]. Although the UVIs in Singapore and Aracati were almost the same, the prevalence of myopia in Singapore was very high [47–49] because of differences in the time spent outdoors and genetic backgrounds between Singapore and Aracati. A previous study [50] showed that the average time spent outdoors among Singaporean children was only 61 min/day, although the time spent outdoors in Aracati was 155.9 min/day in the current study. Even though genetic backgrounds affected the rate of myopia prevalence, the time spent outdoors in Aracati, which was almost 2.5 times more than that in Singapore, may also affect ALs and refractive errors. Therefore, environmental factors including both the time spent outdoors and light environment are crucial factors for the prevalence of myopia.

The current multiple regression analysis results indicated that AL was significantly associated with older age and male sex. In the current study, there was no significant relationship between myopia and lifestyle factors. Regarding the time spent sleeping, the average time among the Brazilian children was 507.8 min daily in the current study, and the time among Japanese school children was 525.2 min daily, which we reported previously [4]. Thus, the time spent sleeping among Brazilian students was less than that of Japanese students by about 20 min daily. A previous study reported that high myopia was significantly correlated with short sleep duration in Japan [51], although the time spent sleeping among Brazilian children was shorter; nevertheless, their ALs were shorter than those of the Japanese school children. These investigations imply that lifestyle factors are not associated with myopia in the equatorial area of Brazil because of the light environment including the illuminance, annual daylight hours, and violet light irradiance. Thus, the current study indicates that the intensity of the sunlight may play an important role in the low prevalence of myopia and short AL among the Brazilian schoolchildren in equatorial regions.

The current study had some limitations. First, we did not use cycloplegia. The non-cycloplegic refraction was a big limitation of this study, especially for children because the non-cycloplegic refraction masked the real refraction as a result of their accommodative ability. Considering that, the prevalence of myopia may have been overestimated. We also might have overestimated the AL because a previous study reported that the AL was 0.009 mm shorter after cycloplegia in children whose mean age was 9.20 years [52]. Since the difference was small, the ALs in Brazilian schoolchildren tended to be short, and measuring the AL was the strength of the current study. Second, there may have been some recall bias and misunderstanding of the questionnaire. Third, we could not obtain accurate information about the participants' races because the percentage of mixed-race individuals was about 43%, according to The Brazilian Institute of Geography and Statistics. It may be better to choose another place in Brazil where the sunlight is less intense because the races in Brazil and Japan differ. Fourth, over half of the students did not completely answer the questionnaire about their lifestyle, and we could perform multiple regression analysis about lifestyle for only 114 participants. We considered that the lack of association between lifestyle factors and myopia could be because of a lack of power. Finally, we measured only the violet light irradiance because we focused on violet light in the current study. We should have measured not only violet light but also other spectral components of light.

5. Conclusions

In summary, the current results reflect the ALs and the prevalence of myopia among Brazilian schoolchildren. There is a possibility that the light environment in addition to other confounding factors including racial differences affects their ALs and refractive errors, and further studies are needed in the future.

6. Patents

Outside the submitted work, but related to myopia prevention, H.T., T.K., and K.T. have been applying internationally for two patents, WO 2015/186723 and WO 2017/094886. The former has been registered in Japan, the U.S., and China, and the latter, in Japan, the U.K., France, Germany, Italy, Hong Kong, and Singapore.

Supplementary Materials: The following are available online at https://www.mdpi.com/2077-0383/10/1/115/s1, Figure S1: The illuminance and violet light irradiance in Tokyo and Aracati.

Author Contributions: Conceptualization, E.Y., H.T., H.O., R.Y.H., T.S., I.C.T., Y.V.B.L.R., C.F.M.d.N., T.K., K.T. and K.N.; methodology, E.Y., H.T., H.O., R.Y.H., T.S., I.C.T., Y.V.B.L.R., C.F.M.d.N., K.M. and M.U.; formal analysis, E.Y., H.O. and T.S.; investigation, R.Y.H., T.S., I.C.T., Y.V.B.L.R. and C.F.M.d.N.; data curation, E.Y., H.T., H.O. and T.S.; project administration, H.T., R.Y.H., T.K., K.T. and K.N.; writing—original draft preparation, E.Y. and H.O.; writing—review and editing, E.Y., H.T., H.O., R.Y.H., T.S., I.C.T., Y.V.B.L.R., C.F.M.d.N., K.M., M.U., T.K., K.T. and K.N.; supervision, T.K., K.T. and K.N. All authors have read and agreed to the published version of the manuscript.

Funding: This research was funded by grant 18K16934 from the Japan Society for the Promotion of Science.

Institutional Review Board Statement: The study was conducted according to the guidelines of the Declaration of Helsinki, and approved by the Keio University School of Medicine Ethics Committee, and the Institutional Review Board and Ethics Committee of Penha Eye Institute. (Approval number 20160092, IOP-100451-06, respectively and date of approval were 11 July 2016 and 25 April 2017, respectively).

Informed Consent Statement: Informed consent was obtained from all subjects involved in the study.

Data Availability Statement: The data presented in this study are available on request from the corresponding author. The data is stored, and it will be discarded as the approved document by Ethics Committee.

Acknowledgments: We thank Raimundo Erandir Lucas, the director of the Professor Antonio Monteiro School, for cooperation; Milton Massato Hida, Leo Satoshi Hida, and Mayumi Suzuki for coordination in Brazil; and Lynda Charters for editing the English of the manuscript.

Conflicts of Interest: Outside the submitted work, K.T. reports that he is the CEO of Tsubota Laboratory, Inc., Tokyo, Japan, a company developing products for the treatment of myopia. The other authors declare no conflict of interest.

References

1. Morgan, I.G.; Ohno-Matsui, K.; Saw, S.-M. Myopia. *Lancet* **2012**, *379*, 1739–1748. [CrossRef]
2. Foster, P.J.; Jiang, Y. Epidemiology of myopia. *Eye* **2014**, *28*, 202–208. [CrossRef] [PubMed]
3. Dolgin, E. The myopia boom. *Nature* **2015**, *519*, 276–278. [CrossRef] [PubMed]
4. Yotsukura, E.; Torii, H.; Inokuchi, M.; Tokumura, M.; Uchino, M.; Nakamura, K.; Hyodo, M.; Mori, K.; Jiang, X.; Ikeda, S.-I.; et al. Current Prevalence of Myopia and Association of Myopia With Environmental Factors Among Schoolchildren in Japan. *JAMA Ophthalmol.* **2019**, *137*, 1233–1239. [CrossRef] [PubMed]
5. Sherwin, J.C.; Reacher, M.H.; Keogh, R.H.; Khawaja, A.P.; Mackey, D.A.; Foster, P.J. The association between time spent outdoors and myopia in children and adolescents: A systematic review and meta-analysis. *Ophthalmology* **2012**, *119*, 2141–2151. [CrossRef] [PubMed]
6. Jones, L.A.; Sinnott, L.T.; Mutti, D.O.; Mitchell, G.L.; Moeschberger, M.L.; Zadnik, K. Parental history of myopia, sports and outdoor activities, and future myopia. *Investig. Ophthalmol. Vis. Sci.* **2007**, *48*, 3524–3532. [CrossRef]
7. Rose, K.A.; Morgan, I.G.; Ip, J.; Kifley, A.; Huynh, S.; Smith, W.; Mitchell, P. Outdoor activity reduces the prevalence of myopia in children. *Ophthalmology* **2008**, *115*, 1279–1285. [CrossRef]
8. Xiong, S.; Sankaridurg, P.; Naduvilath, T.; Zang, J.; Zou, H.; Zhu, J.; Lv, M.; He, X.; Xu, X. Time spent in outdoor activities in relation to myopia prevention and control: A meta-analysis and systematic review. *Acta Ophthalmol.* **2017**, *95*, 551–566. [CrossRef]
9. Ho, C.-L.; Wu, W.-F.; Liou, Y.M. Dose-Response Relationship of Outdoor Exposure and Myopia Indicators: A Systematic Review and Meta-Analysis of Various Research Methods. *Int. J. Environ. Res. Public Health* **2019**, *16*, 2595. [CrossRef]
10. Ashby, R.S.; Ohlendorf, A.; Schaeffel, F. The effect of ambient illuminance on the development of deprivation myopia in chicks. *Investig. Ophthalmol. Vis. Sci.* **2009**, *50*, 5348–5354. [CrossRef]
11. Karouta, C.; Ashby, R.S. Correlation Between Light Levels and the Development of Deprivation Myopia. *Investig. Ophthalmol. Vis. Sci.* **2015**, *56*, 299–309. [CrossRef]
12. Torii, H.; Kurihara, T.; Seko, Y.; Negishi, K.; Ohnuma, K.; Inaba, T.; Kawashima, M.; Jiang, X.; Kondo, S.; Miyauchi, M.; et al. Violet Light Exposure Can Be a Preventive Strategy Against Myopia Progression. *EBioMedicine* **2017**, *15*, 210–219. [CrossRef]
13. Torii, H.; Ohnuma, K.; Kurihara, T.; Tsubota, K.; Negishi, K. Violet Light Transmission is Related to Myopia Progression in Adult High Myopia. *Sci. Rep.* **2017**, *7*, 14523. [CrossRef] [PubMed]
14. Troilo, D.; Smith, E.L., 3rd; Nickla, D.L.; Ashby, R.; Tkatchenko, A.V.; Ostrin, L.A.; Gawne, T.J.; Pardue, M.T.; Summers, J.A.; Kee, C.S.; et al. IMI—Report on Experimental Models of Emmetropization and Myopia. *Investig. Ophthalmol. Vis. Sci.* **2019**, *60*, M31–M88. [CrossRef]
15. Saw, S.-M.; Zhang, M.-Z.; Hong, R.-Z.; Fu, Z.-F.; Pang, M.-H.; Tan, D.T.H. Near-work activity, night-lights, and myopia in the Singapore-China study. *Arch. Ophthalmol.* **2002**, *120*, 620–627. [CrossRef] [PubMed]
16. Lin, Z.; Vasudevan, B.; Jhanji, V.; Mao, G.Y.; Gao, T.Y.; Wang, F.H.; Rong, S.S.; Ciuffreda, K.; Liang, Y.B. Near work, outdoor activity, and their association with refractive error. *Optom. Vis. Sci.* **2014**, *91*, 376–382. [CrossRef]
17. Mutti, D.O.; Mitchell, G.L.; Moeschberger, M.L.; Jones, L.A.; Zadnik, K. Parental myopia, near work, school achievement, and children's refractive error. *Investig. Ophthalmol. Vis. Sci.* **2002**, *43*, 3633–3640.
18. Ip, J.M.; Saw, S.-M.; Rose, K.A.; Morgan, I.G.; Kifley, A.; Liew, G.; Mitchell, P. Role of near work in myopia: Findings in a sample of Australian school children. *Investig. Ophthalmol. Vis. Sci.* **2008**, *49*, 2903–2910. [CrossRef]
19. Pan, C.-W.; Ramamurthy, D.; Saw, S.-M. Worldwide prevalence and risk factors for myopia. *Ophthalmic. Physiol. Opt.* **2012**, *32*, 3–16. [CrossRef]
20. Yang, M.-L.; Huang, C.-Y.; Hou, C.-H.; Lin, K.-K.; Lee, J.-S. Relationship of lifestyle and body stature growth with the development of myopia and axial length elongation in Taiwanese elementary school children. *Indian J. Ophthalmol.* **2014**, *62*, 865–869. [CrossRef] [PubMed]
21. Schaal, L.F.; Schellini, S.A.; Pesci, L.T.; Galindo, A.; Padovani, C.R.; Corrente, J.E. The Prevalence of Strabismus and Associated Risk Factors in a Southeastern Region of Brazil. *Semin. Ophthalmol.* **2018**, *33*, 357–360. [CrossRef] [PubMed]
22. Lira, R.P.C.; Santo, I.F.D.E.; Astur, G.L.D.V.; Maziero, D.; Passos, T.H.M.; Arieta, C.E.L. Refractive error in school children in Campinas, Brazil. *Arq. Bras. Oftalmol.* **2014**, *77*, 203–204. [CrossRef]
23. Ferraz, F.H.; Corrente, J.E.; Opromolla, P.A.; Padovani, C.R.; Schellini, S.A. Refractive errors in a Brazilian population: Age and sex distribution. *Ophthalmic. Physiol. Opt.* **2015**, *35*, 19–27. [CrossRef]
24. Saw, S.-M.; Chua, W.-H.; Hong, C.-Y.; Wu, H.-M.; Chia, K.-S.; A Stone, R.; Tan, D. Height and its relationship to refraction and biometry parameters in Singapore Chinese children. *Investig. Ophthalmol. Vis. Sci.* **2002**, *43*, 1408–1413.
25. Lu, T.L.; Wu, J.F.; Ye, X.; Hu, Y.Y.; Wu, H.; Sun, W.; Guo, D.D.; Wang, X.R.; Bi, H.; Jonas, J.B. Axial Length and Associated Factors in Children: The Shandong Children Eye Study. *Ophthalmologica* **2016**, *235*, 78–86. [CrossRef] [PubMed]
26. Rusnak, S.; Salcman, V.; Hecova, L.; Kasl, Z. Myopia Progression Risk: Seasonal and Lifestyle Variations in Axial Length Growth in Czech Children. *J. Ophthalmol.* **2018**, *2018*, 5076454. [CrossRef] [PubMed]

7. Lira, R.P.C.; Arieta, C.E.L.; Passos, T.H.M.; Maziero, D.; Astur, G.L.D.V.; Santo Ítalo, F.D.E.; Bertolani, A.C.; Pozzi, L.F.; De Castro, R.S.; Ferraz, Á.B. Distribution of Ocular Component Measures and Refraction in Brazilian School Children. *Ophthalmic. Epidemiol.* **2017**, *24*, 29–35. [CrossRef] [PubMed]
8. French, A.N.; Morgan, I.G.; Mitchell, P.; Rose, K.A. Risk factors for incident myopia in Australian schoolchildren: The Sydney adolescent vascular and eye study. *Ophthalmology* **2013**, *120*, 2100–2108. [CrossRef]
9. Li, S.-M.; Li, S.-Y.; Kang, M.-T.; Zhou, Y.; Liu, L.-R.; Li, H.; Wang, Y.-P.; Zhan, S.-Y.; Gopinath, B.; Mitchell, P.; et al. Anyang Childhood Eye Study, Near Work Related Parameters and Myopia in Chinese Children: The Anyang Childhood Eye Study. *PLoS ONE* **2015**, *10*, e0134514. [CrossRef]
10. You, Q.S.; Wu, L.J.; Duan, J.L.; Luo, Y.X.; Liu, L.J.; Li, X.; Gao, Q.; Wang, W.; Xu, L.; Jonas, J.B.; et al. Factors Associated with Myopia in School Children in China: The Beijing Childhood Eye Study. *PLoS ONE* **2012**, *7*, e52668. [CrossRef]
11. Gong, Y.; Zhang, X.; Tian, D.; Wang, D.; Xiao, G. Parental myopia, near work, hours of sleep and myopia in Chinese children. *Health* **2014**, *6*, 64–70. [CrossRef]
12. Huang, H.-M.; Chang, D.S.-T.; Wu, P.-C. The Association between Near Work Activities and Myopia in Children-A Systematic Review and Meta-Analysis. *PLoS ONE* **2015**, *10*, e0140419. [CrossRef] [PubMed]
13. Bucksch, J.; Sigmundova, D.; Hamrik, Z.; Troped, P.J.; Melkevik, O.; Ahluwalia, N.; Borraccino, A.; Tynjälä, J.; Kalman, M.; Inchley, J.C. International Trends in Adolescent Screen-Time Behaviors From 2002 to 2010. *J. Adolesc. Health* **2016**, *58*, 417–425. [CrossRef] [PubMed]
14. Bassett, D.R.; John, D.; Conger, S.A.; Fitzhugh, E.C.; Coe, D.P. Trends in Physical Activity and Sedentary Behaviors of United States Youth. *J. Phys. Act. Health* **2015**, *12*, 1102–1111. [CrossRef] [PubMed]
15. Read, S.A.; Collins, M.J.; Vincent, S.J. Light exposure and physical activity in myopic and emmetropic children. *Optom. Vis. Sci.* **2014**, *91*, 330–341. [CrossRef]
16. Guo, Y.; Liu, L.J.; Xu, L.; Lv, Y.Y.; Tang, P.; Feng, Y.; Meng, M.; Jonas, J.B. Outdoor activity and myopia among primary students in rural and urban regions of Beijing. *Ophthalmology* **2013**, *120*, 277–283. [CrossRef]
17. French, A.N.; Ashby, R.S.; Morgan, I.G.; Rose, K.A. Time outdoors and the prevention of myopia. *Exp. Eye Res.* **2013**, *114*, 58–68. [CrossRef]
18. Guggenheim, J.A.; Northstone, K.; McMahon, G.; Ness, A.R.; Deere, K.; Mattocks, C.; Pourcain, B.S.; Williams, C. Time outdoors and physical activity as predictors of incident myopia in childhood: A prospective cohort study. *Investig. Ophthalmol. Vis. Sci.* **2012**, *53*, 2856–2865. [CrossRef]
19. Dirani, M.; Tong, L.; Gazzard, G.; Zhang, X.; Chia, A.; Young, T.L.; Rose, K.A.; Mitchell, P.; Saw, S.-M. Outdoor activity and myopia in Singapore teenage children. *Br. J. Ophthalmol.* **2009**, *93*, 997–1000. [CrossRef]
20. Jones-Jordan, L.A.; Sinnott, L.T.; Graham, N.D.; Cotter, S.A.; Kleinstein, R.N.; Manny, R.E.; Mutti, D.O.; Twelker, J.D.; Zadnik, K. The contributions of near work and outdoor activity to the correlation between siblings in the Collaborative Longitudinal Evaluation of Ethnicity and Refractive Error (CLEERE) Study. *Investig. Ophthalmol. Vis. Sci.* **2014**, *55*, 6333–6339. [CrossRef]
21. Wu, P.-C.; Tsai, C.-L.; Wu, H.-L.; Yang, Y.-H.; Kuo, H.-K. Outdoor activity during class recess reduces myopia onset and progression in school children. *Ophthalmology* **2013**, *120*, 1080–1085. [CrossRef]
22. Jin, J.-X.; Hua, W.; Jiang, X.; Wu, J.; Yang, J.-W.; Gao, G.; Fang, Y.; Pei, C.-L.; Wang, S.; Zhang, J.-Z.; et al. Effect of outdoor activity on myopia onset and progression in school-aged children in northeast China: The Sujiatun Eye Care Study. *BMC Ophthalmol.* **2015**, *15*, 73. [CrossRef]
23. He, M.; Xiang, F.; Zeng, Y.; Mai, J.; Chen, Q.; Zhang, J.; Smith, W.; Rose, K.; Morgan, I.G. Effect of Time Spent Outdoors at School on the Development of Myopia Among Children in China: A Randomized Clinical Trial. *JAMA* **2015**, *314*, 1142–1148. [CrossRef]
24. Tkatchenko, T.V.; Shen, Y.; Braun, R.D.; Bawa, G.; Kumar, P.; Avrutsky, I.; Tkatchenko, A.V. Photopic visual input is necessary for emmetropization in mice. *Exp. Eye Res.* **2013**, *115*, 87–95. [CrossRef]
25. Norton, T.T.; Siegwart, J.T., Jr. Light levels, refractive development, and myopia—A speculative review. *Exp. Eye Res.* **2013**, *114*, 48–57. [CrossRef]
26. World Weather Online. Available online: https://www.worldweatheronline.com/ (accessed on 23 September 2020).
27. Saw, S.-M.; Tong, L.; Chua, W.-H.; Chia, K.-S.; Koh, D.; Tan, D.T.H.; Katz, J. Incidence and progression of myopia in Singaporean school children. *Investig. Ophthalmol. Vis. Sci.* **2005**, *46*, 51–57. [CrossRef]
28. Saw, S.-M.; Tan, S.-B.; Fung, D.; Chia, K.-S.; Koh, D.; Tan, D.T.H.; Stone, R.A. Stone, IQ and the association with myopia in children. *Investig. Ophthalmol. Vis. Sci.* **2004**, *45*, 2943–2948. [CrossRef]
29. Quek, T.P.L.; Chua, C.G.; Chong, C.S.; Chong, J.H.; Hey, H.W.; Lee, J.; Lim, Y.F.; Saw, S.-M. Prevalence of refractive errors in teenage high school students in Singapore. *Ophthalmic. Physiol. Opt.* **2004**, *24*, 47–55. [CrossRef]
30. Read, S.A.; Vincent, S.J.; Tan, C.-S.; Ngo, C.; Collins, M.J.; Saw, S.-M. Patterns of Daily Outdoor Light Exposure in Australian and Singaporean Children. *Transl. Vis. Sci. Technol.* **2018**, *7*, 8. [CrossRef]
31. Ayaki, M.; Torii, H.; Tsubota, K.; Negishi, K. Decreased sleep quality in high myopia children. *Sci. Rep.* **2016**, *6*, 33902. [CrossRef]
32. Hashemi, H.; Asharlous, A.; Khabazkhoob, M.; Iribarren, R.; Khosravi, A.; Yekta, A.; Emamian, M.H.; Fotouhi, A. The Effect of Cyclopentolate on Ocular Biometric Components. *Optom. Vis. Sci.* **2020**, *97*, 440–447. [CrossRef] [PubMed]

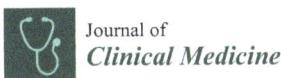

Article

Subjective Happiness and Satisfaction in Postoperative Anisometropic Patients after Refractive Surgery for Myopia

Kazuno Negishi [1,*,†], Ikuko Toda [2,†], Masahiko Ayaki [1,3,*,†], Hidemasa Torii [1] and Kazuo Tsubota [1,4]

1. Department of Ophthalmology, Keio University School of Medicine, Tokyo 1608582, Japan; hidemasatorii@yahoo.co.jp (H.T.); tsubota@z3.keio.jp (K.T.)
2. Minamiaoyama Eye Clinic, Tokyo 1070061, Japan; toda@minamiaoyama.or.jp
3. Otake Clinic Moon View Eye Center, Kanagawa 2420001, Japan
4. Tsubota Laboratory, Inc., Tokyo 1070061, Japan
* Correspondence: kazunonegishi@keio.jp (K.N.); mayaki@olive.ocn.ne.jp (M.A.)
† These authors contributed equally to this work.

Received: 20 October 2020; Accepted: 27 October 2020; Published: 28 October 2020

Abstract: Laser-assisted in situ keratomileusis (LASIK) contributes to increased patient happiness one month after surgery; however, longer term effects are unknown. We performed a retrospective cross-sectional study on 472 patients who underwent bilateral LASIK surgery to measure happiness and satisfaction with LASIK, and to identify affecting factors. Patients completed questionnaires on satisfaction with the surgery and the subjective happiness scale (SHS) before, and 1, 3, 6, and 12 months after surgery. Multiple regression analyses were performed to determine independent predictors of SHS and satisfaction scores. Mean SHS increased at one month but was similar to baseline levels by six months. The SHS of older patients was greater than younger ones at baseline and at one and three months, while satisfaction among the older group was poorer at one and three months. Multiple regression analyses revealed that the decrease in SHS score from one month to three months correlated with baseline SHS, SHS at one month, uncorrected distance visual acuity (UDVA), and age. Regression analysis revealed SHS at six months correlated with preoperative SHS, SHS at one month, and satisfaction at six months. Satisfaction at final visit correlated with age, UDVA, anisometropia, and with SHS at each visit. We conclude that happiness and satisfaction were age- and UDVA-dependent, and anisometropic patients report poorer satisfaction scores.

Keywords: myopia; LASIK; happiness; satisfaction; anisometropia

1. Introduction

Surgical correction of refractive errors restores uncorrected visual acuity and quality of life (QOL). Ophthalmic surgery drastically improves vision, even on the same day as the procedure, and patients experience the benefits of surgery. Cataract surgery is the most common surgical procedure for the elderly to improve vision and its effects on cognitive function, sleep and motor function [1–3]. Laser-assisted in situ keratomileusis (LASIK) for myopia correction is another established vision-restoring surgery, and beneficial for unaided vision and QOL in all generations [4–7]. Recent investigations described improved subjective happiness after LASIK [8] and cataract surgery [9] and a decline in dry eye symptoms [10]. Happiness is associated with health and disease, including longevity, QOL, cardiovascular diseases, and the neuroendocrine system [11–14]. Happiness or positive emotions are now regarded as a critical component of health [15–17], and subjective happiness can be measured with a validated questionnaire—the subjective happiness scale (SHS) [18,19].

Psychometric parameters may not remain stable for a long time, despite constantly normalized or improved physical status according to response shift theory [20]. Response shift theory has been applied to patient-reported outcomes when there are changes to the patients' internal standards after the event. Likewise, happiness may not be stable after LASIK under constant ocular conditions in terms of visual acuity, refraction, and accommodation [21–24]. Despite the satisfactory surgical outcome of LASIK, such as spectacle independence, happiness may be autoregressive depending on individual life events [25,26] and happiness after LASIK has not been fully investigated.

Numerous repeats have associated satisfaction with LASIK and age, complications, and uncorrected distance visual acuity (UDVA) [21–24]. We hypothesized that anisometropia could be another factor contributing to the decline of satisfaction and happiness that may happen in some patients due to ocular conditions, surgical complications, and intentional monovision for presbyopic LASIK [27–30]. Anisometropia after LASIK could be a significant issue, both in unexpected and expected cases. One magnetic resonance imaging (MRI) study described cortical changes in anisometropic adults after LASIK, and the authors discussed improved fixational instability [31].

The aim of this study was to track changes in SHS and satisfaction after LASIK and explore predictors that affect psychological parameters. We focused on postoperative anisometropia, in addition to conventionally assessed age, refraction, visual acuity and presbyopia. The measurement of subjective happiness with the validated questionnaire "SHS" is a novel aspect of the current study.

2. Experimental Section

2.1. Patients and Ethical Approval

This study was a retrospective chart review of patients who underwent bilateral LASIK procedures at the Minamiaoyama Eye Clinic, Tokyo, between September 2011 and August 2014. Subjects completed preoperative and postoperative (1, 3, 6 and 12 months after surgery) questionnaires of SHS and satisfaction with surgery. The Institutional Review Board of the Minamiaoyama Eye Clinic approved the research protocol, and the study was conducted in accordance with the tenets of the Declaration of Helsinki. Informed consent was obtained with an opt-out option.

2.2. Surgical Procedure and Ocular Examinations

Bilateral LASIK procedures were performed in succession on each patient using identical procedures. The corneal flap was created using an MK-2000 microkeratome (Nidek Co., Ltd., Aichi, Japan), an IntraLase FS60 (Abbott Medical Optics, Inc., Tokyo, Japan), or an IntraLase iFS laser (Abbott Medical Optics, Inc., Tokyo, Japan). Laser ablation was performed using the EC-5000 CXII excimer laser (Nidek Co., Ltd., Aichi, Japan). Detailed procedures, examinations, and postoperative medications have been described previously [8].

2.3. Outcome Measures

Outcome measures included UDVA, uncorrected near visual acuity (UNVA), manifest spherical and cylindrical powers, SHS, and satisfaction score. SHS was measured with the validated Japanese version of the SHS [19]. The scale is a four-item questionnaire of subjective happiness where each item requires patients to rate the statements on a seven-point Likert scale. Question and answers were: 1. "In general, I consider myself, (not a very happy person) 1-2-3-4-5-6-7 (a very happy person)"; 2. "Compared with most of my peers, I consider myself, (less happy) 1-2-3-4-5-6-7 (more happy)"; 3. "Some people are generally very happy. They enjoy life regardless of what is going on, getting the most out of everything. To what extent does this characterization describe you? (not at all) 1-2-3-4-5-6-7 (a great deal)"; 4. "Some people are generally not very happy. Although they are not depressed, they never seem as happy as they might be. To what extent does this characterization describe you? (not at all) 1-2-3-4-5-6-7 (a great deal)". The overall SHS score was calculated by taking the mean of the responses of the four items after a rescaling was carried out for question 4. The possible scores ranged from one to seven and higher values corresponded to higher subjective happiness. A one-item questionnaire rated on a four-point Likert scale ranging from 1 (very satisfied), 2 (satisfied), 3 (less satisfied), to 4 (least satisfied) was used to measure patient satisfaction with surgery. A lower score indicated a higher level of satisfaction. Satisfaction score has been used in many studies with a Likert scale, visual analogue scale (VAS), and specific questions. For example, participants answered how strongly they agreed with the statement "I would recommend my current method of vision correction to a close friend or family members" for comparison of satisfaction between LASIK and contact lens prescription [22]. The SHS and satisfaction questionnaires were routinely employed for all patients scheduled for refractive surgery to aid in decision-making and we offered it at every visit before and after LASIK in our practice. However, some patients refused to complete the questionnaire, and sometimes appointments were cancelled after LASIK.

2.4. Statistical Analysis

The data obtained from the right eyes were used for all statistical analyses. Visual acuity was converted to the logarithm of the minimum angle of resolution (logMAR). Differences between the preoperative and postoperative SHS scores and satisfaction scores were tested using the Dunnett multiple comparison test. We then performed a multiple regression analysis to assess factors affecting SHS and patient satisfaction with LASIK surgery. Finally, we conducted a multiple regression analysis to investigate predictors of postoperative SHS, delta SHS (final SHS—SHS at one month), and possible predictors of satisfaction scores (SHS and satisfaction score at each visit, UDVA and UNVA at each visit, near add power, presence of anisometropia at one month after LASIK, sex, and age). Patients were stratified by age: <40 years of age (y) as the younger group, and ≥40 y as the older group. Anisometropia after LASIK was defined as anisometropia ≥ 0.75 D and/or UDVA in under-corrected (anisometropia ≥ 0.50 D) eye < 20/20. p-value < 0.05 was considered significant. All statistical analyses were performed using SPSS version 24 for Windows (SPSS Inc., Chicago, IL, USA).

3. Results

There were 472 participants (175 men, 37.1%) and mean age was 34.5 ± 9.7 y. Postoperative UDVA and refraction were stable up to six months (Table 1). Postoperative UDVA of ≥20/20 was achieved in 90.7% of participants, and a refractive error ≤ 0.5 D was achieved in 92.7% of participants. The number of returning participants was 331 at one month, 175 at three months, 123 at six months, and 34 at 12 months; therefore, we used data at 12 months for the results at final visit. The mean SHS of all participants increased one month after surgery († p = 0.002, vs. baseline, Dunnett test) and thereafter decreased to values similar to baseline at three months (p = 0.999) and at six months (p = 0.999), whereas satisfaction was unchanged at three and six months (Table 1, Figure 1).

Table 1. Ophthalmological and psychometric results.

	Baseline	Time after LASIK		
		1 m	3 m	6 m
Subjective Happiness Scale	5.20 ± 0.94	5.35 ± 0.94 (0.002)	5.30 ± 0.97 (0.999)	5.16 ± 1.01 (0.999)
Satisfaction		1.58 ± 0.66	1.57 ± 0.71 (0.999)	1.47 ± 0.62 (0.999)
Uncorrected Distance Visual Acuity	1.14 ± 0.31	−0.09 ± 0.15	−0.09 ± 0.15	−0.10 ± 0.13
Spherical equivalent (D)	−4.96 ± 2.32	0.02 ± 0.41	−0.03 ± 0.40	−0.06 ± 0.39
Cylindrical error (D)	0.84 ± 0.75	0.12 ± 0.29	0.11 ± 0.26	0.11 ± 0.27

p-value of multiple comparison in parentheses (Dunnett test vs. baseline for subjective happiness scale and vs. 1 month for satisfaction). Abbreviations: D, diopter; m, month(s).

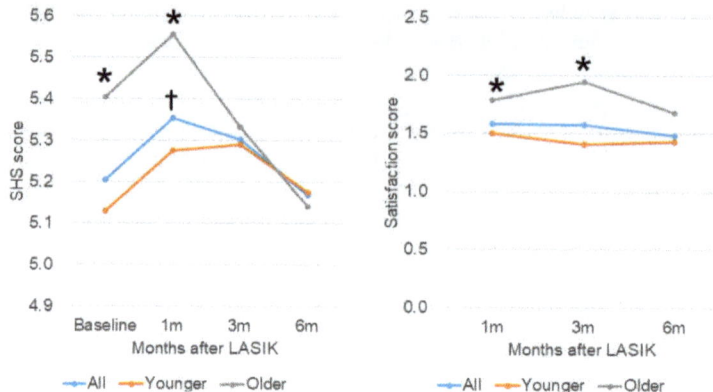

Figure 1. Subjective happiness score (left) and satisfaction scores (right) in patients stratified by age. (Left) Mean Subjective Happiness Score (SHS) of all participants (blue symbol) peaked at one month after surgery († $p = 0.002$, vs. baseline), but then decreased at three months ($p = 0.999$) and returned to baseline at six months ($p = 0.999$). SHS was greater in the older group (grey symbol) compared with the younger group (red symbol) at baseline (* $p = 0.005$) and at one month (* $p < 0.001$), but were similar at three months ($p = 0.155$) and at six months ($p = 0.103$). (Right) Mean satisfaction score of all participants (blue symbol) improved slightly but did not reach statistical significance. Satisfaction score was significantly worse in the older group (grey symbol) than the younger group (red symbol) at one month (* $p = 0.003$), at three months (* $p = 0.017$), but not at six months ($p = 0.128$).

Participants were next stratified by age according to a previous study [8]—342 patients were in the younger group (<40 y) and 130 in the older group (≥40 y). The number of patients in younger/older groups were 342/130 at baseline, 235/91 at one month, 119/54 at three months, and 94/23 at six months. The mean age of the younger/older groups was 29.7 ± 5.8 y/47.3 ± 5.4 y, and the preoperative refraction of the younger/older groups was −5.44 ± 2.41 D/−4.46 ± 2.91 D ($p < 0.001$). There was no difference in postoperative refraction and UDVA. The SHS scores of the older group were much greater than the younger group at baseline (* $p = 0.005$, unpaired t-test) and at one month (* $p < 0.001$), but decreased at three and six months, with no difference between the two groups, ($p = 0.155$ and $p = 0.103$, respectively). There was no significant change in SHS scores in the younger group (Figure 1). Satisfaction score was worse in the older group than the younger group at one ($p = 0.003$) and three months ($p = 0.017$), but not at six months ($p = 0.128$; Figure 1).

Multiple regression analysis revealed that the delta SHS ((SHS at final visit) − (SHS at 1 month)) correlated with SHS at one month ($p = 0.018$), preoperative SHS ($p = 0.029$), postoperative UDVA ($p = 0.021$), and age ($p = 0.041$; Table 2). Satisfaction with surgery at six months correlated with age ($p = 0.047$), preoperative SHS ($p = 0.022$), SHS at six months ($p = 0.001$), satisfaction at one month ($p < 0.001$), UDVA at six months ($p < 0.001$), and presence of isometropia ($p = 0.020$; Table 3). Preoperative and postoperative UNVA were not correlated with SHS or satisfaction scores.

Participants were next stratified by isometropia ($n = 413$, mean age 33.7 ± 9.5 y) and anisometropia ($n = 60$, mean age 40.3 ± 9.4 y). The mean anisometropia of the anisometropia group at final visit was 1.13 ± 0.53D in the monovision group and 0.58 ± 0.44 in the other anisometropia group ($p = 0.367$, unpaired t-test). The final satisfaction score of the isometropia/anisometropia group was one for 243 (59.7%)/15 (25.9%), two for 133 (32.7%)/27 (46.6%), three for 20 (4.9%)/12 (20.7%), and four for 1 (0.2%)/4 (6.9%; $p < 0.001$, Mann–Whitney U test; Figure 2). Satisfaction in the isometropic group was greater than in the anisometropic group at one month ($p = 0.002$, unpaired t-test), three months ($p < 0.001$), and six months ($p < 0.001$), whereas the SHS was similar between the two groups (Table 4). The final satisfaction score was 1.39 ± 0.58 in the younger isometropic group, 1.96 ± 0.92 in the younger anisometropic group, 1.79 ± 0.75 in the older isometropic group, and 2.19 ± 0.82 in the older anisometropic group (Figure 3). Among younger patients, there was a significant difference in satisfaction between isometropic and anisometropic groups (p = 0.002, Mann-Whitney U test, Bonferroni correction), but not among older patients (p = 0.098). SHS and satisfaction with surgery was similar between participants with monovision and anisometropia (Table 4).

Table 2. The results of linear and multiple regression analyses on factors associated with postoperative subjective happiness (SHS).

	Time after LASIK							
	1 m		3 m		6 m		DeltaSHS [A]	
Independent Variables	β	P	β	P	β	P	β	P
Age	0.123	0.026	0.024	0.750	0.008	0.929	−0.166	0.051
	0.124	0.024 *	0.020	0.791	0.017	0.847	−0.176	0.041 *
Sex	−0.043	0.437	0.071	0.349	−0.125	0.178	0.041	0.629
	−0.047	0.391	0.070	0.359	−0.126	0.176	0.068	0.427
Preoperative SHS	0.749	<0.001 *	0.795	<0.001 *	0.460	<0.001 *	−0.217	0.010 *
	0.751	<0.001 *	0.706	<0.001 *	0.477	<0.001 *	−0.188	0.029 *
SHS at 1 m	–	–	0.795	<0.001 *	0.555	<0.001 *	−0.209	0.014 *
	–	–	0.771	<0.001 *	0.562	<0.001 *	−0.199	0.018 *
Satisfaction	−0.200	<0.001 *	−0.087	0.278	−0.234	0.011	−0.093	0.277
	−0.249	<0.001 *	−0.104	0.198	−0.242	0.001 *	0.032	0.722
Preoperative UDVA	−0.018	0.745	−0.188	0.013 *	0.104	0.264	0.067	0.428
	0.012	0.825	−0.196	0.010 *	0.119	0.208	0.031	0.714
Postoperative UDVA	−0.078	0.156	0.999	0.996	−0.121	0.191	−0.032	0.702
	−0.159	0.008 *	0.001	0.989	−0.142	0.141	−0.195	0.021 *
Preoperative UNVA	−0.059	0.292	0.100	0.193	−0.109	0.249	−0.092	0.289
	0.060	0.278	−0.118	0.128	0.085	0.380	0.029	0.741
Postoperative UNVA	−0.159	0.177	0.013	0.866	−0.241	0.266	0.197	0.242
	0.300	0.092	−0.003	0.978	0.386	0.189	0.170	0.504
Near add power	−0.097	0.477	−0.318	0.055	−0.003	0.991	−0.298	0.189
	−0.251	0.164	−0.394	0.106	−0.335	0.347	−0.322	0.229
Isometropia	0.005	0.928	0.004	0.957	−0.109	0.239	−0.013	0.876
	0.028	0.607	0.006	0.936	−0.108	0.253	−0.044	0.606

Dependent variable: postoperative SHS at each visit. * p < 0.05. The results of linear regression, upper rows; the results of multiple regression adjusted for age and sex, lower rows. men = 1, women = 0; isometropia = 1, anisometropia = 0. Delta SHS [A] = (value at final visit) − (value at 1 month). m, month(s); UDVA, uncorrected distance visual acuity; UNVA, uncorrected near visual acuity.

Table 3. The results of linear and multiple regression analyses on factors associated with satisfaction with the surgery.

	Time after LASIK					
	1 m		3 m		6 m	
Independent Variables	β	P	β	P	β	P
Age	0.268	<0.001 *	0.305	<0.001 *	0.180	0.045
	0.269	<0.001 *	0.304	<0.001 *	0.180	0.047 *
Sex	−0.017	0.746	0.045	0.551	0.023	0.794
	−0.029	0.583	0.028	0.699	0.009	0.920

Table 3. Cont.

	Time after LASIK					
	1 m		3 m		6 m	
Independent Variables	β	P	β	P	β	P
Preoperative SHS	−0.160	0.003 *	0.026	0.726	−0.160	0.075
	−0.208	<0.001 *	−0.008	0.905	−0.209	0.022 *
SHS	−0.200	<0.001 *	−0.083	0.278	−0.234	0.011
	−0.234	<0.001 *	−0.095	0.198	−0.239	0.001 *
Satisfaction at 1 m	–	–	0.577	<0.001 *	0.451	<0.001 *
	–	–	0.555	<0.001 *	0.436	<0.001 *
Preoperative UDVA	−0.060	0.272	0.070	0.355	−0.059	0.524
	−0.004	0.928	0.0817	0.263	−0.029	0.749
Postoperative UDVA	0.445	<0.001 *	0.403	<0.001 *	0.368	<0.001 *
	0.409	<0.001 *	0.352	<0.001 *	0.350	<0.001 *
Preoperative UNVA	−0.062	0.259	−0.087	0.253	−0.005	0.956
	0.078	0.146	0.027	0.708	0.047	0.611
Postoperative UNVA	−0.366	0.001 *	−0.309	<0.001 *	−0.175	0.402
	−0.007	0.963	0.163	0.116	0.089	0.741
Near add power	0.192	0.158	0.101	0.549	−0.074	0.776
	−0.044	0.786	0.012	0.960	−0.119	0.743
Isometropia	−0.171	0.001 *	−0.284	<0.001 *	−0.302	<0.001 *
	−0.125	0.020 *	−0.218	0.004 *	−0.280	0.002 *

Dependent variable: satisfaction score at each visit. * $p < 0.05$. The results of linear regression, upper rows; the results of multiple regression adjusted for age and sex, lower rows. men = 1, women = 0; isometropia = 1, anisometropia = 0. m, month(s); SHS, subjective happiness scale; UDVA, uncorrected distance visual acuity; UNVA, uncorrected near visual acuity.

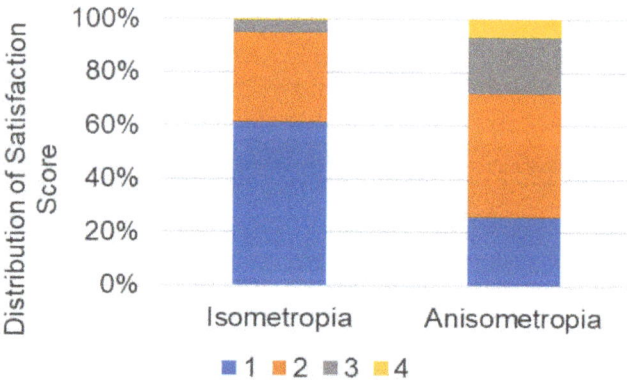

Figure 2. Distribution of final satisfaction score stratified by isometropia/anisometropia. Final satisfaction scores were significantly poorer in the anisometropia group ($p < 0.001$, Mann-Whitney U test).

Table 4. Subjective happiness scale and satisfaction in isometropic and anisometropic participants.

Subjective Happiness Scale	Baseline	1 m	3 m	6 m
		Time after LASIK		
Isometropia	5.18 ± 0.95	5.35 ± 0.95	5.30 ± 0.96	5.12 ± 1.01
Anisometropia	5.37 ± 0.84	5.34 ± 0.80	5.29 ± 1.02	5.48 ± 0.98
p-value	0.140	0.928	0.957	0.239
Satisfaction score				
Isometropia	–	1.53 ± 0.62	1.49 ± 0.65	1.41 ± 0.54
Anisometropia	–	1.89 ± 0.83	2.08 ± 0.84	2.00 ± 0.87
p-value	–	0.002 *	<0.001*	<0.001 *
Subjective Happiness	Baseline	1 m	3 m **	Final Visit
Monovision ($n = 10$)	5.44 ± 0.88	6.05 ± 0.89	–	5.54 ± 1.06
Other anisometropia ($n = 50$)	5.39 ± 0.87	5.28 ± 0.80	–	5.27 ± 0.91
p-value	0.870	0.128	–	0.426
Satisfaction				
Monovision		1.80 ± 1.30	–	2.08 ± 0.90
Other anisometropia		1.91 ± 0.76	–	2.09 ± 0.86
p-value		0.863	–	0.990

* $p < 0.05$, Unpaired t-test. The numbers of subjects are final visit. ** No analysis due to small sample size. m, month(s).

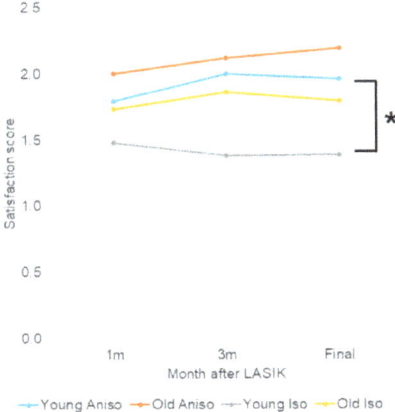

Figure 3. Satisfaction score stratified by anisometropia. The final satisfaction scores of the younger anisometropic group was poorer than the score of the younger isometropic group (* $p = 0.002$), whereas there was no difference between the older groups. Blue, younger anisotropic group; red, older anisometropic group; grey, younger isometropic group; yellow, older isometropic group.

4. Discussion

The present study successfully identified a subjective happiness increase at one month after LASIK using a validated questionnaire and then a subsequent decrease; this satisfaction remained stable after LASIK. Both psychometric parameters were age- and UDVA-dependent, and, in particular, satisfaction was poorer in participants with anisometropia. Multiple regression analysis revealed that the delta SHS correlated with age, preoperative SHS, satisfaction and UDVA, being consistent with a previous study for SHS at one month [8]. The current study indicates that patients with a greater improvement in SHS tended to regress to baseline, despite constant satisfaction. SHS and satisfaction were not correlated with UNVA, and this result confirmed that even older patients exclusively expected LASIK to be more useful for UDVA than UNVA.

We speculate that most of the younger patients without presbyopia fully enjoyed the benefits of improved UDVA and spectacle independence. In contrast, some of the older patients with decreased UNVA may struggle to adapt and accept the visual compromises inherent in presbyopia. This group also eventually need driving glasses and daily glasses, even after successful surgery due to declining visual function with age [27–37]. Older patients may also experience response shifts [20]; their SHS score was greater than that of the younger group at baseline, initially increasing, but then continuously decreasing until there was no difference with the younger group. Lensectomy with implantation of multifocal intraocular lens is sometimes a suitable option for the elderly with high myopia with early cataract [21]. Aged eyes may suffer dry eye symptoms, which is more prevalent in older populations [38,39], and a common pathology of decreased visual function with increased aberration and increased scattering originally induced by tear film instability on the ocular surface [40,41]. Dry eye symptoms may be newly developed after LASIK [42], and the loss of corneal innervation caused by flap making has been suggested as the major cause, affecting the corneal-lacrimal gland, corneal-blinking, and blinking meibomian gland reflexes, resulting in decreased aqueous and lipid tear secretion and mucin expression. Dry eye measurements, including the Schirmer test, conjunctivocorneal staining, tear film break-up time, as well as dry eye symptoms, should be evaluated in future studies.

Post-LASIK anisometropia can be classified as monovision and other anisometropia. Monovision is a planned anisometropia in which the dominant eye is corrected for distant vision, and the nondominant eye is corrected for near vision. Even after simulation with contact lenses, the acceptance by patients is unpredictable. The present study revealed satisfaction was poorer in anisometropic patients, even in cases of monovision, whereas SHS was similar in anisometropic and isometropic groups. We speculate that anisometropic patients may be happier with improved UDVA, and simultaneously disappointed by fixational instability and insufficient binocular vision. In particular, younger patients with anisometropia were dissatisfied at final visit compared with younger isometropic patients who may be sensitive to anisometropia or insufficient UDVA due to under- or overcorrection [31,43].

This study had several limitations. A questionnaire for reporting detailed QOL would be more helpful to assess participants' happiness and satisfaction, as with the Refractive Status and Visual Profile (RSVF) [37], SF-36(MOS 36-Item Short-Form Health Survey) [44], and VFQ-25 (NEI Visual Function Questionnaire-25) [45], for example. Future studies would also benefit from including questionnaires for quality of life related to daily vision (such as night vision, vision for driving, vision for reading) to more comprehensively assess subjective happiness and satisfaction. Presbyopic examinations and dry eye examinations should be conducted for further evaluation of visual function in aged eyes. Finally, happiness should be linked to lifestyle-related parameters, and could be further confirmed with integrated regression analyses. A prospective study with a longer observation period is warranted to minimize drop-out cases and achieve more conclusive results for SHS after LASIK.

5. Conclusions

SHS was maximal one month after LASIK and thereafter regressed to baseline at three months. Satisfaction was stable between 1 and 12 months after LASIK. Both parameters were age- and UDVA-dependent, and younger anisometropic patients reported poorer satisfaction scores at their final visit. As is conventionally addressed, surgeons should be careful of indication and explanation for older patients. Special attention should be paid to postoperative younger anisometropic patients.

Author Contributions: Conceptualization, I.T. and K.T.; methodology, I.T.; software, M.A.; validation, K.N., I.T. and K.T.; formal analysis, M.A.; investigation, M.A.; resources, I.T.; data curation, I.T.; writing—original draft preparation, M.A.; writing—review and editing, K.N., I.T., M.A., H.T., and K.T.; visualization, K.N.; supervision, K.T.; project administration, I.T.; funding acquisition, K.N. All authors have read and agreed to the published version of the manuscript.

Funding: This research received no external funding.

Acknowledgments: We thank Matsuguma and Ogawa for their scientific contribution.

Conflicts of Interest: The authors declare no conflict of interest.

Abbreviations

C: cylindrical power; D, diopter; LASIK, Laser-assisted in situ keratomileusis; MRI, magnetic resonance imaging; QOL, quality of life; S, spherical power; SE, spherical equivalent of subjective manifest refraction; SHS, Subjective Happiness Scale; UDVA, uncorrected distance visual acuity; UNVA, uncorrected near visual acuity.

References

1. Miyata, K.; Yoshikawa, T.; Morikawa, M.; Mine, M.; Okamoto, N.; Kurumatani, N.; Ogata, N. Effect of cataract surgery on cognitive function in elderly: Results of Fujiwara-kyo Eye Study. *PLoS ONE* **2018**, *13*, e0192677. [CrossRef] [PubMed]
2. Zheng, L.; Wu, X.H.; Lin, H.T.; Zheng, L. The effect of cataract surgery on sleep quality: A systematic review and Meta-analysis. *Int. J. Ophthalmol.* **2017**, *10*, 1734–1741. [PubMed]
3. Ayaki, M.; Nagura, T.; Toyama, Y.; Negishi, K.; Tsubota, K. Motor function benefits of visual restoration measured in age-related cataract and simulated patients: Case-control and clinical experimental studies. *Sci. Rep.* **2015**, *5*, 14595. [CrossRef] [PubMed]
4. Garamendi, E.; Pesudovs, K.; Elliott, D.B. Changes in quality of life after laser in situ keratomileusis for myopia. *J. Cataract Refract. Surg.* **2005**, *31*, 1537–1543. [CrossRef] [PubMed]
5. Morse, J.S.; Schallhorn, S.C.; Hettinger, K.; Tanzer, D. Role of depressive symptoms in patient satisfaction with visual quality after laser in situ keratomileusis. *J. Cataract Refract. Surg.* **2009**, *35*, 341–346. [CrossRef] [PubMed]
6. Lazon de la Jara, P.; Erickson, D.; Erickson, P.; Stapleton, F. Visual and non-visual factors associated with patient satisfaction and quality of life in LASIK. *Eye* **2011**, *25*, 1194–1201. [CrossRef]
7. De la Jara, P.L.; Erickson, D.; Erickson, P.; Stapleton, F. Pre-operative quality of life and psychological factors that influence patient decision making in LASIK. *Eye* **2010**, *24*, 270–275. [CrossRef]
8. Matsuguma, S.; Negishi, K.; Kawashima, M.; Toda, I.; Ayaki, M.; Tsubota, K. Patients' satisfaction and subjective happiness after refractive surgery for myopia. *Patient Prefer. Adherence* **2018**, *12*, 1901–1906. [CrossRef]
9. Yotsukura, E.; Ayaki, M.; Nezu, N.; Torii, H.; Arai, H.; Sakatani, K.; Tsubota, K.; Negishi, K. Changes in patient subjective happiness and satisfaction with cataract surgery. *Sci. Rep.* **2020**, *10*, 1–8, in press. [CrossRef]
10. Kawashima, M.; Uchino, M.; Yokoi, N.; Uchino, Y.; Dogru, M.; Komuro, A.; Sonomura, Y.; Kato, H.; Kinoshita, S.; Mimura, M.; et al. Associations between subjective happiness and dry eye disease: A new perspective from the Osaka study. *PLoS ONE* **2015**, *10*, e0123299. [CrossRef]
11. Frey, B.S. Happy people live longer. *Science* **2011**, *331*, 542–543. [CrossRef]
12. Hirosaki, M.; Ishimoto, Y.; Kasahara, Y.; Konno, A.; Kimura, Y.; Fukutomi, E. Self-rated happiness is associated with functional ability, mood, quality of life and income, but not with medical condition in community-dwelling elderly in Japan. *Geriatr. Gerontol. Int.* **2011**, *11*, 531–533. [CrossRef]
13. Shirai, K.; Iso, H.; Ohira, T.; Ikeda, A.; Noda, H.; Honjo, K.; Inoue, M.; Tsugane, S. Japan public health center-based study group. Perceived level of life enjoyment and risks of cardiovascular disease incidence and mortality: The Japan public health center-based study. *Circulation* **2009**, *120*, 956–963. [CrossRef]
14. Matsunaga, M.; Isowa, T.; Yamakawa, K.; Tsuboi, H.; Kawanishi, Y.; Kaneko, H.; Kasugai, K.; Yoneda, M.; Ohira, H. Association between perceived happiness levels and peripheral circulating pro-inflammatory cytokine levels in middle-aged adults in Japan. *Neuro. Endocrinol. Lett.* **2011**, *32*, 458–463. [PubMed]
15. Seligman, M.E.; Csikszentmihalyi, M. Positive psychology. An introduction. *Am. Psychol.* **2000**, *55*, 5–14. [PubMed]
16. Lyubomirsky, S.; King, L.; Diener, E. The benefits of frequent positive affect: Does happiness lead to success? *Psychol. Bull.* **2005**, *131*, 803–855. [CrossRef] [PubMed]
17. Steptoe, A.; Dockray, S.; Wardle, J. Positive affect and psychobiological processes relevant to health. *J. Pers.* **2009**, *77*, 1747–1776. [CrossRef]
18. Lyubomirsky, S.; Lepper, H.S. A measure of subjective happiness: Preliminary reliability and construct validation. *Soc. Indic. Res.* **1999**, *46*, 137–155. [CrossRef]

19. Shimai, S.; Otake, K.; Utsuki, N.; Ikemi, A.; Lyubomirsky, S. Development of a Japanese version of the Subjective Happiness Scale (SHS), and examination of its validity and reliability (authors' translation). *Nihon Koshu Eisei Zasshi* **2004**, *51*, 845–853. (In Japanese)
20. Howard, J.S.; Mattacola, C.G.; Howell, D.M.; Lattermann, C. Response shift theory: An application for health-related quality of life in rehabilitation research and practice. *J. Allied. Health* **2011**, *40*, 31–38.
21. Hieda, O.; Nakamura, Y.; Wakimasu, K.; Yamamura, K.; Suzukamo, Y.; Kinoshita, S.; Sotozono, C. Patient-reported vision-related quality of life after laser in situ keratomileusis, surface ablation, and phakic intraocular lens: The 5-year follow-up study. *Medicine* **2020**, *99*, e19113. [CrossRef] [PubMed]
22. Price, M.O.; Price, D.A.; Bucci, F.A.J.; Durrie, D.S.; Bond, W.I.; Price, F.W.J. Three-year longitudinal survey comparing visual satisfaction with LASIK and contact lenses. *Ophthalmology* **2016**, *123*, 1659–1666. [CrossRef]
23. Schallhorn, S.C.; Venter, J.A.; Teenan, D.; Hannan, S.J.; Hettinger, K.A.; Pelouskova, M.; Schallhorn, J.M. Patient-reported outcomes 5 years after laser in situ keratomileusis. *J. Cataract Refract. Surg.* **2016**, *42*, 879–889. [CrossRef] [PubMed]
24. Cumberland, P.M.; Chianca, A.; Rahi, J.S. Laser refractive surgery in the UK Biobank study: Frequency, distribution by sociodemographic factors, and general health, happiness, and social participation outcomes. *J. Cataract Refract. Surg.* **2015**, *41*, 2466–2475. [CrossRef] [PubMed]
25. Lucas, R.E.; Donnellan, M.B. How stable is happiness? Using the STARTS model to estimate the stability of life satisfaction. *J. Res. Pers.* **2007**, *41*, 1091–1098. [PubMed]
26. Lucas, R.E.; Clark, A.E.; Georgellis, Y.; Diener, E. Reexamining adaptation and the set point model of happiness: Reactions to changes in marital status. *J. Pers. Soc. Psychol.* **2003**, *84*, 527–539. [CrossRef] [PubMed]
27. Stival, L.R.; Figueiredo, M.N.; Santhiago, M.R. Presbyopic excimer laser ablation: A review. *J. Refract. Surg.* **2018**, *34*, 698–710. [CrossRef]
28. Lim, D.H.; Chung, E.S.; Kim, M.J.; Chung, T.Y. Visual quality assessment after presbyopic laser in-situ keratomileusis. *Int. J. Ophthalmol.* **2018**, *11*, 462–469.
29. Verdoorn, C. Comparison of a hydrogel corneal inlay and monovision laser in situ keratomileusis in presbyopic patients: Focus on visual performance and optical quality. *Clin. Ophthalmol.* **2017**, *11*, 1727–1734. [CrossRef]
30. Wilkinson, J.M.; Cozine, E.W.; Kahn, A.R. Refractive eye surgery: Helping patients make informed decisions about LASIK. *Am. Fam. Physician.* **2017**, *95*, 637–644.
31. Vuori, E.; Vanni, S.; Henriksson, L.; Tervo, T.M.; Holopainen, J.M. Refractive surgery in anisometropic adult patients induce plastic changes in primary visual cortex. *Acta Ophthalmol.* **2012**, *90*, 669–676. [CrossRef] [PubMed]
32. Sandoval, H.P.; Donnenfeld, E.D.; Kohnen, T.; Lindstrom, R.L.; Potvin, R.; Tremblay, D.M.; Solomon, K.D. Modern laser in situ keratomileusis outcomes. *J. Cataract Refract. Surg.* **2016**, *42*, 1224–1234. [CrossRef]
33. Pasquali, T.A.; Smadja, D.; Savetsky, M.J.; Reggiani Mello, G.H.; Alkhawaldeh, F.; Krueger, R.R. Long-term follow-up after laser vision correction in physicians: Quality of life and patient satisfaction. *J. Cataract Refract. Surg.* **2014**, *40*, 395–402. [CrossRef]
34. Messmer, J.J. LASIK: A primer for family physicians. *Am. Fam. Physician.* **2010**, *81*, 42–47. [PubMed]
35. Bailey, M.D.; Mitchell, G.L.; Dhaliwal, D.K.; Brian, S.; Wachler, B.; Zadnik, K. Patient satisfaction and visual symptoms after laser in situ keratomileusis. *Ophthalmology* **2003**, *110*, 1371–1378. [CrossRef]
36. McGhee, C.N.; Craig, J.P.; Sachdev, N.; Weed, K.H.; Brown, A.D. Functional, psychological, and satisfaction outcomes of laser in situ keratomileusis for high myopia. *J. Cataract Refract. Surg.* **2000**, *26*, 497–509. [CrossRef]
37. Schein, O.D.; Vitale, S.; Cassard, S.D.; Steinberg, E.P. Patient outcomes of refractive surgery. The refractive status and vision profile. *J. Cataract Refract. Surg.* **2001**, *27*, 665–673. [CrossRef]
38. Stapleton, F.; Alves, M.; Bunya, V.Y.; Jalbert, I.; Lekhanont, K.; Malet, F.; Na, K.S.; Schaumberg, D.; Uchino, M.; Vehof, J.; et al. TFOS DEWS II Epidemiology Report. *Ocul. Surf.* **2017**, *15*, 334–365. [CrossRef] [PubMed]
39. Wang, M.T.M.; Muntz, A.; Lim, J.; Kim, J.S.; Lacerda, L.; Arora, A.; Craig, J.P. Ageing and the natural history of dry eye disease: A prospective registry-based cross-sectional study. *Ocul. Surf.* **2020**, *18*, 736–741. [CrossRef]
40. Kaido, M.; Toda, I.; Oobayashi, T.; Kawashima, M.; Katada, Y.; Tsubota, K. Reducing short-wavelength blue light in dry eye patients with unstable tear film improves performance on tests of visual acuity. *PLoS ONE* **2016**, *11*, e0152936. [CrossRef]

41. Koh, S. Irregular astigmatism and higher-order aberrations in eyes with dry eye disease. *Investig. Vis. Sci.* **2018**, *59*, DES36–DES40. [CrossRef] [PubMed]
42. Toda, I. Dry eye after LASIK. *Investig. Ophthalmol. Vis. Sci.* **2018**, *59*, DES109–DES115. [CrossRef] [PubMed]
43. Garcia-Gonzalez, M.; Teus, M.A.; Hernandez-Verdejo, J.L. Visual outcomes of LASIK-induced monovision in myopic patients with presbyopia. *Am. J. Ophthalmol.* **2010**, *150*, 381–386. [CrossRef] [PubMed]
44. Suzukamo, Y.; Fukuhara, S.; Green, J.; Kosinski, M.; Gandek, B.; Ware, J.E. Validation testing of a three-component model of Short Form-36 scores. *J. Clin. Epidemiol.* **2011**, *64*, 301–308. [CrossRef]
45. Mangione, C.M.; Lee, P.P.; Gutierrez, P.R.; Spritzer, K.; Berry, S.; Hays, R.D. Development of the 25-item national eye institute visual function questionnaire. *Arch. Ophthalmol. (Chicago Ill 1960)* **2001**, *119*, 1050–1058. [CrossRef]

Publisher's Note: MDPI stays neutral with regard to jurisdictional claims in published maps and institutional affiliations.

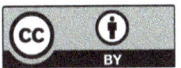

© 2020 by the authors. Licensee MDPI, Basel, Switzerland. This article is an open access article distributed under the terms and conditions of the Creative Commons Attribution (CC BY) license (http://creativecommons.org/licenses/by/4.0/).

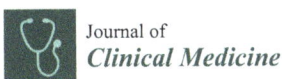 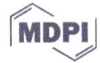

Article

Effect of Instrument Design and Technique on the Precision and Accuracy of Objective Refraction Measurement

Alberto Domínguez-Vicent *, Loujain Al-Soboh, Rune Brautaset and Abinaya Priya Venkataraman

Section of Eye and Vision, Department of Clinical Neuroscience, Karolinska Institute, 171 77 Stockholm, Sweden; loujain.al-soboh@stud.ki.se (L.A.-S.); rune.brautaset@ki.se (R.B.); abinaya.venkataraman@ki.se (A.P.V.)
* Correspondence: alberto.dominguez.vicent@ki.se; Tel.: +46-700-915-398; Fax: +46-86-723-846

Received: 17 August 2020; Accepted: 21 September 2020; Published: 23 September 2020

Abstract: Background: To evaluate the precision and accuracy of objective refraction measurement obtained with combinations of instrument design and technique. We also compared the performance of the instruments with subjective refraction measurements. Method and analysis: The objective refraction was measured in 71 subjects with three autorefractometers that have different designs and measurement principles (binocular with fogging, binocular without fogging, and monocular with fogging). Repeatability and reproducibility metrics were calculated for the objective refraction measurements. The agreement of the objective refraction measurements between the three instruments and the agreement with the subjective refraction measurements were evaluated. Results: All three autorefractometers had repeatability and reproducibility limits smaller than 0.70D. The smallest difference (0.10D) in the spherical equivalent was seen between the two binocular instruments. Compared with the subjective refraction, the binocular without fogging technique had the smallest mean difference in spherical equivalent (<0.20D) whereas the binocular fogging technique had the smallest limit of agreement interval (1.00D). For all comparisons, the mean difference and limit of agreement interval for the cylindrical components were lower than 0.10D and 0.75D, respectively. Conclusion: All three instruments evaluated had good repeatability and reproducibility. The binocular fogging technique provided the best agreement with subjective refraction.

Keywords: refraction; fogging; monocular/binocular view; precision

---

1. Introduction

Autorefractometers provide fast and accurate starting points for subjective refraction and are extensively used in both clinical practice and research. Refraction without the use of cycloplegic agents to paralyze the ciliary muscles is known to show higher myopic values [1–4]. From the age of 20 years, this effect was not seen and hence cycloplegic refraction is suggested to be of less clinical relevance [4,5]. There are different autorefractors available, each varying in measurement principle and optical design. Depending on the autorefractometer used, the objective refraction measurements can be performed either with or without fogging, monocular or binocular, through the central or the whole pupil, and with or without open-field viewing. The results of objective refraction measurements vary among autorefractors, and those differences are in most cases clinically significant [6–8]. This could be explained due to the measurement principle and design of each.

As new autorefractometers are developed, the reliability of such instruments needs to be assessed. This is done by comparing the objective refraction values obtained from the new instruments with the standard subjective refraction [9]. The subjective refraction is the gold standard method to determine the optical correction needed, as this takes into account both the optical and neural factors.

The differences between the objective and subjective refraction values can be due to the instrument design and its measuring principle. For example, proximal myopia can be induced in closed-field autorefractometers [10], and when the built-in fogging system is not used more myopic values can be obtained [5,11].

With continuous development in the measurement principles and designs in the new autorefractors, it is important to assess which combinations provide the most accurate objective refraction values. In the present study, we evaluated the precision and agreement of three autorefractometers that have different measurement principles (monocular/binocular and fogging/no fogging). We also compared the performance of these three instruments with subjective refraction.

2. Methods and Materials

2.1. Subjects

A total of 71 healthy participants (15 men and 56 women; mean age of 26.6 ± 4.6 years, range 19–40 years) were included in this study. Data from only the right eye per participant were analyzed in order not to artificially reduce the confidence interval around the limits of agreement [12]. This study was approved by the Regional Ethical Committee and adhered to the tenets of the Declaration of Helsinki. The informed consent was obtained from each participant after explaining the purpose, nature, and possible consequences of the study.

The inclusion criteria to participate in this study were no ocular dysfunctions that could affect the refraction, no history of ocular disease or refractive surgery procedure, best corrected visual acuity (BCVA) of 0.0 logMAR or better, intraocular pressure below 21 mmHg, no pregnancy or lactation, and no use of any systemic or ocular medication that could have any impact on the refraction.

2.2. Instrumentation

Three different autorefractometers were used in this study: the NVision-K 5001 (Shin-Nippon, Japan), the Eye Refract (Visionix, France), and the WaveAnalyzer 700 (Essilor, France). These instruments, that have different designs and measurement principles, were used to measure the objective refraction of each participant. The main differences among the autorefractometers are summarized in Table 1.

Table 1. Summary of the main differences among the autorefractometers.

Characteristics	Eye Refract	NVision-K 5001	WaveAnalyzer 700
Measurement principle	Wavefront	Retinal image size	Wavefront
Open/Binocular view	Yes	Yes	No
Simultaneous binocular measurement	Yes	No	No
Fogging	Yes	No	Yes
Acronym used in the text	B+ F+	B+ F−	B− F+

B+ F+: binocular with fogging. B+ F−: binocular without fogging. B− F+: monocular with fogging.

The Eye Refract is a binocular refractor that measures the objective refraction simultaneously on both eyes and provides a semi-open-field view. This instrument combines a digital phoropter with a dual Hartman-Shack sensor and uses fogging while measuring the objective refraction. The Eye Refract has been reported to provide similar refraction and BCVA than a conventional subjective refraction [13]. In this study, the participants were instructed to look at a fixation target displayed on a digital screen at 4.5 m from the instrument.

The NVision-K 5001 is an open-field autorefractor in which the objective refraction is measured monocularly without fogging. This instrument has been reported to provide repeatable [14] and accurate [15] measurements of the refractive error. During the measurement, the participants fixated binocularly to a Maltese Cross placed at 4 m from the instrument.

The WaveAnalyzer 700 combines a Hartmann-Shack sensor, a Scheimpflug camera, and a Placido disc ring to measure objective refraction and anterior segment parameters. This is a closed-field autorefractometer that measures the objective refraction monocularly with fogging technique.

2.3. Measurements

All the objective refraction measurements were performed by a single experienced examiner. In total, three objective measurements were performed with each instrument on each participant. The measurements were performed on two consecutive days. On the first day, two measurements were performed in succession with each instrument under repeatability conditions. These measurements were used to calculate the repeatability metrics and assess the agreement among the autorefractometers. On the next day, a third measurement was performed between 23 and 25 h after the last measurement of the previous day. This measurement was used together with the first measurement from day 1 to calculate the reproducibility metrics. On both days, the instrument order was randomized for all participants, and the room illumination was the same.

Another experienced observer measured the subjective refraction on a different day in a subgroup of 40 participants (8 men and 32 women; mean age of 26.3 ± 4.7 years) that were chosen randomly from the study population. The objective refraction measured from the WaveAnalyzer 700 was used as a starting value for the subjective refraction. The subjective refraction was performed with conventional fogging method with the aim of finding the maximum positive/minimum negative spherical value that gives the maximum visual acuity. The cylinder was refined using the Jackson Cross cylinder technique. From the binocular refraction performed, only the values from the right eyes were included in the analysis.

2.4. Statistical Analysis

The objective and subjective refractions were measured using the spherocylindrical notation, and were converted into power-vector notation for analysis purposes, using the following Equations [16]:

$$M = S + \frac{C}{2}$$

$$J0 = -\frac{C}{2} \cdot \cos 2\cdot\alpha$$

$$J45 = -\frac{C}{2} \cdot \sin 2\cdot\alpha$$

In these equations, M represents the spherical equivalent, $J0$ and $J45$ represent the cylindrical vectors, S, C, and α represent the spherical power, the negative value of the cylindrical power, and the cylinder axis, respectively. All statistical calculations were done using the M, $J0$, and $J45$.

Descriptive statistics were used to summarize the baseline demographics of the results obtained from each measurement and autorefractor. The precision of each instrument was described in terms of repeatability and reproducibility metrics. For this, the within subject standard deviation (S_w) was calculated using the respective measurements for repeatability and reproducibility. The S_w was estimated from the square root of the residual mean square from the one-way analysis of variance (ANOVA) with the subjects as a factor [12]. The repeatability and reproducibility limits were then calculated as $1.96 \cdot \sqrt{2} \cdot S_w$ and represent the expected limits that 95% of the measurements should be within. The Pearson correlation coefficient was calculated to determine the relation between the precision of the measurements and M.

A Bland-Altman analysis for repeated measurements was used to assess the agreement among the instruments [17]. The 95% limits of agreement were also calculated. The agreement between the subjective and objective refraction was assessed using a Bland-Altman for non-repeated measurements. An ANOVA was also performed to find whether the differences among the autorefractometers and subjective refraction were statistically significant. In all cases, the statistical significance limit was set to a p-value < 0.05.

3. Results

3.1. Precision

The refractive outcomes obtained with each measurement and autorefractor are summarized in Table 2. On average, the differences among the three measurements taken with the same autorefractor were smaller than 0.10D for M, J0, and J45. These differences were not statistically significant ($p > 0.05$) for any of the components.

Table 2. Refractive values obtained with each autorefractor.

Measurements	M			J0			J45		
	1	2	3	1	2	3	1	2	3
B+ F+	−1.30 ± 2.44	−1.31 ± 2.47	−1.26 ± 2.45	0.15 ± 0.36	0.16 ± 0.35	0.16 ± 0.36	−0.05 ± 0.19	−0.05 ± 0.20	−0.05 ± 0.18
B+ F−	−1.20 ± 2.40	−1.21 ± 2.42	−1.14 ± 2.35	0.08 ± 0.34	0.09 ± 0.35	0.06 ± 0.35	−0.09 ± 0.17	−0.10 ± 0.18	−0.09 ± 0.16
B− F+	−1.44 ± 2.73	−1.45 ± 2.64	−1.38 ± 2.62	0.14 ± 0.37	0.15 ± 0.37	0.15 ± 0.36	−0.02 ± 0.20	−0.01 ± 0.21	−0.03 ± 0.21

The values represent average ±1 standard deviation. All values are expressed in dioptres. B+ F+: binocular with fogging. B+ F−: binocular without fogging. B− F+: monocular with fogging. M: spherical equivalent. J0 and J45: cylindrical vectorial components.

Figure 1 shows the repeatability and reproducibility limits of each autorefractor for the M (Figure 1A), J0 (Figure 1B), and J45 (Figure 1C). For all the instruments, the repeatability limits were smaller than the reproducibility limits for each vectorial component. However, the differences never exceeded 0.07D for both fogging instruments. For the B− F+, the maximum difference between the repeatability and reproducibility limits was 0.10D.

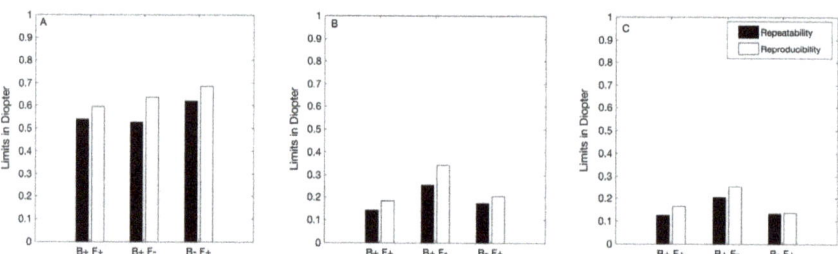

Figure 1. Repeatability and reproducibility limits of objective refraction measurement with the three instruments. The repeatability and reproducibility limits were calculated as $1.96 \cdot \sqrt{2} \cdot S_w$ where Sw is the within subject standard deviation. (**A**) spherical equivalent, (**B**) cylindrical vector J0, (**C**) cylindrical vectors J45. B+ F+: binocular instrument with fogging, B+ F−: binocular instrument without fogging, and B− F+: monocular instrument with fogging.

The repeatability limits of all instruments for M (Figure 1A) were smaller than 0.65D and similar among each other (differences smaller than 0.10D). For the astigmatic components (Figure 1B,C), the repeatability limits of all the fogging instruments were smaller than 0.25D. The reproducibility limits obtained for M were larger than or equal to 0.60D for the three instruments, and those values were similar among them. For the cylindrical components, the non-fogging instrument showed the largest value for both J0 and J45 (reproducibility limit larger than 0.25D).

Figure 2 shows the relation between the repeatability (Figure 2A–C) and reproducibility (Figure 2D–F) of the measurements against the M for the three instruments. For B− F+ (Figure 2C,F), the Sw for the reproducibility has a significant negative correlation to M ($r = -0.36$, $p = 0.0023$). The other parameters did not show a significant correlation to M.

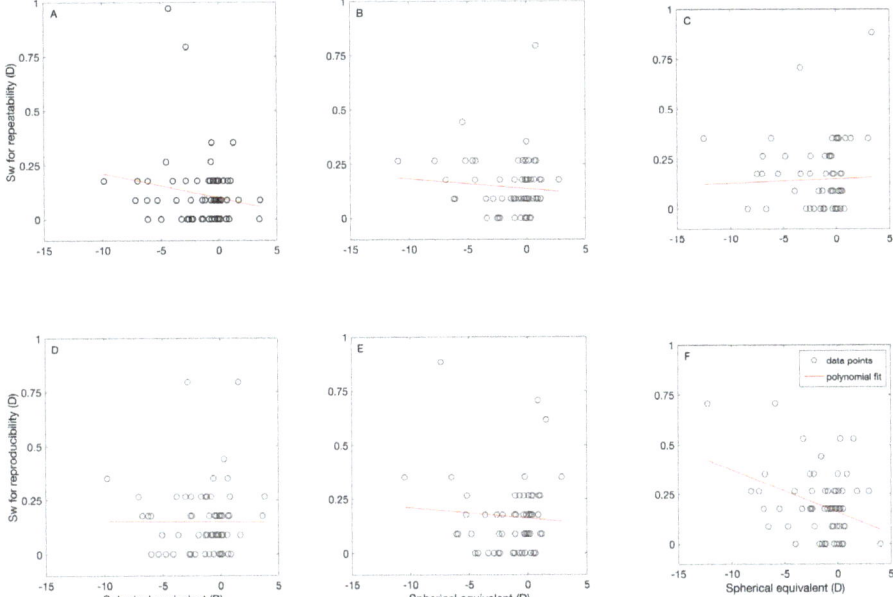

Figure 2. Correlation between spherical equivalent and within subject standard deviation for repeatability (**A–C**) and reproducibility (**D,E**) for each instrument. The results for the binocular instrument with fogging are shown in (**A,D**), for the binocular instrument without fogging are shown in (**B,E**), and for the monocular instrument with fogging are shown in (**C,F**).

3.2. Agreement among Autorefractors

Figure 3A summarizes the agreement values between the autorefractors. In this figure, the symbols and error bars represent the mean difference and 95% limits of agreement, respectively. On average, the smallest (0.10D) and largest (0.25D) difference in M was seen between the two binocular instruments, and between B+ F− and B− F+, respectively. The limit of agreement interval was about 2.00D for each comparison.

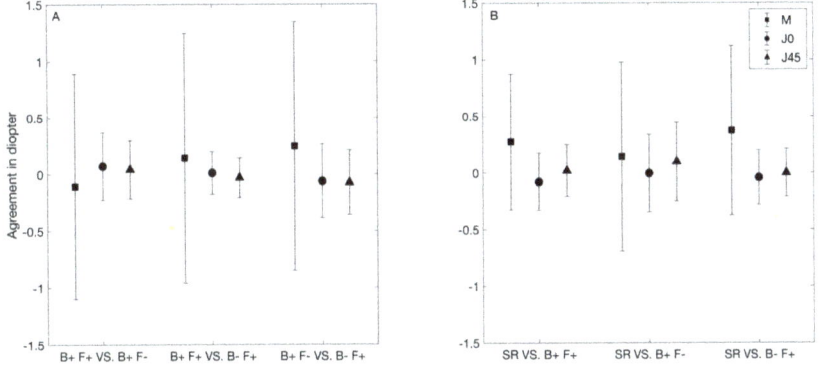

Figure 3. Agreement between different refractive methods. (**A**) Agreement between the objective refraction measurements. (**B**) Agreement between the subjective refraction and the objective refraction measurement by each instrument. The filled symbols denote the mean difference and the error bars

denote the 95% agreement limits. M, J0, and J45 represent the spherical equivalent and the two cylindrical vectorial components. B+ F+: binocular instrument with fogging, B+ F−: binocular instrument without fogging, and B− F+: binocular instrument with fogging. SR: subjective refraction.

The agreement among the autorefractors was similar for both J0 and J45. The mean difference and limit of agreement interval were always lower than 0.10D and 0.75D, respectively. The lowest limit of agreement interval was obtained between the two fogging instruments (about 0.35D), and that interval was about 0.50 to 0.60D for the other two comparisons.

Figure 4A–C show the relationship between the differences and the mean M for the autorefractor comparisons. The red line represents the quadratic polynomial curve fit of the data. The B+F+ showed a "U" shaped curve with the other two autorefractors. Compared to B+ F+, B+ F− tends to provide less myopic values for mean M between −7.00 D to +0.25 D. Whereas, B− F+ tends to provide more myopic values in general. A trend was seen between the difference and mean M of the comparison of B+F− and B−F+. The B−F+ showed more myopic values as the mean M becomes more myopic.

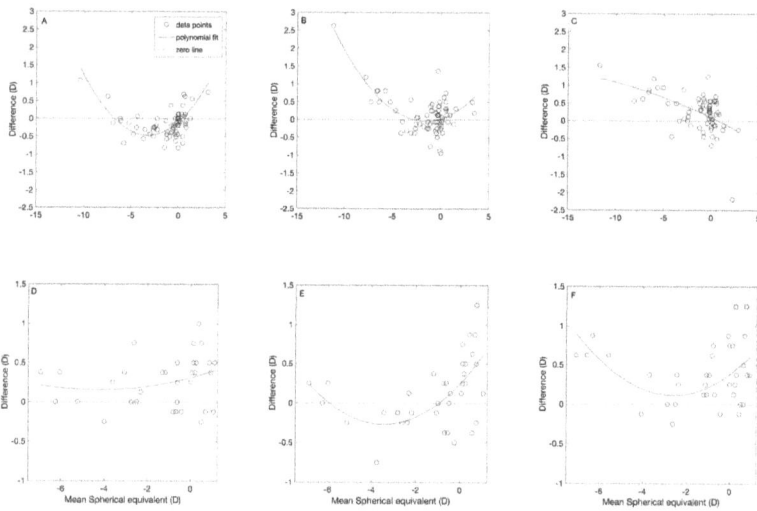

Figure 4. Relation between spherical equivalent and the mean difference among different refractive methods. (**A–C**) Relation between the spherical equivalent and the mean difference of each instrument. (**A**) Relation between the binocular instrument with fogging (B+ F+) and the binocular instrument without fogging (B+ F−); (**B**) relation between the B+ F+ and the monocular instrument with fogging (B− F+); (**C**) relation between the B+F− and B−F+. (**D–F**): relation between spherical equivalent and the mean difference for the comparison between the subjective refraction and the objective refraction measurement by each instrument. (**D**) relation between the subjective refraction (SR) and the B+ F+; (**E**) relation between the SR and B+ F−; (**F**) relation between the SR and B− F+. For all figures, the open circles denote the mean difference and the red lines represent the quadratic polynomial curve fit.

3.3. Agreement between the Subjective and Objective Refraction

Figure 3B summarizes the agreement values between the subjective and the objective refraction measured with each autorefractor. In this figure, the symbols and error bars represent the mean difference and limits of agreement, respectively. On average, the M was positive and lower than 0.50D for each comparison between the subjective and objective refraction. The narrowest and widest limits of agreement interval were about 1.00D (obtained for B+ F+) and 1.75D (obtained for B+ F−).

The agreement between the subjective and each objective refraction was similar for both J0 and J45. For all comparisons, the mean difference and limit of agreement interval were lower than 0.10D and 0.75D, respectively. The narrowest limit of agreement interval was obtained for both B+F+ and B−F+ (about 0.50D in both cases), and the widest interval was obtained for B+ F− (about 0.70D).

Figure 4D–F show the relationship between the differences and the mean M for all three comparisons. The red line in each graph represents the quadratic polynomial curve fit of the data. There is no trend seen for the comparison of subjective refraction with the B+ F+. The B+ F− and B− F+ showed a "U" shaped curve. For the comparison of the subjective refraction and B+ F−, the former provided more myopic values for the mean M between −6.00D and −1.00D. For the comparison of the subjective refraction and B− F+, the entire curve was above zero difference line (dashed line), and the least difference was seen at −2.50D mean M.

4. Discussion

We evaluated the precision and agreement of three autorefractometers and compared their performance with the subjective refraction. This was done in order to find the measurement principle and technique (monocular/binocular and fogging/no fogging) that provides the best objective refraction values. All three autorefractometers evaluated had good repeatability and reproducibility parameters. Comparing the objective refraction measurements, the mean difference in M was lower than 0.25D among all the instruments. Compared to the subjective refraction, the limit of agreement intervals were lower than 1.75D for all instruments.

Our precision results showed good repeatability and reproducibility outcomes, and the limits never exceeded 0.70D for M and 0.40D for the cylindrical components. The autorefractometers available for clinical use have been shown to have good repeatability and reproducibility for measuring the objective refraction [7,14,18–20]. With the introduction of new instruments, the intra- and inter-session precision needs to be evaluated, although the objective refraction measurements are automated and are seldom influenced by the examiner. There are other factors like patient's accommodation that can influence the measurements. These could the reason why the precision parameters are worse for M than for the cylindrical components. The repeatability limits were slightly better than the reproducibility limits for all three components measured with each autorefractometer. This could also be due to subject factors such as accommodation and fixation.

The relation between the repeatability and reproducibility of the measurements against M for each autorefractometer (Figure 2) was weak for all instruments, although the correlation for B−F+ was significant ($r = -0.36$). These results show that the repeatability and reproducibility of these autorefractometers do not depend on the patient's refractive error. We calculated the measurement tolerance, MT ($MT = (1.96 \cdot S_w)/\sqrt{N}$) for N number of measurements [21,22]. For 1, 2, and 3 number of measurements, the MT for M is 0.44D, 0.31D, and 0.25D for measurements taken under repeatability conditions, and 0.49D, 0.34D, and 0.28D for measurements taken under reproducibility conditions. In all cases, one measurement is enough to ensure a MT less than 0.50D.

Comparing the objective refraction measurements among the three different instruments, we found that the limit of agreement interval was about 2.00D. This interval is considerably large clinically and thus these instruments cannot be used interchangeably. Many of the previous studies have also shown similar large limits of agreement intervals [7,10,23,24]. The difference in the objective refraction values obtained with different autorefractometers are suggested to be caused by the fixation target, viewing conditions, fogging system, and wavefront sensors for measurements [23,24].

Comparing the two binocular vision systems used in the present study, the open-view instrument (B+ F−) provided less myopic values than the semi-open-view instrument (B+ F+). Similarly, the B+ F− provided less myopic values than the B− F+ instrument. Though the fogging system is shown to provide less myopic values [5,11], the open/closed view also seem to impact the measurement accuracy. This might be different while measuring in children where accommodation plays a major role [1,4,5]. Comparing the two fogging instruments, the monocular instrument provided more myopic values in general, highlighting the importance of binocular view.

In order to assess the clinical accuracy of the objective refraction measurements, we have to compare it with the subjective refraction. Our results show that on average, the M from all three autorefractometers provide more myopic values than subjective refraction, and the limits of agreement interval was lower than 1.75D. Similar limits of agreement intervals were reported in previous literature using different autorefractometers [13,14,25,26]. Based on the relationship between the differences and the mean M for all three comparisons (Figure 4D–F), the open-view instrument (B+ F−) measured less myopic values compared to the subjective refraction in a range of mean M between −6.00D and −1.00D. This instrument also provided a mean difference close to zero for M (Figure 3B). The other two instruments provided more myopic values in general compared to the subjective refraction.

This also supports the importance of binocular open-view instruments for the measurement of objective refraction. It is essential to know the instrument with the best precision and accuracy in order to optimize the time spent during the subjective refraction, especially in situations where only objective refraction measurements are used and in longitudinal measurements.

The findings from this study cannot be applicable for children since it is known that the accommodation plays a major role in the accuracy of refraction measurements. Our study population had fewer hyperopic subjects and the accuracy in such a case might also be affected due to accommodation in non-presbyopic subjects.

In conclusion, all three autorefractometers had good repeatability and reproducibility parameters. The binocular instruments were more comparable to subjective refraction and the binocular fogging technique had the best agreement.

Author Contributions: Conceptualization—A.D.-V., R.B., A.P.V.; methodology—A.D.-V., L.A.-S., A.P.V.; formal analysis—A.D.-V., A.P.V.; writing–original draft preparation—A.D.-V., A.P.V.; writing—review and editing—A.D.-V., L.A.-S., R.B., A.P.V.; supervision—A.D.-V., A.P.V. All authors have read and agreed to the published version of the manuscript.

Funding: This research received no external funding.

Conflicts of Interest: The authors declare no conflict of interest.

References

1. Fotedar, R.; Rochtchina, E.; Morgan, I.; Wang, J.J.; Mitchell, P.; Rose, K.A. Necessity of cycloplegia for assessing refractive error in 12-year-old children: A population-based study. *Am. J. Ophthalmol.* **2007**, *144*, 307–309. [CrossRef] [PubMed]
2. Jorge, J.; Queiros, A.; González-Méijome, J.; Fernandes, P.; Almeida, J.B.; Parafita, M.A. The influence of cycloplegia in objective refraction. *Ophthalmic Physiol. Opt. J. Br. Coll. Ophthalmic Opt.* **2005**, *25*, 340–345. [CrossRef] [PubMed]
3. Morgan, I.G.; Iribarren, R.; Fotouhi, A.; Grzybowski, A. Cycloplegic refraction is the gold standard for epidemiological studies. *Acta Ophthalmol.* **2015**, *93*, 581–585. [CrossRef]
4. Sanfilippo, P.G.; Chu, B.-S.; Bigault, O.; Kearns, L.S.; Boon, M.-Y.; Young, T.L.; Hammond, C.J.; Hewitt, W.; Mackey, A. What is the appropriate age cut-off for cycloplegia in refraction? *Acta Ophthalmol.* **2014**, *92*, e458–e462. [CrossRef] [PubMed]
5. Wesemann, W.; Dick, B. Accuracy and accommodation capability of a handheld autorefractor. *J. Cataract. Refract. Surg.* **2000**, *26*, 62–70. [CrossRef]
6. Yassa, E.T.; Ünlü, C. Comparison of Autorefraction and Photorefraction with and without Cycloplegia Using 1% Tropicamide in Preschool Children. *J. Ophthalmol.* **2019**, *2019*, 1487013. [CrossRef]
7. Carracedo, G.; Carpena-Torres, C.; Batres, L.; Serramito, M.; Gonzalez-Bergaz, A. Comparison of Two Wavefront Autorefractors: Binocular Open-Field versus Monocular Closed-Field. *J. Ophthalmol.* **2020**, *2020*, 8580471. [CrossRef]
8. Xiong, S.; Lv, M.; Zou, H.; Zhu, J.; Lu, L.; Zhang, B.; Deng, J.; Yao, C.; He, X.; Xu, X.; et al. Comparison of Refractive Measures of Three Autorefractors in Children and Adolescents. *Optom. Vis. Sci. Off. Publ. Am. Acad. Optom.* **2017**, *94*, 894–902. [CrossRef]
9. Elliott, D.B. What is the appropriate gold standard test for refractive error? *Ophthalmic Physiol. Opt. J. Br. Coll. Ophthalmic Opt.* **2017**, *37*, 115–117. [CrossRef]

10. Gwiazda, J.; Weber, C. Comparison of spherical equivalent refraction and astigmatism measured with three different models of autorefractors. *Optom. Vis. Sci. Off. Publ. Am. Acad. Optom.* **2004**, *81*, 56–61. [CrossRef]
11. Zhao, J.; Mao, J.; Luo, R.; Li, F.; Pokharel, G.P.; Ellwein, L.B. Accuracy of noncycloplegic autorefraction in school-age children in China. *Optom. Vis. Sci. Off. Publ. Am. Acad. Optom.* **2004**, *81*, 49–55. [CrossRef] [PubMed]
12. McAlinden, C.; Khadka, J.; Pesudovs, K. Statistical methods for conducting agreement (comparison of clinical tests) and precision (repeatability or reproducibility) studies in optometry and ophthalmology. *Ophthalmic Physiol. Opt. J. Br. Coll. Ophthalmic Opt.* **2011**, *31*, 330–338. [CrossRef] [PubMed]
13. Carracedo, G.; Carpena-Torres, C.; Serramito, M.; Batres-Valderas, L.; Gonzalez-Bergaz, A. Comparison Between Aberrometry-Based Binocular Refraction and Subjective Refraction. *Transl. Vis. Sci. Technol.* **2018**, *7*, 11. [CrossRef]
14. Davies, L.N.; Mallen, E.A.H.; Wolffsohn, J.S.; Gilmartin, B. Clinical Evaluation of the Shin-Nippon NVision-K 5001/Grand Seiko WR-5100K Autorefractor. *Optom. Vis. Sci.* **2003**, *80*. Available online: https://journals.lww.com/optvissci/Fulltext/2003/04000/Clinical_Evaluation_of_the_Shin_Nippon_NVision_K.11.aspx (accessed on 22 September 2020). [CrossRef] [PubMed]
15. Wolffsohn, J.S.; Davies, L.N.; Naroo, S.A.; Buckhurst, P.J.; Gibson, G.A.; Gupta, N.; Craig, J.P.; Shah, S. Evaluation of an open-field autorefractor's ability to measure refraction and hence potential to assess objective accommodation in pseudophakes. *Br. J. Ophthalmol.* **2011**, *95*, 498–501. [CrossRef]
16. Thibos, L.N.; Wheeler, W.; Horner, D. Power vectors: An application of Fourier analysis to the description and statistical analysis of refractive error. *Optom. Vis. Sci. Off. Publ. Am. Acad. Optom.* **1997**, *74*, 367–375. [CrossRef]
17. Tiland, J.; Altman, D. Measuring agreement in method comparison studies. *Stat Methods Med. Res.* **1999**, *8*, 135–160.
18. Allen, P.M.; Radhakrishnan, H.; O'Leary, D.J. Repeatability and validity of the PowerRefractor and the Nidek AR600-A in an adult population with healthy eyes. *Optom. Vis. Sci. Off. Publ. Am. Acad. Optom.* **2003**, *80*, 245–251. [CrossRef] [PubMed]
19. Ogbuehi, K.C.; Almaliki, W.H.; AlQarni, A.; Osuagwu, U.L. Reliability and reproducibility of a handheld videorefractor. *Optom. Vis. Sci. Off. Publ. Am. Acad. Optom.* **2015**, *92*, 632–641. [CrossRef]
20. Paudel, N.; Adhikari, S.; Thakur, A.; Shrestha, B.; Loughman, J. Clinical Accuracy of the Nidek ARK-1 Autorefractor. *Optom. Vis. Sci. Off. Publ. Am. Acad. Optom.* **2019**, *96*, 407–413. [CrossRef]
21. ISO. *Probability and General Statistical Terms. Statistics: Vocabulary and Symbols*; ISO 3534-1:2006; International Organization for Standardization: Geneva, Switzerland, 2006.
22. ISO. *Accuracy (Trueness and Precision) of Measurement Methods and Results—Part 1: General Principles and Definitions*; ISO 5725-1:1994; International Organization for Standardization: Geneva, Switzerland, 1994.
23. McCullough, S.J.; Little, J.-A.; Breslin, K.M.; Saunders, K.J. Comparison of Refractive Error Measures by the IRX3 Aberrometer and Autorefraction. *Optom. Vis. Sci.* **2014**, *91*. Available online: https://journals.lww.com/optvissci/Fulltext/2014/10000/Comparison_of_Refractive_Error_Measures_by_the_9.aspx (accessed on 22 September 2020). [CrossRef] [PubMed]
24. Wosik, J.; Patrzykont, M.; Pniewski, J. Comparison of refractive error measurements by three different models of autorefractors and subjective refraction in young adults. *J. Opt. Soc. Am. A* **2019**, *36*, B1–B6. Available online: http://josaa.osa.org/abstract.cfm?URI=josaa-36-4-B1 (accessed on 22 September 2020). [CrossRef] [PubMed]
25. Bennett, J.R.; Stalboerger, G.M.; Hodge, D.O.; Schornack, M.M. Comparison of refractive assessment by wavefront aberrometry, autorefraction, and subjective refraction. *J. Optom.* **2015**, *8*, 109–115. [CrossRef] [PubMed]
26. Choong, Y.-F.; Chen, A.-H.; Goh, P.-P. A comparison of autorefraction and subjective refraction with and without cycloplegia in primary school children. *Am. J. Ophthalmol.* **2006**, *142*, 68–74. [CrossRef] [PubMed]

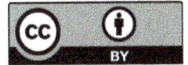 © 2020 by the authors. Licensee MDPI, Basel, Switzerland. This article is an open access article distributed under the terms and conditions of the Creative Commons Attribution (CC BY) license (http://creativecommons.org/licenses/by/4.0/).

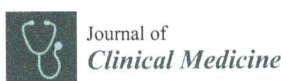

Article

Improvement in Contrast Sensitivity Function after Lacrimal Passage Intubation in Eyes with Epiphora

Sujin Hoshi *, Kuniharu Tasaki, Takahiro Hiraoka and Tetsuro Oshika

Department of Ophthalmology, Faculty of Medicine, University of Tsukuba, Ibaraki 305-8575, Japan; k.tasaki1986@gmail.com (K.T.); thiraoka@md.tsukuba.ac.jp (T.H.); oshika@eye.ac (T.O.)
* Correspondence: hoshisujin@md.tsukuba.ac.jp; Tel.: +81-298-53-3148

Received: 4 July 2020; Accepted: 24 August 2020; Published: 26 August 2020

Abstract: This prospective case series aimed to investigate the contrast sensitivity function before and after lacrimal passage intubation (LPI) in eyes with epiphora due to lacrimal passage obstruction. We included 58 eyes of 51 patients who underwent LPI for lacrimal passage obstruction. The best-corrected visual acuity (BCVA), contrast sensitivity function, and lower tear meniscus were compared before LPI and one month after lacrimal duct stent removal. The area under the log contrast sensitivity function (AULCSF) was calculated for the analyses. Lower tear meniscus was assessed using anterior segment optical coherence tomography. The BCVA was comparable ($p = 0.61$) before and after LPI, while AULCSF increased significantly after treatment (before LPI: 1.29 ± 0.17, after LPI: 1.37 ± 0.14, $p < 0.0001$). Treatment resulted in a significant increase in contrast sensitivity at all spatial frequencies, 3–18 cycles/degree ($p < 0.01$ for 3, $p < 0.01$ for 6, $p < 0.0005$ for 12, $p < 0.05$ for 18 cycles/degree). The lower tear meniscus parameters improved significantly after treatment ($p < 0.005$); however, no correlation between the changes in the tear meniscus and those of the AULCSF was found. The contrast sensitivity significantly improved after LPI in eyes with epiphora due to lacrimal passage obstruction.

Keywords: contrast sensitivity function; epiphora; lacrimal passage obstruction; lacrimal passage intubation

1. Introduction

Patients with epiphora owing to lacrimal passage obstruction often complain of physical discomfort, such as unwilling tearing, skin eczema, and vision-related discomfort. Although visual acuity is maintained, it is reported that contrast sensitivity function [1], optical quality [2], and quality of life (QoL) are compromised in eyes with epiphora owing to lacrimal passage obstruction [3–5].

Lacrimal passage intubation (LPI) is a well-established and effective method used for treating lacrimal passage obstruction to recanalize and recover the patency of lacrimal passage; this method has been employed as an alternative to dacryocystorhinostomy [6–12]. Moreover, dacryoendoscope and dacryoendoscopic techniques, which have recently been developed, have allowed for the improvement of the success rate and safety of LPI by facilitating direct visualization [13–17].

Although patients often experience an improvement in the quality of their vision, it is unknown whether the deteriorated contrast sensitivity function of eyes with epiphora owing to nasolacrimal passage obstruction recovers after LPI. It is important to assess the effect of LPI on contrast sensitivity, as contrast sensitivity is widely used for the clinical assessment of quality of vision in various diseases. As a fall in contrast sensitivity affects the quality of vision, this may be an indication for LPI in patients with epiphora due to lacrimal passage obstruction. This study aimed to investigate contrast sensitivity function in eyes with epiphora owing to lacrimal passage obstruction before and after LPI using different methods.

2. Experimental Section

This study was a single-institutional prospective case series that was approved by the Institutional Review Board of University of Tsukuba Hospital (H27-153) and adhered to the tenets of the Declaration of Helsinki. After the nature and possible consequences of the study were explained in detail, informed consent was obtained from all patients.

2.1. Patient Population

Patients with lacrimal passage obstruction who received LPI between November 2015 and July 2019 at the University of Tsukuba Hospital and had a distance best-corrected visual acuity (BCVA) of 20/20 or better, as determined by Snellen testing, were considered for enrollment. The inclusion criteria were the presence of symptoms of epiphora and at least one of the following dacryoendoscopic findings: nasolacrimal duct obstruction (NLDO), canalicular obstruction, or punctal obstruction. The exclusion criteria were congenital lacrimal duct obstruction, acute dacryocystitis, and a history of ocular surface surgery. Patients with cortical cataract formation in the central lens, intraocular lens only in one eye, other ocular diseases, or a history of treatment that might affect contrast sensitivity were excluded. In total, 58 eyes of 51 patients (men: 17, women: 34; mean age: 62.3 ± 9.6 years; range: 37–80 years) with lacrimal passage obstruction participated in our study. Table 1 categorizes the type of obstruction diagnosed in all our participants. Thirty-two eyes showed NLDO alone, and 26 eyes showed the involvement of proximal obstruction, i.e., punctal and/or canalicular obstruction with/without NLDO. Of 32 eyes with NLDO alone, 14 had complete NLDO and the remaining 18 had partial obstruction. Of 26 eyes with proximal obstruction, five had complete NLDO, nine had proximal NLDO, and the remaining 12 were without NLDO.

Table 1. Type of obstruction as determined using dacryoendoscopy.

Underlying Disease	Eyes (N)
Nasolacrimal duct obstruction only	32
Proximal involved	26
Common canalicular obstruction combined with nasolacrimal duct obstruction	14
Common canalicular obstruction	10
Upper and/or lower punctal obstruction	2

2.2. Surgical Technique and Postoperative Follow-Up

All surgeries were performed by three surgeons (TH, SH, KT). The surgical procedure of LPI performed in the current study was a combination of sheath-guided endoscopic probing (SEP) and sheath-guided intubation (SGI). This technique enables surgeons to perform lacrimal passage reconstruction under dacryoendoscopic guidance without blind manipulation [16,17]. The lacrimal passage anesthesia protocol involved an infratrochlear nerve block with 1% lidocaine and canalicular system irrigation with a 4% lidocaine solution, followed by the dilation of both puncta. Prior to SEP, a dacryoendoscope (LAC-06NZ-HS; MACHIDA Endoscope Co., Ltd., Chiba, Japan) was covered with a sheath that was prepared with an 18-gauge plastic cannula (SurFlash Polyurethane IV Catheters; Terumo Corporation, Tokyo, Japan). After a dacryoendoscope equipped with a sheath was inserted into the punctum, SEP was performed by widening the blocked section. The outer diameter of the dacryoendoscope was 0.9 mm (20 gauge). After the removal of the dacryoendoscope, the sheath was temporarily retained in the lacrimal passage and used as a guide for tube insertion during SGI. An 11-cm-long polyurethane Nunchaku-style lacrimal duct stent tube (LACRIFAST; KANEKA Corporation, Tokyo, Japan) was connected with the sheath. By retrieving the sheath through the nasal cavity, the surgeon was able to draw the lacrimal tube into the recanalized passage. The same steps were repeated for the other punctum using a combination of SEP and SGI. During this operation, the precise location of the lacrimal passage obstruction was recorded and utilized for diagnosing the type of obstruction in each case.

A lacrimal passage lavage with saline was performed every month postoperatively. The lacrimal duct stent tube was removed 2 to 3 months postoperatively, which is similar to the periods in previous reports [3,5,9,12]. In addition, a dacryoendoscopic investigation was performed to confirm whether the obstructed lacrimal passage was successfully recanalized.

2.3. Examination Protocol

Assessment of lower tear meniscus using anterior segment optical coherence tomography (OCT) and contrast sensitivity was performed preoperatively and 1 month after the removal of lacrimal duct stent tube to avoid the possible effects of intubation-associated ductal inflammation on the meniscus and visual function.

2.4. Assessment of Tear Meniscus

Cross-sectional images of the lower tear meniscus were captured vertically across the central cornea using swept-source anterior segment optical coherence tomography (OCT; SS-1000, CASIA; Tomey Corp., Nagoya, Japan). The OCT images were processed using in-built software. The principles, technique, and reproducibility of evaluating tear meniscus using this device have been described previously [18,19].

Lower tear meniscus height (TMH) and lower tear meniscus area (TMA) were calculated from the cross-sectional OCT images of the lower tear meniscus. The measurement was performed 4–5 s after blinking, with spontaneous eye opening.

2.5. Assessment of Contrast Sensitivity

The CSV-1000E chart (Vector Vision CO., Greenville, OH, USA) was used to measure contrast sensitivity function. The test was performed monocularly when the pupils of the eyes were undilated, and the testing distance was 2.5 m with best spectacle correction. Background illumination of the translucent chart was provided using a fluorescent luminance source of the instrument and was automatically calibrated to 85 cd/m^2.

The CSV-1000E chart presents vertical sine-wave gratings at four spatial frequencies, i.e., 3, 6, 12, and 18 cycles/degree; each spatial frequency has eight different levels of contrast. Each row consists of eight pairs of circular patches and includes sine waves of a single spatial frequency. In each pair, one patch presents a grating, and the other patch is blank. The patients were asked to identify the patch with the grating, and the contrast level of the last correct response was defined as the contrast threshold in logarithmic values for each frequency [20]. From these data, the area under the log contrast sensitivity function (AULCSF) was calculated according to the method described by Applegate et al. [21]. In brief, the AULCSF was determined as the integration of the fitted third-order polynomials of the log contrast sensitivity units between the fixed limits of 0.48 (corresponding to 3 cycles/degree) and 1.26 (18 cycles/degree) on the log spatial frequency scale. This provides contrast sensitivity data as one number and makes statistical analysis easier. The AULCSF calculated by the average levels of contrast in each spatial frequency as described by the supplier (http://www.vectorvision.com/educational-resources/) is 1.24 in people aged 50–75 years.

2.6. Statistical Analyses

Normally distributed data before and after LPI were compared using a paired *t*-test (two-tailed test). Data that were not normally distributed were compared using the Wilcoxon signed-rank test. Analysis of the correlation between the difference in tear meniscus dimension (TMH and TMA) and the difference in quality of vision (BCVA and contrast sensitivity) before and after LPI were evaluated using Pearson's correlation coefficient.

The AULCSF was compared between eyes with only NLDO and those with the involvement of proximal obstruction using an unpaired *t*-test (Student's *t*-test).

The p values of < 0.05 were considered statistically significant for all analyses. Statistical analyses were performed using Statcel (add-in software for Microsoft Excel), version 4 (Microsoft Corp., Redmond, WA, USA).

3. Results

3.1. Comparison of Parameters before and after LPI

Table 2 shows the comparison of BCVA, AULCSF, TMH, and TMA before and after LPI. The BCVA was comparable ($p = 0.61$) before and after surgery, while AULCSF increased significantly after surgery ($p < 0.0001$). The lower tear meniscus parameters, TMH and TMA, decreased significantly after surgery ($p < 0.005$).

Table 2. Comparison between measured parameters before and after lacrimal passage intubation.

Parameters	Before LPI	After LPI	p Value
BCVA (logMAR)	−0.10 ± 0.06 (−0.08, −0.18 to −0.08)	−0.10 ± 0.05 (−0.08, −0.18 to −0.08)	[a] 0.61
AULCSF	1.29 ± 0.17 (1.31, 1.17 to 1.44)	1.37 ± 0.14 (1.39, 1.28 to 1.49)	[b] <0.0001
Tear meniscus height (mm)	0.46 ± 0.20 (0.46, 0.31 to 0.58)	0.34 ± 0.11 (0.33, 0.24 to 0.42)	[b] <0.005
Tear meniscus area (mm^2)	0.09 ± 0.07 (0.07, 0.04 to 0.11)	0.04 ± 0.03 (0.04, 0.03 to 0.06)	[a] <0.005

Data are presented as the mean ± standard deviation (median, interquartile range). The [a] p value, evaluated using the Wilcoxon signed-rank test. The [b] p value, evaluated using a paired t-test. LPI, lacrimal passage obstruction; BCVA, best-corrected visual acuity; AULCSF, area under the log contrast sensitivity function.

3.2. Comparison of Contrast Sensitivity at Four Specific Frequencies before and after LPI

Treatment resulted in significant increases in contrast sensitivity at all spatial frequencies from 3 to 18 cycles/degree ($p < 0.01$ for 3, $p < 0.01$ for 6, $p < 0.0005$ for 12, $p < 0.05$ for 18 cycles/degree; Figure 1).

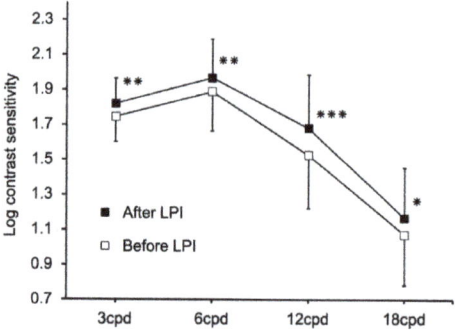

Figure 1. Contrast sensitivity at four specific frequencies before and after lacrimal passage obstruction. Treatment resulted in significant increases in contrast sensitivity at all spatial frequencies from 3 to 18 cycles/degree ($p < 0.01$ for 3 cycles/degree, $p < 0.01$ for 6 cycles/degree, $p < 0.0005$ for 12 cycles/degree, $p < 0.05$ for 18 cycles/degree). Values are expressed as the mean ± standard deviation. * $p < 0.05$, ** $p < 0.01$, *** $p < 0.0005$

3.3. Correlations between Changes in Tear Meniscus and Changes in AULCSF

The changes in AULCSF did not correlate with the changes in TMH ($r = 0.009$, $p = 0.95$) or TMA ($r = 0.109$, $p = 0.41$). The changes in log contrast sensitivity at each frequency were correlated with the changes in neither TMH (3 cycles/degree: r = −0.108, p = 0.41; 6 cycles/degree; r = 0.108, p = 0.42; 12 cycles/degree; r = −0.014, p = 0.91, 18 cycles/degree; r = −0.001, p = 0.99) nor TMA (3 cycles/degree: r = 0.026, p = 0.84; 6 cycles/degree: r = 0.082, p = 0.54; 12 cycles/degree: r = 0.114, p = 0.39; 18 cycles/degree: r = 0.016, p = 0.91).

3.4. Changes and Comparison of AULCSF in Eyes with NLDO Only and Those with the Involvement of Proximal Obstruction before and after LPI

Figure 2 shows changes in AULCSF in eyes with NLDO only and those with the involvement of proximal obstruction. The AULCSF significantly improved after LPI in both the groups (NLDO only group: 1.26 ± 0.17 to 1.36 ± 0.16, $p < 0.001$; proximal involvement group: 1.33 ± 0.16 to 1.38 ± 0.13, $p < 0.05$). Before LPI, there was a significant difference in AULCSF between the two groups ($p < 0.05$); however, the difference became insignificant after LPI ($p = 0.32$).

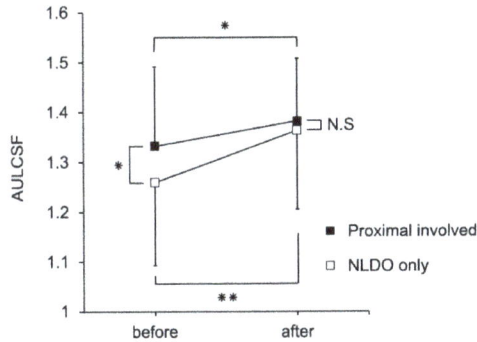

Figure 2. Changes and comparison of AULCSF in eyes with NLDO only and those with the involvement of proximal obstruction before and after LPI. The AULCSF improved significantly after LPI in both groups (NLDO only group, $p < 0.001$; proximal involvement group, $p < 0.05$). Before LPI, there was a significant difference in AULCSF between the two groups ($p < 0.05$); however, the difference became insignificant after LPI ($p = 0.32$). Values are expressed as the mean ± standard deviation. LPI, lacrimal passage obstruction; AULCSF, area under the log contrast sensitivity function; NLDO, nasolacrimal duct obstruction. * $p < 0.05$, ** $p < 0.001$

There were no significant differences in TMH or TMA between the two groups before and after LPI (TMH before LPI: $p = 0.11$, TMH after LPI: $p = 0.24$, TMA before LPI: $p = 0.37$, TMA after LPI: $p = 0.22$).

4. Discussion

Contrast sensitivity tests are more sensitive for investigating the quality of vision than are standard visual acuity tests, which capture high spatial frequency channels well but do not necessarily predict vision at middle and lower frequencies [22]. Therefore, contrast sensitivity tests are useful for evaluating the quality of vision in eyes without or with slight decline in visual acuity. For example, dry eyes or eyes that underwent LASIK intervention show deterioration of contrast sensitivity, while their visual acuity remains unaffected [23,24]. In line with these findings, we previously reported a reduction in contrast sensitivity in eyes with epiphora caused by lacrimal passage obstruction, in which conventional visual acuity is maintained [1]. A contrast sensitivity test is also useful for evaluating the quality of vision before and after treatment in various anterior segment disease of the eyes, such as dry eye [25,26], ptosis and dermatochalasis [27], conjunctivochalasis [28], and cataract [29], as well as posterior segment eye diseases such as retinal detachment [30], epiretinal membrane [31], and posterior vitreous detachment [32], among others [33]. To the best of our knowledge, this is the first study to report improvement in the contrast sensitivity of the eyes after LPI for epiphora owing to lacrimal passage obstruction.

Regarding dry eyes—another common disease characterized by abnormalities in the tear film on the ocular surface—Koh et al. reported that AULCSF of dry eyes decreased to 1.24 ± 0.16, while that of normal eyes was 1.35 ± 0.11 [23]. Asano et al. revealed that eye drop treatment with diquafosol ophthalmic solution improves AULCSF from 1.26 ± 0.12 to 1.35 ± 0.14 in patients with SCL-related dry eyes [34]. In our study, LPI improved AULCSF from 1.29 ± 0.16 to 1.37 ± 0.14, which was comparable to the findings of the two above-mentioned reports, i.e., treatment for lacrimal passage obstruction with treatment for dry eye brings the same level of improvement in contrast sensitivity.

In this study, we found that AULCSF before LPI was significantly worse in the NLDO only group than in the proximal involvement group. When we performed lacrimal passage system irrigation, reflux fluid often contained mucus and/or pus in the eyes with NLDO alone but not in those with proximal involvement. Differences in the turbidity of tear meniscus between eyes with NLDO alone and those with proximal involvement may affect the difference in contrast sensitivity. Hiraoka et al. reported that increased light scattering after instillation of brinzolamide causes deterioration of contrast sensitivity [35]. In patients with NLDO, it is possible that light scattering may increase because of excessive retention of proteins in tear film that is not excreted into the nasal fossa, while this is less common in the eyes with proximal involvement. In contrast, tear meniscus volume did not seem to directly affect contrast sensitivity because there were no significant differences in TMH or TMA between the NLDO only and proximal involvement groups. The AULCSF improved after LPI in both the groups, and there was no difference in AULCSF between both groups after LPI. This may suggest that LPI leads to normalization of tear content, resulting in the improvement of contrast sensitivity to the same level in both cases. Although it is not volume-dependent, excessive tear meniscus volume can lead to instability of the tear film on the corneal surface, which can affect contrast sensitivity in eyes with lacrimal passage obstruction.

Improvement in AULCSF was not correlated with changes in tear meniscus parameters in this study. Our previous study including unilateral lacrimal passage obstruction cases also revealed no correlation between AULCSF and tear meniscus parameters [1]. Similarly, Koh et al. reported that tear meniscus parameters were not correlated to the quality of vision or optical quality in patients with epiphora owing to nasolacrimal passage obstruction [2]. From these results, tear meniscus volume does not seem to affect visual quality in patients with lacrimal passage obstruction. One possible explanation would be that the tear film varies and has different phases with blinking; therefore, the condition of tear meniscus is not constant between OCT measurement of the tear meniscus and the visual quality tests.

This study had some limitations. Contrast sensitivity and the other parameters were not recorded with the stent in place, since postoperative measurements were performed one month after removal of the stent. As many patients are aware of improvement in their visual performance soon after LPI, with the stent in place, contrast sensitivity and the other parameters should also be investigated at that stage, to precisely describe the effect of LPI on vision. Another limitation was the rather short follow-up period in the study. Patency decreases with follow-up, and long-term results of LPI are not always satisfactory [7,36]. Recurrence of stenosis and obstruction of the lacrimal passage during longer follow-up may affect the quality of vision. Further investigations are needed to clarify the long-term effects of LPI on visual function including contrast sensitivity.

5. Conclusions

In conclusion, contrast sensitivity significantly improved after LPI in eyes with epiphora owing to lacrimal passage obstruction. Contrast sensitivity measurement before and after LPI might aid in our understanding of the effectiveness of treatment on the recovery of visual function in eyes that underwent LPI.

Author Contributions: Conceptualization, S.H. and T.H.; methodology, S.H., K.T., and T.H.; software, S.H. and K.T.; validation, S.H. and T.H.; formal analysis, S.H., K.T., and T.H.; investigation, S.H., K.T., and T.H.; resources, S.H., K.T., T.H., and T.O.; data curation, S.H., K.T., and T.H.; writing—original draft preparation, S.H.; writing—review and editing, S.H., T.H., and T.O.; visualization, S.H. and T.H.; supervision, S.H., T.H., and T.O.; project administration, S.H., T.H., and T.O. All authors have read and agreed to the published version of the manuscript.

Funding: This research received no external funding.

Conflicts of Interest: The authors declare no conflict of interest.

References

1. Tasaki, K.; Hoshi, S.; Hiraoka, T.; Oshika, T. Deterioration of contrast sensitivity in eyes with epiphora due to lacrimal passage obstruction. *PLoS ONE* **2020**, *15*, e0233295. [CrossRef] [PubMed]
2. Koh, S.; Inoue, Y.; Ochi, S.; Takai, Y.; Maeda, N.; Nishida, K. Quality of vision in eyes with epiphora undergoing lacrimal passage intubation. *Am. J. Ophthalmol.* **2017**, *181*, 71–78. [CrossRef] [PubMed]
3. Kabata, Y.; Goto, S.; Takahashi, G.; Tsuneoka, H. Vision-related quality of life in patients undergoing silicone tube intubation for lacrimal passage obstructions. *Am. J. Ophthalmol.* **2011**, *152*, 147–150. [CrossRef]
4. Oh, J.R.; Chang, J.H.; Yoon, J.S.; Jang, S.Y. Change in quality of life of patients undergoing silicone stent intubation for nasolacrimal duct stenosis combined with dry eye syndrome. *Br. J. Ophthalmol.* **2015**, *99*, 1519–1522. [CrossRef] [PubMed]
5. Kamao, T.; Takahashi, N.; Zheng, X.; Shiraishi, A. Changes of visual symptoms and functions in patients with and without dry eye after lacrimal passage obstruction treatment. *Curr. Eye Res.* **2020**. [CrossRef] [PubMed]
6. Demirci, H.; Elner, V.M. Double silicone tube intubation for the management of partial lacrimal system obstruction. *Ophthalmology* **2008**, *115*, 383–385. [CrossRef] [PubMed]
7. Connell, P.P.; Fulcher, T.P.; Chacko, E.; O'Connor, M.J.; Moriarty, P. Long term follow up of nasolacrimal intubation in adults. *Br. J. Ophthalmol.* **2006**, *90*, 435–436. [CrossRef]
8. Liu, D.; Bosley, T.M. Silicone nasolacrimal intubation with mitomycin-C: A prospective, randomized, double-masked study. *Ophthalmology* **2003**, *110*, 306–310. [CrossRef]
9. Inatani, M.; Yamauchi, T.; Fukuchi, M.; Denno, S.; Miki, M. Direct silicone intubation using Nunchaku-style tube (NST-DSI) to treat lacrimal passage obstruction. *Acta Ophthalmol. Scand.* **2000**, *78*, 689–693. [CrossRef]
10. Fulcher, T.; O'Connor, M.; Moriarty, P. Nasolacrimal intubation in adults. *Br. J. Ophthalmol.* **1998**, *82*, 1039–1041. [CrossRef]
11. Khoubian, J.F.; Kikkawa, D.O.; Gonnering, R.S. Trephination and silicone stent intubation for the treatment of canalicular obstruction: Effect of the level of obstruction. *Ophthalmic Plast. Reconstr. Surg.* **2006**, *22*, 248–252. [CrossRef] [PubMed]
12. Mimura, M.; Ueki, M.; Oku, H.; Sato, B.; Ikeda, T. Indications for and effects of Nunchaku-style silicone tube intubation for primary acquired lacrimal drainage obstruction. *Jpn. J. Ophthalmol.* **2015**, *59*, 266–272. [CrossRef]
13. Sasaki, T.; Sounou, T.; Sugiyama, K. Dacryoendoscopic surgery and tube insertion in patients with common canalicular obstruction and ductal stenosis as a frequent complication. *Jpn. J. Ophthalmol.* **2009**, *53*, 145–150. [CrossRef] [PubMed]
14. Matsumura, N.; Suzuki, T.; Goto, S.; Fujita, T.; Yamane, S.; Maruyama-Inoue, M.; Kadonosono, K. Transcanalicular endoscopic primary dacryoplasty for congenital nasolacrimal duct obstruction. *Eye* **2019**, *33*, 1008–1013. [CrossRef] [PubMed]
15. Sasaki, T.; Nagata, Y.; Sugiyama, K. Nasolacrimal duct obstruction classified by dacryoendoscopy and treated with inferior meatal dacryorhinotomy. Part I: Positional diagnosis of primary nasolacrimal duct obstruction with dacryoendoscope. *Am. J. Ophthalmol.* **2005**, *140*, 1065–1069. [CrossRef]
16. Sugimoto, M. New sheath-assisted dacryoendoscopic surgery. *J. Eye* **2007**, *24*, 1219–1222. (In Japanese)
17. Inoue, Y. New method of lacrimal passage intubation using Teflon sheath as guide. *J. Eye* **2008**, *25*, 1131–1133. (In Japanese)
18. Fukuda, R.; Usui, T.; Miyai, T.; Yamagami, S.; Amano, S. Tear meniscus evaluation by anterior segment swept-source optical coherence tomography. *Am. J. Ophthalmol.* **2013**, *155*, 620–624. [CrossRef]
19. Ohtomo, K.; Ueta, T.; Fukuda, R.; Usui, T.; Miyai, T.; Shirakawa, R.; Amano, S.; Nagahara, M. Tear meniscus volume changes in dacryocystorhinostomy evaluated with quantitative measurement using anterior segment optical coherence tomography. *Investig. Ophthalmol. Vis. Sci.* **2014**, *55*, 2057–2061. [CrossRef]
20. Pomerance, G.N.; Evans, D.W. Test-retest reliability of the CSV-1000 contrast test and its relationship to glaucoma therapy. *Investig. Ophthalmol. Vis. Sci.* **1994**, *35*, 3357–3361.

21. Applegate, R.A.; Howland, H.C.; Sharp, R.P.; Cottingham, A.J.; Yee, R.W. Corneal aberrations and visual performance after radial keratotomy. *J. Refract. Surg.* **1998**, *14*, 397–407. [CrossRef] [PubMed]
22. Richman, J.; Spaeth, G.L.; Wirostko, B. Contrast sensitivity basics and a critique of currently available tests. *J. Cataract. Refract. Surg.* **2013**, *39*, 1100–1106. [CrossRef] [PubMed]
23. Koh, S.; Maeda, N.; Ikeda, C.; Asonuma, S.; Ogawa, M.; Hiraoka, T.; Oshika, T.; Nishida, T. The effect of ocular surface regularity on contrast sensitivity and straylight in dry eye. *Investig. Ophthalmol. Vis. Sci.* **2017**, *58*, 2647–2651. [CrossRef]
24. Oshika, T.; Tokunaga, T.; Samejima, T.; Miyata, K.; Kawana, K.; Kaji, Y. Influence of pupil diameter on the relation between ocular higher-order aberration and contrast sensitivity after laser in situ keratomileusis. *Investig. Ophthalmol. Vis. Sci.* **2006**, *47*, 1334–1338. [CrossRef]
25. Akin, T.; Karadayi, K.; Aykan, U.; Certel, I.; Hamdi Bilge, A. The effects of artificial tear application on contrast sensitivity in dry and normal eyes. *Eur. J. Ophthalmol.* **2006**, *16*, 785–790. [CrossRef]
26. Ridder, W.H., III; Tomlinson, A.; Paugh, J. Effect of artificial tears on visual performance in subjects with dry eye. *Optom. Vis. Sci.* **2005**, *82*, 835–842. [CrossRef] [PubMed]
27. Fowler, B.T.; Pegram, T.A.; Cutler-Peck, C.; Kosko, M.; Tran, Q.T.; Fleming, J.C.; Oester, A.E., Jr. Contrast sensitivity testing in functional ptosis and dermatochalasis surgery. *Ophthalmic Plast. Reconstr. Surg.* **2015**, *31*, 272–274. [CrossRef]
28. Qiu, W.; Zhang, M.; Xu, T.; Liu, Z.; Lv, H.; Wang, W.; Li, X. Evaluation of the effects of conjunctivochalasis excision on tear stability and contrast sensitivity. *Sci. Rep.* **2016**, *6*, 37570. [CrossRef]
29. Oshika, T.; Arai, H.; Fujita, Y.; Inamura, M.; Inoue, Y.; Noda, T.; Miyata, K. One-year clinical evaluation of rotationally asymmetric mutifocal intraocular lens with +1.5 diopters near addition. *Sci. Rep.* **2019**, *9*, 13117. [CrossRef]
30. Okamoto, F.; Sugiura, Y.; Okamoto, Y.; Hiraoka, T.; Oshika, T. Changes in contrast sensitivity after surgery for macula-on rhegmatogenous retinal detachment. *Am. J. Ophthalmol.* **2013**, *156*, 667–672. [CrossRef] [PubMed]
31. Sugiura, Y.; Okamoto, F.; Okamoto, Y.; Hiraoka, T.; Oshika, T. Contrast sensitivity and foveal microstructure following vitrectomy for epiretinal membrane. *Investig. Ophthalmol. Vis. Sci.* **2014**, *55*, 7594–7600. [CrossRef] [PubMed]
32. Mano, F.; LoBue, S.A.; Eno, A.; Chang, K.C.; Mano, T. Impact of posterior vitreous detachment on contrast sensitivity in patients with multifocal intraocular lens. *Graefe's Arch. Clin. Exp. Ophthalmol.* **2020**. [CrossRef] [PubMed]
33. Okamoto, F.; Okamoto, Y.; Fukuda, S.; Hiraoka, T.; Oshika, T. Vision-related quality of life and visual function after vitrectomy for various vitreoretinal disorders. *Investig. Ophthalmol. Vis. Sci.* **2010**, *51*, 744–751. [CrossRef] [PubMed]
34. Asano, H.; Ogami, T.; Iguchi, A.; Sano, M.; Yamada, Y.; Hiraoka, T.; Oshika, T. Efficacy and safety of diquafosol ophthalmic solution for soft contact lens-related dry eye. *Investig. Ophthalmol. Vis. Sci.* **2018**, *59*, 1788.
35. Hiraoka, T.; Daito, M.; Okamoto, F.; Kiuchi, T.; Oshika, T. Contrast sensitivity and optical quality of the eye after instillation of timolol maleate gel-forming solution and brinzolamide ophthalmic suspension. *Ophthalmology* **2010**, *117*, 2080–2087. [CrossRef]
36. Pinilla, I.; Fernandez-Prieto, A.F.; Asencio, M.; Arbizu, A.; Pelaez, N.; Frutos, R. Nasolacrimal stents for the treatment of epiphora: Technical problems and long-term results. *Orbit* **2006**, *25*, 75–81. [CrossRef]

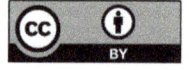

© 2020 by the authors. Licensee MDPI, Basel, Switzerland. This article is an open access article distributed under the terms and conditions of the Creative Commons Attribution (CC BY) license (http://creativecommons.org/licenses/by/4.0/).

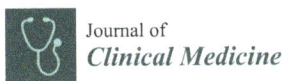

Article

Difference in Pupillary Diameter as an Important Factor for Evaluating Amplitude of Accommodation: A Prospective Observational Study

Miyuki Kubota [1,2,3,*], Shunsuke Kubota [1,2,3], Hidenaga Kobashi [1,3], Masahiko Ayaki [1,4], Kazuno Negishi [1,*] and Kazuo Tsubota [1,5]

1. Department of Ophthalmology, Keio University School of Medicine, Tokyo 160-8582, Japan; shun_kubota@keio.jp (S.K.); hidenaga_kobashi@keio.jp (H.K.); mayaki@olive.ocn.ne.jp (M.A.); tsubota@z3.keio.jp (K.T.)
2. Department of Ophthalmology, Shonan Keiiku Hospital, Kanagawa 252-0816, Japan
3. Graduate School of Media and Governance, Keio University, Kanagawa 252-0882, Japan
4. Department of Ophthalmology, Otake Clinic Moon View Eye Center, Kanagawa 224-0001, Japan
5. Tsubota Laboratory, Inc., Tokyo 160-0016, Japan
* Correspondence: myu.kubota@keio.jp (M.K.); kazunonegishi@keio.jp (K.N.)

Received: 8 July 2020; Accepted: 15 August 2020; Published: 18 August 2020

Abstract: Presbyopia is increasing globally due to aging and the widespread use of visual display terminals. Presbyopia is a decrease in the eye's amplitude of accommodation (AA) due to loss of crystalline lens elasticity. AA differs widely among individuals. We aimed to determine the factors that cause presbyopia, other than advanced age, for early medical intervention. We examined 95 eyes of 95 healthy volunteers (33 men, 62 women) aged 22–62 years (mean: 37.22 ± 9.77 years) with a corrected visual acuity of ≥1.0 and without other eye afflictions except ametropia. Subjective refraction, AA, maximum and minimum pupillary diameters during accommodation, axial length of the eye, and crystalline lens thickness were measured. AA was measured using an auto refractometer/keratometer/tonometer/pachymeter. The difference between maximum and minimum pupillary diameters was calculated. On multiple regression analysis, age and difference in pupillary diameter were both significantly and independently associated with AA in participants aged <44 years, but not in those aged ≥45 years. Our results suggest that the difference in pupillary diameter could be an important age-independent factor for evaluating AA in healthy individuals without cataract. Thus, improving the difference in pupillary diameter values could be an early treatment target for presbyopia.

Keywords: amplitude of accommodation; pupillary diameter; presbyopia; cataract; crystalline lens; subjective refraction; axial length of the eye

1. Introduction

Presbyopia is defined as a decrease in the amplitude of accommodation (AA) of the eye resulting from the loss of elasticity in the crystalline lens. The aging of society has increased the number of people with presbyopia to 1.37 billion in 2020, which is predicted to reach 1.8 billion by 2050 [1]. The number of patients with asthenopia, neck stiffness, and headache due to the non-correction or under-correction of presbyopia has also been increasing [2–6], likely in part because of the widespread use of visual display terminals (VDTs) [7]. Furthermore, the worldwide loss in gross domestic product (GDP) due to the non-correction or under-correction of presbyopia in individuals younger than 65 years old was reported to be $25 billion in 2011, which is equivalent to 0.037% of the GDP [1]. This attests to the gravity of this social problem.

AA gradually decreases from early childhood, with a linear decline observed from 20 to 50 years of age [8,9]. Although subjective symptoms of presbyopia are confirmed from around the age of 40 years, large individual variations are known to occur [10–12]. In addition to aging, which is the greatest risk factor for the decline in AA, hypermetropia [13], temperature [14,15], female sex [13,16,17], diabetes [15], alcohol intake [13], smoking [18,19], and laser-assisted in situ keratomileusis [20] have also been implicated.

Methods for presbyopia correction include reading glasses, multifocal or monovision contact lenses, and refractive surgeries. In terms of medical treatments, pirenoxine was reported to be useful in preventing progression of presbyopia [19]. There have also been reports of supplements such as Enkin® (a food product containing lutein), astaxanthin [21], docosahexaenoic acid, and composite antioxidants [22] as well as thermotherapy [23] for presbyopia correction. However, no perfect treatment has yet been developed.

Pupillary diameter is an important optical factor in accommodation. However, it has not been fully evaluated in presbyopia. We hypothesized that the dynamics of pupillary diameter may be associated with the AA in addition to conventionally recognized parameters including age, sex, lens thickness, axial length, and refraction. In this study, we aimed to identify factors affecting AA in the normal population by analyzing the data of various ocular examinations.

2. Materials and Methods

2.1. Participants

In this prospective observational study, the left eyes of 95 healthy participants aged 22–62 years, with no ocular complications other than ametropia, were studied from August 2019 until January 2020. Participants with a corrected distance visual acuity (CDVA) in the logarithm of minimal angle resolution [logMAR (CDVA)] worse than 0.0 were excluded from the study. The participants were further divided according to age, with those 45 years of age and over in one group (older group) and those under 45 years of age in the other group (young group), since most people are aware of presbyopia by the age of 45 as their AA drops to 3 diopter level [10]. This study was approved by the ethics committee at Shonan Keiiku Hospital and was conducted with the written consent of all participants, in accordance with the Declaration of Helsinki.

2.2. Ocular Examinations

The subjective refraction, CDVA, AA, maximum and minimum pupillary diameters during accommodation, axial length of the eye, and crystalline lens thickness were measured for all participants. AA was measured using an auto refractometer/keratometer/tonometer/pachymeter (TONOREF III®; NIDEK, Tokyo, Japan). The maximum and minimum pupillary diameters were also measured simultaneously using the same device. The subjects were instructed to look at the internal target of TONOREF III® monocularly without the aid of contact lenses or glasses. While the target was moving closer from the initial position, continuous measurement of refraction and pupil size was performed concomitantly, at up to 30 s. All measurements were obtained firstly from the right and then from the left eye. Since the measurement values of the left eye were determined to be optimal based on a preliminary study, the analysis was performed using the results of the left eye. The difference in pupillary diameter (DPD) was defined as the difference between the maximum and minimum pupillary diameters during the measurement of AA. Axial length and crystalline lens thickness were measured using the IOL Master 700® (Carl Zeiss Meditec AG, Jena, Germany).

2.3. Measurement of AA and Pupillary Diameter by TONOREF III®

The subjects were instructed to look at the internal target of TONOREF III® monocularly, and the objective refraction was measured first. Next, the target was moved from the initial position closer to the eye, and the continuous measurement of refraction and pupil size was performed concomitantly. At up to 30 s the accommodation amplitude (AA) was calculated automatically by subtracting the initial objective refraction (i.e., the minimum refraction) from the maximum refraction during measurement. Therefore, AA could be measured using this device regardless of the subject's refractive error. The representative results of AA and pupillary diameters using TONOREF III® are shown in Figure 1.

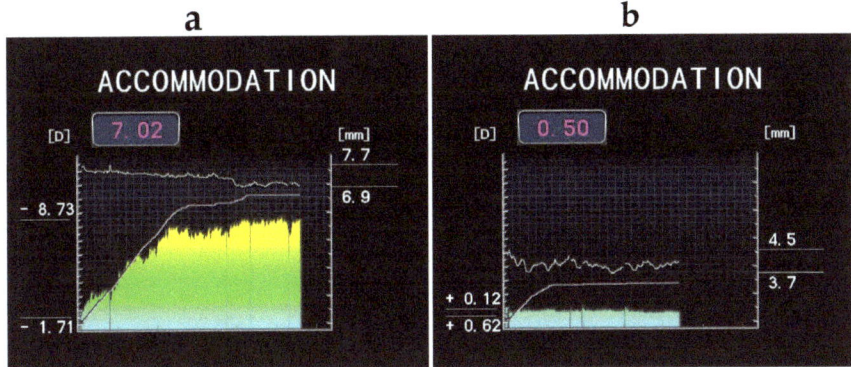

Figure 1. Representative results of the amplitude of accommodation (AA) and pupillary diameters measured by TONOREF III®; (**a**) 25-year-old female, 7.02 D of AA; (**b**) 53-year-old female, 0.50 D of AA. The X-axis represents an examination time of up to 30 s. The left Y-axis represents refraction, and the right Y-axis represents the pupil diameter during measurement. The upper wave is a continuously recorded pupillary diameter. The colored bars represent the real-time refraction, and the line chart represents the internal target position. The values on the left Y-axis are the maximum and minimum refraction values, and the magnitude calculated as AA (D) is shown in the upper square. The minimum refraction value represents refraction when the visual target is located in the initial position. The values on the right Y-axis are the maximum and minimum pupillary diameters.

2.4. Statistical Analysis

The distributions of the continuous variables are presented as mean ± standard deviations. Student's *t*-test was used to compare differences in normally distributed clinical parameters including age, CDVA, crystalline lens thickness, maximum pupillary diameter, and minimum pupillary diameter between the young and old groups. The Mann-Whitney U test was used to compare the non-normally distributed clinical parameters, such as subjective refraction, AA, axial length, and DPD, between the young and older groups. The chi-square test was used to compare sex between the young and older groups [24–26]. For these 10 factors, our null hypothesis was that there is no difference between the younger and older group. A single regression analysis was used to investigate the correlation between age and AA, DPD and AA, age and DPD. For multiple regression analysis, AA was used as the dependent variable, and age, sex, axial length, crystalline lens thickness, subjective refraction, and DPD were used as explanatory variables. Multiple regression analysis with interaction term was used to indicate whether the multiple significant factors obtained from a multivariate analysis were independent. If the significant factors were independent, the two items indicated by x are $p \geq 0.05$ in interaction term. All analyses were conducted using SPSS version 25 for Windows (IBM Corp., Armonk, NY, USA). A *p*-value of <0.05 was considered statistically significant.

3. Results

3.1. Participant Profiles and Results of Ocular Examinations

The participant profiles and results of the ocular examinations are presented in Table 1. There were significant differences in age, AA, crystalline lens thickness, maximum pupillary diameter, minimum pupillary diameter, and DPD between the two groups. Subjective refraction, CDVA, and axial length were not significantly different between the two groups.

Table 1. Participant profiles and results of ocular examinations.

	All	Young Group (<45 Years Old)	Older Group (≥45 Years Old)	p-Value (Young vs. Old)
Number of eyes	95	70	25	-
Age (range)	22–62	22–44	45–62	<0.01 *
Sex (male/female)	33/62	30/40	3/22	<0.01 ***
Subjective refraction (D)	−2.85 ± 2.53	−2.88 ± 2.33	−2.77 ± 3.10	0.333 **
AA (D)	3.19 ± 2.27	4.04 ± 2.00	0.74 ± 0.50	<0.01 **
CDVA	−0.10 ± 0.05	−0.11 ± 0.06	−0.10 ± 0.04	0.359 *
Axial length (mm)	24.53 ± 2.65	24.74 ± 1.23	23.94 ± 4.64	0.745 **
Crystalline lens thickness (mm)	3.93 ± 0.37	3.81 ± 0.31	4.27 ± 0.29	<0.01 *
Maximum pupillary diameter (mm)	5.65 ± 0.91	5.94 ± 0.74	4.93 ± 0.81	<0.01 *
Minimum pupillary diameter (mm)	4.58 ± 1.02	4.76 ± 1.01	4.06 ± 0.92	<0.01 *
DPD (mm)	1.07 ± 0.55	1.17 ± 0.58	0.87 ± 0.59	<0.01 **

AA, amplitude of accommodation; CDVA, corrected distance visual acuity in the logarithm of minimal angle resolution (logMAR (CDVA)); DPD, difference in pupillary diameter; *, p-value in Student's t test; **, p-value in Mann-Whitney U test; ***, p-value in chi-square test; -, not calculated. From the test based on the null hypothesis, age, AA, crystalline lens thickness, maximum pupillary diameter, minimum pupillary diameter, and DPD were rejected since they were significant between the two groups.

3.2. Single Regression Analyses among AA, Age, and DPD in All Participants

The results of the single regression analyses among AA, age, and DPD are presented in Figure 2. There were significant correlations between age and AA (Figure 2a; correlation coefficient: −0.771, $p < 0.001$), age and DPD (Figure 2b; correlation coefficient: −0.420, $p < 0.001$), and DPD and AA (Figure 2c; correlation coefficient: 0.634, $p < 0.001$).

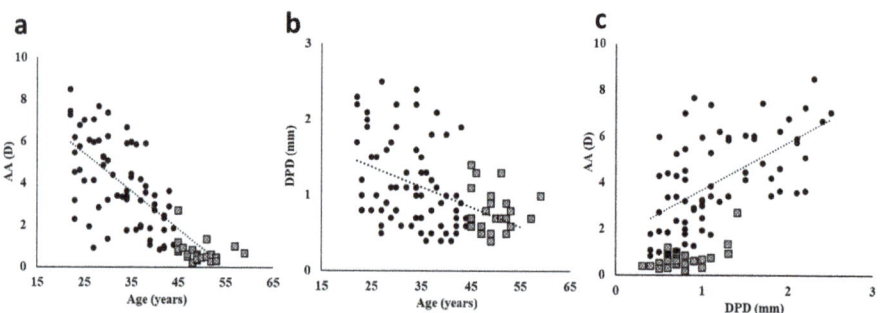

Figure 2. Single correlation curve of age and accommodation in 95 participants. (**a**) AA vs age (correlation coefficient, −0.771; $p \leq 0.01$; (**b**) AA vs. DPD (correlation coefficient, −0.420; $p \leq 0.01$); and (**c**) DPD vs. age (correlation coefficient, 0.634; $p \leq 0.01$). AA: amplitude of accommodation, DPD: difference in pupillary diameter. ●, young group; □, older group.

3.3. Factors Affecting AA in All Participants

Table 2 shows the results of the multiple regression analysis in all 95 participants. We found that DPD correlated positively with AA (standardized β coefficient (Std β) = 0.365, $t = 5.885$, $p < 0.001$), while age had a significant negative correlation with AA (Std β = −0.543, t = −6.046, p < 0.001). Table 3 shows the results of the multiple regression analysis with interaction term. The results show that DPD and age did not interact with each other (p = 0.506); i.e., they were significant and independent factors influencing AA.

Table 2. Multiple regression analysis in all participants (n = 95 and adjusted R^2 = 0.712).

	Unstandardized		Standardized			95% CI	
	B	SE	Beta	t	p	Lower	Upper
(Constant)	7.345	2.113		3.476	0.001	3.145	11.546
Age	−0.126	0.021	−0.543	−6.046	<0.01 **	−0.168	−0.085
Sex	0.277	0.291	0.058	0.951	0.344	−0.302	0.856
Axial length	−0.058	0.052	−0.065	−1.116	0.268	−0.163	0.046
Crystalline lens thickness	0.049	0.049	0.056	0.990	0.325	−0.049	0.147
Subjective refraction	−0.672	0.536	−0.109	−1.255	0.213	−1.738	0.393
DPD	1.513	0.257	0.365	5.885	<0.01 **	1.002	2.024

Dependent variable: amplitude of accommodation. CI, confidence interval; B, partial regression coefficient; SE, standard error; DPD, difference in pupillary diameter; **, p < 0.01.

Table 3. Multiple regression analysis with interaction term (adjusted R^2 = 0.703).

Source	Type III Sum of Squares	df	Mean Square	F	p
Corrected model	344.983	3	114.994	75.098	0.000
Intercept	43.455	1	43.455	28.379	0.000
Age	26.344	1	26.344	17.204	0.000
DPD	7.691	1	7.691	5.023	0.027
Age × DPD	0.682	1	0.682	0.446	0.506
Error	139.344	86	1.531		
Total	1440.115	94			

df, degree of freedom; F, the ratio of mean square for each factor to that of the error; DPD, difference in pupillary diameter.

3.4. Factors Affecting AA in the Young and Older Groups

Table 4 shows the results of the multiple regression analysis in the 70 participants who were under 45 years of age. The results showed that DPD had a significant positive correlation with AA (Std β = 0.438, t = 5.246, p < 0.001), meaning that people with greater differences in pupil size during accommodation also have a higher amplitude of accommodation. On the other hand, age had a significant negative correlation with AA (Std β = −0.395, t = −3.729, p < 0.001). Table 5 shows the results of the interaction term. The results showed that age and DPD were significant and independent factors that influenced AA in participants under 45 years of age.

Table 4. Multiple regression analysis in the young group (22–44 years old, $n = 70$ and adjusted $R^2 = 0.579$).

	Unstandardized		Standardized			95% CI	
	B	SE	Beta	t	p	Lower	Upper
(Constant)	5.581	3.833		1.456	0.150	−2.080	13.242
Age	−0.120	0.032	−0.395	−3.729	<0.01 **	−0.185	−0.056
Sex	0.596	0.349	0.148	1.709	0.092	−0.101	1.293
Axial length	−0.090	0.072	−0.104	−1.246	0.217	−0.233	0.054
Crystalline lens thickness	0.174	0.137	0.106	1.271	0.209	−0.100	0.448
Subjective refraction	−1.129	0.659	−0.176	−1.714	0.091	−2.446	0.187
DPD	1.513	0.288	0.438	5.246	<0.01 **	0.937	2.090

Dependent variable: amplitude of accommodation. CI, confidence interval; B, partial regression coefficient; SE, standard error; DPD, difference in pupillary diameter; **, $p < 0.01$.

Table 5. Multiple regression analysis with interaction term (adjusted $R^2 = 0.523$).

Source	Type III Sum of Squares	df	Mean Square	F	p
Corrected model	150.366a	3	50.122	26.212	0.000
Intercept	23.866	1	23.866	12.481	0.001
Age	12.427	1	12.427	6.499	0.013
DPD	1.676	1	1.676	0.876	0.353
Age × DPD	0.054	1	0.054	0.028	0.867
Error	126.203	66	1.912		
Total	1420.617	70			
Corrected total	276.570	69			

df, degree of freedom; F, the ratio of mean square for each factor to that of the error; DPD, difference in pupillary diameter. Age significantly correlated with the amplitude of accommodation, and the age variables were independent of each other.

Table 6 shows the results of the multiple regression analysis in the 25 participants aged 45 years and over. The results showed that DPD had a significant positive correlation with AA (Std β = 0.589, $t = 3.285$, $p < 0.01$), indicating that a greater difference in pupil size during accommodation is present in individuals with a higher amplitude of accommodation. Unlike the results presented in Tables 2–5, age did not have a negative correlation with AA (Std β = −0.013, $t = −0.069$, $p = 0.946$).

Table 6. Multiple regression analysis in the older group (45–62 years old, $n = 25$ and adjusted $R^2 = 0.427$).

	Unstandardized		Standardized			95% CI	
	B	SE	Beta	t	p	Lower	Upper
(Constant)	3.027	1.628		1.859	0.079	−0.394	6.447
Age	−0.001	0.021	−0.013	−0.069	0.946	−0.046	0.043
Sex	−0.483	0.265	−0.319	−1.823	0.085	−1.040	0.074
Axial length	−0.025	0.029	−0.155	−0.873	0.394	−0.087	0.036
Crystalline lens thickness	−0.008	0.017	−0.073	−0.461	0.650	−0.044	0.028
Subjective refraction	−0.581	0.380	−0.330	−1.526	0.144	−1.380	0.219
DPD	1.043	0.317	0.589	3.285	< 0.01 **	0.376	1.710

Dependent variable: amplitude of accommodation. CI, confidence interval; B, partial regression coefficient; SE, standard error; DPD, difference in pupillary diameter; **, $p < 0.01$.

4. Discussion

Conventionally, age was thought to be the sole factor affecting AA in normal populations. In this study, we found that DPD correlated significantly with AA, and this relationship was independent of age. Therefore, we believe that DPD can be a new indicator of AA in addition to age.

The pupil has two functional roles. The first role is the light reflex, characterized by pupil constriction in response to light, which adjusts the amount of light that enters the eyeball. The second role is miosis, which is one element of the near reflex (consisting of miosis, convergence, and lens accommodation). The latency of the light reflex increases with advancing age [27]. Conversely, miotic latency associated with the near reflex does not increase with age [28,29]. Even when presbyopia has completely developed, accommodative reaction to near stimuli is maintained [29]. The pupillary sphincter, which is responsible for miosis, is controlled by the parasympathetic nervous system. Like the ciliary ring muscles that tense during accommodation, this muscle has muscarinic M3 receptors. The function of the ciliary muscles is preserved in elderly individuals [30]. It has been reported that even in cases of intraocular lens (IOL) insertion in elderly individuals, the ciliary muscle function is maintained [30]. Other reports have indicated that the force of contraction of the ciliary muscle increases until the fifth decade of life [31].

Although most people worldwide are susceptible to age-related changes of presbyopia, certain ethnicities seem to have some inherent advantages. The Moken people of southeast Asia have good visual acuity, even while diving in the dark ocean [32]. Normally, the corneal refractive power is lost underwater, and objects appear blurry. However, it appears that the Moken people can deepen their focal length by constricting their pupils for focus adjustment. Gislen et al. [33] reported that the underwater visual acuity of European children improved after they engaged in training sessions to constrict their pupils underwater. In addition, Weng et al. recently reported that the change in pupillary diameter was correlated with AA [34]. However, the number of subjects in Weng's study was small (35 subjects), and the interaction or dependence between age and the change in pupillary diameter is not yet elucidated [34]. The current study is the first study enrolling a large number of cases to reveal that pupillary diameter is strongly correlated with AA and that individual differences are involved in presbyopia, independent of age.

Importantly, we found that age did not correlate with AA in the older group, probably because the decrease in AA had almost plateaued in this group (Figure 2a, closed square plots). In contrast, DPD strongly correlated with AA in the older group. These results suggested that DPD is a key factor for determining AA, especially in older individuals. Future research should address the treatment of presbyopia to develop a method to increase DPD, considering that an accommodative reaction to near stimuli is maintained even when presbyopia has completely developed [29], and the function of the ciliary muscles is preserved in elderly individuals [30]. Individual differences in AA are large [10–12], but the reason remains unknown. Furthermore, it has been reported that the use of digital devices decreases AA even in young individuals [5,35,36]. The differences in DPD might be a reasonable explanation of those cases, and this should be addressed in future studies.

Our study has some limitations. We measured AA monocularly, and we did not check convergence. DPD and AA are considered to be a part of the near reflex, and their relationship might be influenced by abnormal convergence. In addition, the number of subjects with fully developed presbyopia, i.e., over age 50, was small. These subjects warrant further investigation. Furthermore, DPD in Table 5 was not significant in the interaction term; however, it was significant on multiple regression analysis. When the main effect in a general multiple regression analysis is not significant, the interaction term cannot be subsequently examined. The results of the main effect in multiple regression analysis are adopted in covariance analysis, which is used to examine the interaction term. Table 4 shows the results of the multiple regression analysis, while Table 5 shows those of the covariance analysis. Since the statistical methods used for these results differ slightly, it is possible that the results may vary. In any case, the data in Tables 4–6 are still auxiliary to the main results in Tables 2 and 3. In conclusion, this study revealed that DPD is an important independent factor other than age that affects AA in all age groups. Therefore, increasing DPD using various methods, such as exercises or medications, might be a new option for the treatment of presbyopia.

Author Contributions: Conceptualization, M.K., K.N. and K.T.; Methodology, M.K., K.N. and S.K.; Software, M.K.; Validation, M.K. and K.N.; Formal Analysis, M.K. and K.N.; Investigation, M.K. and S.K.; Resources, K.T.; Data Curation, M.K., H.K., and K.N.; Writing—Original Draft Preparation, M.K.; Writing—Review & Editing, K.N. and M.A.; Visualization, M.K. and K.N.; Supervision, K.N. and K.T.; Project Administration, M.K. and S.K.; Funding Acquisition, K.T. All authors have read and agreed to the published version of the manuscript.

Funding: This research received no external funding.

Acknowledgments: We are grateful to Ryo Takemura, for the statistical suggestions.

Conflicts of Interest: K.T. reports he is CEO of Tsubota Laboratory, Inc., Tokyo, Japan, a company developing products for the treatment for presbyopia. The reward for participants and the rendering service of a certified orthoptist were provided by Tsubota Lab Inc. The sponsors had no role in the design, execution, interpretation, or writing of the study. The remaining authors declare that they have no conflict of interests.

References

1. Fricke, T.R.; Tahhan, N.; Resnikoff, S.; Papas, E.; Burnett, A.; Ho, S.M.; Naduvilath, T.; Naidoo, K.S. Global Prevalence of Presbyopia and Vision Impairment from Uncorrected Presbyopia: Systematic Review, Meta-analysis, and Modelling. *Ophthalmology* **2018**, *125*, 1492–1499. [CrossRef]
2. Coles-Brennan, C.; Sulley, A.; Young, G. Management of digital eye strain. *Clin. Exp. Optom.* **2019**, *102*, 18–29. [CrossRef]
3. Rosenfield, M. Computer vision syndrome: A review of ocular causes and potential treatments. *Ophthalmic. Physiol. Opt.* **2011**, *31*, 502–515. [CrossRef]
4. Blehm, C.; Vishnu, S.; Khattak, A.; Mitra, S.; Yee, R.W. Computer vision syndrome: A review. *Surv. Ophthalmol.* **2005**, *50*, 253–262. [CrossRef]
5. Kosehira, M.; Machida, N.; Kitaichi, N. A 12-Week-Long Intake of Bilberry Extract (*Vaccinium myrtillus* L.) Improved Objective Findings of Ciliary Muscle Contraction of the Eye: A Randomized, Double-Blind, Placebo-Controlled, Parallel-Group Comparison Trial. *Nutrients* **2020**, *12*, 600. [CrossRef]
6. Jaschinski, W.; Konig, M.; Mekontso, T.M.; Ohlendorf, A.; Welscher, M. Computer vision syndrome in presbyopia and beginning presbyopia: Effects of spectacle lens type. *Clin. Exp. Optom.* **2015**, *98*, 228–233. [CrossRef]
7. Ministry of Internal Affairs and Communications of Japan 2019. Available online: https://www.soumu.go.jp/main_sosiki/joho_tsusin/eng/Releases/Telecommunications/2019_07_09_2.html (accessed on 1 July 2020).
8. Anderson, H.A.; Glasser, A.; Manny, R.E.; Stuebing, K.K. Age-related changes in accommodative dynamics from preschool to adulthood. *Investig. Ophthalmol. Vis. Sci.* **2010**, *51*, 614–622. [CrossRef] [PubMed]
9. Charman, W.N. The eye in focus: Accommodation and presbyopia. *Clin. Exp. Optom.* **2008**, *91*, 207–225. [CrossRef] [PubMed]
10. Duane, A. Studies in Monocular and Binocular Accommodation, with Their Clinical Application. *Trans. Am. Ophthalmol. Soc.* **1922**, *20*, 132–157. [CrossRef]
11. Jackson, E. Amplitude of Accommodation at Different Periods of Life. *Cal. State. J. Med.* **1907**, *5*, 163–166. [PubMed]
12. Lopez-Alcon, D.; Marin-Franch, I.; Fernandez-Sanchez, V.; Lopez-Gil, N. Optical factors influencing the amplitude of accommodation. *Vis. Res.* **2016**, *141*, 16–22. [CrossRef] [PubMed]
13. Nirmalan, P.K.; Krishnaiah, S.; Shamanna, B.R.; Rao, G.N.; Thomas, R. A population-based assessment of presbyopia in the state of Andhra Pradesh, south India: The Andhra Pradesh Eye Disease Study. *Investig. Ophthalmol. Vis. Sci.* **2006**, *47*, 2324–2328. [CrossRef] [PubMed]
14. Jain, I.S.; Ram, J.; Gupta, A. Early onset of presbyopia. *Am. J. Optom. Physiol. Opt.* **1982**, *59*, 1002–1004. [CrossRef] [PubMed]
15. Weale, R.A. Epidemiology of refractive errors and presbyopia. *Surv. Ophthalmol.* **2003**, *48*, 515–543. [CrossRef]
16. Pointer, J.S. The presbyopic add. II. Age-related trend and a gender difference. *Ophthalmic. Physiol. Opt.* **1995**, *15*, 241–248. [CrossRef]
17. Hickenbotham, A.; Roorda, A.; Steinmaus, C.; Glasser, A. Meta-analysis of sex differences in presbyopia. *Investig. Ophthalmol. Vis. Sci.* **2012**, *53*, 3215–3220. [CrossRef]
18. Andualem, H.B.; Assefa, N.L.; Weldemichael, D.Z.; Tefera, T.K. Prevalence and associated factors of presbyopia among school teachers in Gondar city, Northwest Ethiopia, 2016. *Clin. Optom.* **2017**, *9*, 85–90. [CrossRef]

19. Tsuneyoshi, Y.; Higuchi, A.; Negishi, K.; Tsubota, K. Suppression of presbyopia progression with pirenoxine eye drops: Experiments on rats and non-blinded, randomized clinical trial of efficacy. *Sci. Rep.* **2017**, *7*, 6819. [CrossRef]
20. Tsuneyoshi, Y.; Negishi, K.; Saiki, M.; Toda, I.; Tsubota, K. Apparent progression of presbyopia after laser in situ keratomileusis in patients with early presbyopia. *Am. J. Ophthalmol.* **2014**, *158*, 286–292. [CrossRef]
21. Kono, K.; Shimizu, Y.; Takahashi, S.; Matsuoka, S.; Yui, K. Effect of Multiple Dietary Supplement Containing Lutein, Astaxanthin, Cyanidin-3-glucoside, and DHA on Accommodative Ability. *Immunol. Endocr. Metab. Agent Med. Chem.* **2014**, *14*, 114–125. [CrossRef]
22. Uchino, Y.; Uchino, M.; Dogru, M.; Fukagawa, K.; Tsubota, K. Improvement of accommodation with anti-oxidant supplementation in visual display terminal users. *J. Nutr. Health Aging* **2012**, *16*, 478–481. [CrossRef] [PubMed]
23. Takahashi, Y.; Igaki, M.; Suzuki, A.; Takahashi, G.; Dogru, M.; Tsubota, K. The effect of periocular warming on accommodation. *Ophthalmology* **2005**, *112*, 1113–1118. [CrossRef] [PubMed]
24. Neely, J.G.; Hartman, J.M.; Forsen, J.W., Jr.; Wallace, M.S. Tutorials in clinical research: VII. Understanding comparative statistics (contrast)–part B: Application of T-test, Mann-Whitney U, and chi-square. *Laryngoscope* **2003**, *113*, 1719–1725. [CrossRef] [PubMed]
25. De Muth, J.E. Overview of biostatistics used in clinical research. *Am. J. Health Syst. Pharm.* **2009**, *66*, 70–81. [CrossRef] [PubMed]
26. Negishi, K.; Hayashi, K.; Kamiya, K.; Sato, M.; Bissen-Miyajima, H. Survey Working Group of the Japanese Society of, C.; Refractive, S., Nationwide Prospective Cohort Study on Cataract Surgery With Multifocal Intraocular Lens Implantation in Japan. *Am. J. Ophthalmol.* **2019**, *208*, 133–144. [CrossRef]
27. Lobato-Rincon, L.L.; Cabanillas-Campos Mdel, C.; Bonnin-Arias, C.; Chamorro-Gutierrez, E.; Murciano-Cespedosa, A.; Sanchez-Ramos Roda, C. Pupillary behavior in relation to wavelength and age. *Front. Hum. Neurosci.* **2014**, *8*, 221.
28. Kasthurirangan, S.; Glasser, A. Age related changes in the characteristics of the near pupil response. *Vis. Res.* **2006**, *46*, 1393–1403. [CrossRef]
29. Heron, G.; Charman, W.N.; Schor, C. Dynamics of the accommodation response to abrupt changes in target vergence as a function of age. *Vis. Res.* **2001**, *41*, 507–519. [CrossRef]
30. Tabernero, J.; Chirre, E.; Hervella, L.; Prieto, P.; Artal, P. The accommodative ciliary muscle function is preserved in older humans. *Sci. Rep.* **2016**, *6*, 25551. [CrossRef]
31. Fisher, R.F. The force of contraction of the human ciliary muscle during accommodation. *J. Physiol.* **1977**, *270*, 51–74. [CrossRef]
32. Gislen, A.; Dacke, M.; Kroger, R.H.; Abrahamsson, M.; Nilsson, D.E.; Warrant, E.J. Superior underwater vision in a human population of sea gypsies. *Curr. Biol.* **2003**, *13*, 833–836. [CrossRef]
33. Gislen, A.; Warrant, E.J.; Dacke, M.; Kroger, R.H. Visual training improves underwater vision in children. *Vis. Res.* **2006**, *46*, 3443–3450. [CrossRef] [PubMed]
34. Weng, C.C.; Hwang, D.K.; Liu, C.J. Repeatability of the amplitude of accommodation measured by a new generation autorefractor. *PLoS ONE* **2020**, *15*, e0224733. [CrossRef] [PubMed]
35. Jaiswal, S.; Asper, L.; Long, J.; Lee, A.; Harrison, K.; Golebiowski, B. Ocular and visual discomfort associated with smartphones, tablets and computers: What we do and do not know. *Clin. Exp. Optom.* **2019**, *102*, 463–477. [CrossRef]
36. Yeow, P.T.; Taylor, S.P. Effects of long-term visual display terminal usage on visual functions. *Optom. Vis. Sci.* **1991**, *68*, 930–941. [CrossRef]

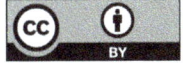

© 2020 by the authors. Licensee MDPI, Basel, Switzerland. This article is an open access article distributed under the terms and conditions of the Creative Commons Attribution (CC BY) license (http://creativecommons.org/licenses/by/4.0/).

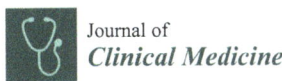 Journal of *Clinical Medicine*

Article

Advancing Digital Workflows for Refractive Error Measurements

Arne Ohlendorf [1,2], Alexander Leube [1,2] and Siegfried Wahl [1,2,*]

1. Institute for Ophthalmic Research, Center for Ophthalmology, Eberhard Karls University of Tuebingen, Elfriede-Aulhorn-Straße 7, 72076 Tuebingen, Germany; arne.ohlendorf@medizin.uni-tuebingen.de (A.O.); alexander.leube@uni-tuebingen.de (A.L.)
2. Technology & Innovation, Carl Zeiss Vision International GmbH, Turnstrasse 27, 73430 Aalen, Germany
* Correspondence: siegfried.wahl@uni-tuebingen.de

Received: 9 June 2020; Accepted: 10 July 2020; Published: 12 July 2020

Abstract: Advancements in clinical measurement of refractive errors should lead to faster and more reliable measurements of such errors. The study investigated different aspects of advancements and the agreement of the spherocylindrical prescriptions obtained with an objective method of measurement ("Aberrometry" (AR)) and two methods of subjective refinements ("Wavefront Refraction" (WR) and "Standard Refraction" (StdR)). One hundred adults aged 20–78 years participated in the course of the study. Bland–Altman analysis of the right eye measurement of the spherocylindrical refractive error (M) identified mean differences (±95% limits of agreement) between the different types of measurements of +0.36 D (±0.76 D) for WR vs. AR (t-test: $p < 0.001$), +0.35 D (± 0.84 D) for StdR vs. AR (t-test: $p < 0.001$), and 0.0 D (± 0.65 D) for StdR vs. WR (t-test: $p < 0.001$). Monocular visual acuity was 0.0 logMAR in 96% of the tested eyes, when refractive errors were corrected with measurements from AR, indicating that only small differences between the different types of prescriptions are present.

Keywords: refractive error; visual acuity; myopia

1. Introduction

Subjective refraction is a key measure in the optometric and ophthalmic field. Typically, the combination of the most positive lenses (spherical and astigmatic) that provides the highest visual acuity is determined in this process that follows a predefined workflow [1]. Since this measurement is by its definition subjective, the repeatability and the precision of the measurement within the same and between different examiner can vary and was reported to have a 95% limit of agreement (LoA) between ±0.27 and ±0.75 D for the spherical equivalent refractive error [2–5]. To improve the repeatability of the technique and to make the process easier and more time efficient, it is common to use either objective data, which are obtained from an autorefractor, or the currently worn prescription as a starting point for the subjective assessment of individual refractive errors. So far, studies examining different objective autorefractors have shown that these are repeatable, under noncycloplegic as well as cycloplegic conditions. In addition, 95% limits of agreement (95% LoA) between ±0.35 and ±0.72 D for the measurement of the spherical refractive error under noncycloplegic conditions were reported [2,6,7]. Nowadays, aberrometers are used to describe the eyes aberrations in more detail. Although lower order aberrations affect vision most and account for approximately 90% of the overall aberrations, [8] also higher order aberrations such as spherical aberration, coma, and trefoil can significantly degrade the quality of the optical image received by the retina [9]. Limits of agreement for the wavefront measurement of the spherical error were found to be between ±0.2 (for a pupil diameter of 4.0 and 6.7 mm) [10] and ±0.55 D [11] (for pupil diameters of 4.0 and 6.0 mm) and did not differ between several measurements, also without the use of an cycloplegic agent to block accommodation [11]. Additionally, e.g., to consider different lighting conditions [12], wavefront sensors allow to compute the refractive errors for different pupil sizes and/or allow the consideration of different higher order aberrations [13].

The purpose of this study was to evaluate the agreement between three different methods to assess the spherocylindrical correction. Method 1 represents an Autorefraction (AR) approach using aberrometry measurements; in Method 2, the sphere of the refractive correction of Method 1 was adjusted; and in Method 3, the sphere, the cylinder, and its axis of the prescription from Method 1 were adjusted. The study investigates the question how much refinement a clinician has to perform subjectively so that the final prescription results in a good and acceptable visual acuity and therefore, saves time.

2. Experimental Section

2.1. Subjects

Correction of spherocylindrical errors was measured in 100 participants, aged 20–78 years (mean: 38.7 ± 13.2 years). Participants had a mean spherical refractive error (computed from the objective wavefront measurement for a 3 mm pupil diameter and a 12 mm vertex distance) of −1.40 ± 2.15 D (−12.75 to +2.5 D) and a range of astigmatic refractive errors between 0 and −3.25 D. Inclusion criterions for participation was (a) refractive error of less than ±13.00 D sphere, ≤ −6.00 D of astigmatism, and (b) best corrected visual acuity of minimum 0.1 logMAR (logarithm of the minimum angle of resolution). Participants with known/reported ocular diseases were not allowed to participate in the course of the study. The study followed the tenets of the Declaration of Helsinki and was approved by the Institutional Review Board of the Medical Faculty of the University of Tubingen (392/2015BO2). Informed consent was obtained from all participants after the content and possible consequences of the study had been explained.

2.2. Experimental Procedures to Measure Refractive Errors Objectively and Subjectively

Objective measurement of the refractive error of each eye was obtained once prior to the subjective measurements by author A.O. using a wavefront aberrometer (i.Profiler plus, Carl Zeiss Vision GmbH, Aalen, Germany). Refractive correction (Sphere, Cylinder, Axis) was calculated from the objectively measured wavefront errors using the lower order Zernike polynomials for a pupil diameter of 3 mm and a vertex distance of 12 mm [14]. Using the lower order terms for the spherical, straight, and oblique astigmatic component of the wavefront shapes, a simple sphere fitting was performed to calculate the best correction [13], based on the purely objective measurements without using higher order terms.

One examiner (author A.L.) subjectively measured the refractive errors using a digital phoropter (ZEISS VISUPHOR 500, Carl Zeiss Vision GmbH, Aalen, Germany) and the two methods "Wavefront Refraction" and "Standard Refraction." The digital phoropter was operated via a tablet PC (iPad Air, Apple, Cupertino, CA, USA). The screen of the tablet PC was covered with black paper in the area where refractive readings were displayed to exclude any influence or bias on the examiner, during the assessment of the spherocylindrical prescriptions with both subjective methods. The sequence of testing of the "Wavefront Refraction" and "Standard Refraction" was randomized between each participant, but the refraction always started with the right eye. As the ZEISS VISUSCREEN 500 also registers the time that is needed for the binocular measurement of the refractive error, time was recorded and analyzed. During the "Wavefront Refraction," only the spherical error of the refractive error was adjusted, whereas during the "Standard Refraction," the spherical error as well as the astigmatism was adjusted. For both methods, the used optotypes (letters) were displayed on an LCD screen (ZEISS VISUSCREEN 500, Carl Zeiss Vision GmbH, Germany) at 6 m distance and followed the EDTRS-layout. Lighting conditions were in the range of 250 cd/m^2 and followed the international standard ISO 8596:2018 [15]. In the case of the assessment of the spherical error under monocular conditions, three lines of letters (each consisting of five single optotypes) were presented on the screen, and the lowest presented acuity was 0.1 logMAR. In case astigmatism was adjusted, also letters were used, but only one line with five letters was presented on the screen, and the letter size was 0.1 logMAR steps bigger than the smallest optotypes visible after correction of the spherical error. A simultaneous cross-cylinder was used to measure the astigmatism and its axis. After both procedures, the dissociated binocular balance was tested, using a single line of letters that was dissociated using a prism (power: right eye 3 D base up, left eye 3 D base down). The size of the presented letters was set to 0.3 logMAR and spherical blur of +0.5 D was added to both eyes. Then, additional plus lenses were induced until the participants perceived the images in both eyes equally blurred. Afterwards, to achieve a binocular balance as endpoint for refraction, the nondissociated binocular best corrected vision was tested using letters, presented in an ETDRS layout and while the blurring lenses from the previous test were removed. The prescription was changed until visual acuity was maximal in both eyes.

2.3. Assessment of Visual Acuity and Subjective Preference

Visual acuity for each eye was assessed after correction of the refractive errors with each of the earlier described methods. As stated above, each acuity line consisted of five optotypes and each correctly identified single letter was scored 0.02 logMAR units [16]. Highest visual acuity describes the smallest optotype for the given test distance that was correctly identified. At the end of the experiment, and in order to not only rely on the subjective prescription determined by an optometrist that corrects the refractive error, the participants were asked, which of the three corrections they preferred most. This was done using the capability of the digital phoropter in conjunction with the tablet PC to store the refractive readings for each single participant and to show these in a fast sequence at the end of an examination. During such comparison, the subjects viewed a line of 5 optotypes with a size of 0.1 logMAR, presented on the described LCD display at the test distance of 6 m. Using this possibility, the subject was able to compare the different corrections that were obtained with one of the three methods. The following direct comparisons were evaluated in a randomized order: (a) Autorefraction vs. Wavefront Refraction, (b) Autorefraction vs. Standard Refraction, (c) Wavefront Refraction vs. Standard Refraction, and (d) Autorefraction vs. Wavefront Refraction vs. Standard Refraction.

2.4. Analysis and Statistics

The right eye of each subject was used for the analysis of the data. Refractive measurements were analyzed for the spherical refractive error (S), the spherical equivalent refractive error (M), and the cross-cylinder components J0 and J45 that were introduced by Thibos, Wheeler, and Horner [17]. The agreement between the different methods for the spherocylindrical correction of the right as well as for the visual acuity was tested using Bland–Altman analysis [18]. The calculated mean difference between two methods represents the estimated bias of one method, and the standard deviation of the differences measures the random fluctuations around this mean. The computation of the 95% limit of agreement (calculated as 1.96*standard deviation) describes how far apart measurements by two methods were more likely to be for most individuals. Statistical analyses were performed with the statistics software package JMP 11.0 (SAS Institute, Cary, USA). In case of the Bland–Altman analysis, a t-test was performed to calculate statistical power between the compared methods. A one-way ANOVA with post hoc Tukey HSD test was used to test whether the used method of refraction had an influence on the measurement of the spherical equivalent refractive error. A t-test was used to compare the time that each of the subjective method needed to assess the spherocylindrical refraction.

3. Results

3.1. Agreement Between Subjective and Objective Refractions

Figure 1a represents the Bland–Altman plots for the comparison of the spherical equivalent refractive error computed from Autorefraction vs. the Wavefront Refraction and Figure 1b represents the comparison between the Autorefraction vs. the Standard Refraction.

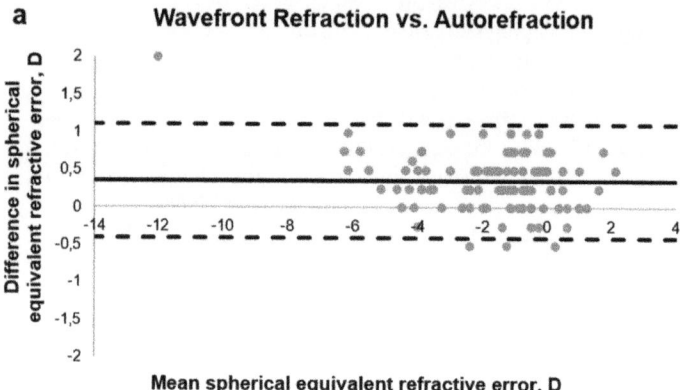
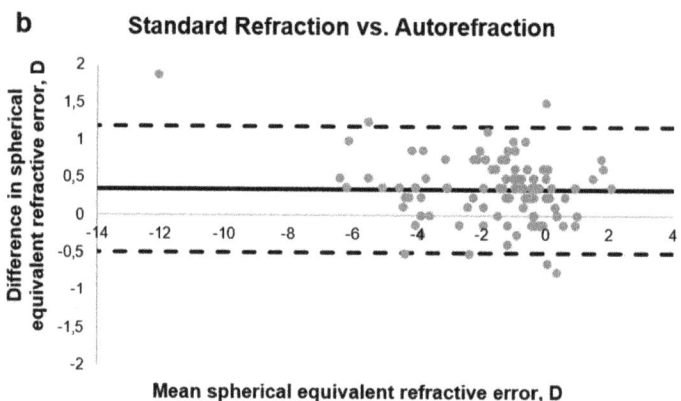
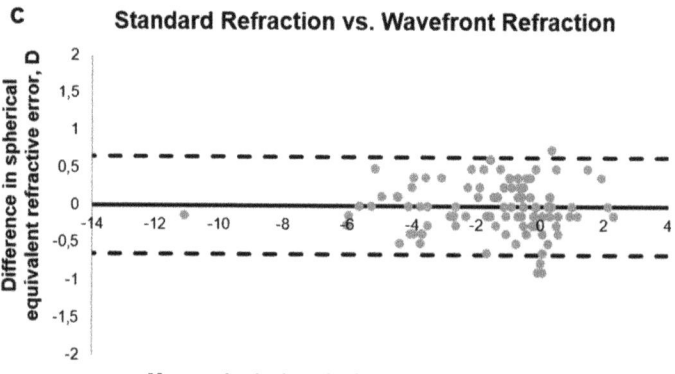

Figure 1. Bland–Altman plot for the comparison of the spherical equivalent refractive error after binocular testing with (**a**) Wavefront Refraction vs. Autorefraction, (**b**) Standard Refraction vs. Autorefraction, and (**c**) Standard Refraction vs. Wavefront Refraction.

When comparing the Wavefront Refraction as well as the Standard Refraction to the objective data obtained with the aberrometer, the calculated bias was around 0.3 D, resulting in too negative readings of the spherical errors when using the aberrometer (for details, see Table 1). The limits of agreement are smaller, in case Autorefraction was compared to the Wavefront Refraction, and this result is attributed to the fact that only the spherical refractive error was adjusted between both methods. In addition, when the cylinder and its axis were rechecked (comparison between Autorefraction and Standard Refraction, Figure 1b), the limits of agreement slightly increased because the power of the cylindrical error may have changed between both methods. The one-way ANOVA with post hoc Tukey HSD test revealed that the used method ($F_{4,13} = 0.89$, $p = 0.4$) did not influenced the measured spherical equivalent error. Table 1 summarizes the mean differences as well as the 95% limits of agreement for all three possible comparisons as well as for the spherical refractive error (S) and the three power vectors M, J0 and J45.

Table 1. Descriptive and statistical analysis for the comparison of the three methods to assess the habitual refractive errors.

		Mean Difference, D	95% Limit of Agreement, D	p
Wavefront Refraction vs. Autorefraction	S *	+0.36	±0.76	< 0.001
	M'	+0.36	±0.76	< 0.001
	J0°		Not assessed	
	J45^		Not assessed	
Standard Refraction vs. Autorefraction	S *	+0.27	±0.88	< 0.001
	M'	+0.35	±0.84	< 0.001
	J0°	−0.05	±0.35	< 0.001
	J45^	+0.02	±0.27	< 0.01
Standard Refraction vs. Wavefront Refraction	S *	0.09	±0.65	= 0.6
	M'	+0.0	±0.65	= 0.3
	J0°	−0.05	±0.36	< 0.001
	J45^	+0.02	±0.27	< 0.01

S * = spherical refractive error; M' = spherical equivalent refractive error; J0° = Jackson cross cylinder at 0°; J45^ = Jackson cross cylinder at 45°.

Comparisons of the power vectors J0 and J45 showed very small mean differences and low 95% limits of agreement, when methods were compared with each other. Since in case of the refractive measurement that was based on the objective Autorefraction and the Wavefront Refraction, the astigmatism and its axis were not changed, the descriptive as well as statistical analysis was not assessed. For the spherical and spherical equivalent refractive error, the statistical analysis revealed a significant difference between the measurements obtained with the objective measurement calculated from the wavefront errors and both subjective refractive measurements (Wavefront Refraction and Standard Refraction).

3.2. Differences in Cylinder and Its Axis

The bias between two methods as well as the 95% limit of agreement were calculated for the power vectors M, J0 and J45. These power vectors lend itself to calculations of sums, differences, and averages and are the correct form for describing refractions for such measures. Nevertheless, especially in case of the cylinder and its axis, these are not the ideal notations to get an overview, if the data obtained with an autorefractor and with a subjective refraction are equal or differ, e.g., depending on the amount of astigmatism or on its axis. Therefore, a comparison between the measured astigmatism and its axis between the autorefraction data and the values from the Standard Refraction was performed, following the analysis by Grein et al. [19]. In Figure 2, the discrepancy for the axis, based on the objective measurement of the wavefront errors and with the Standard Refraction, is analyzed depending on the power of the astigmatic error. It must be noted that in this analysis, an astigmatism was only considered if it was found in both methods of refraction, therefore, only data of 85 eyes were analyzed.

A positive difference means a change of the axis into the clockwise direction, whereas a negative difference is equal to a counterclockwise change.

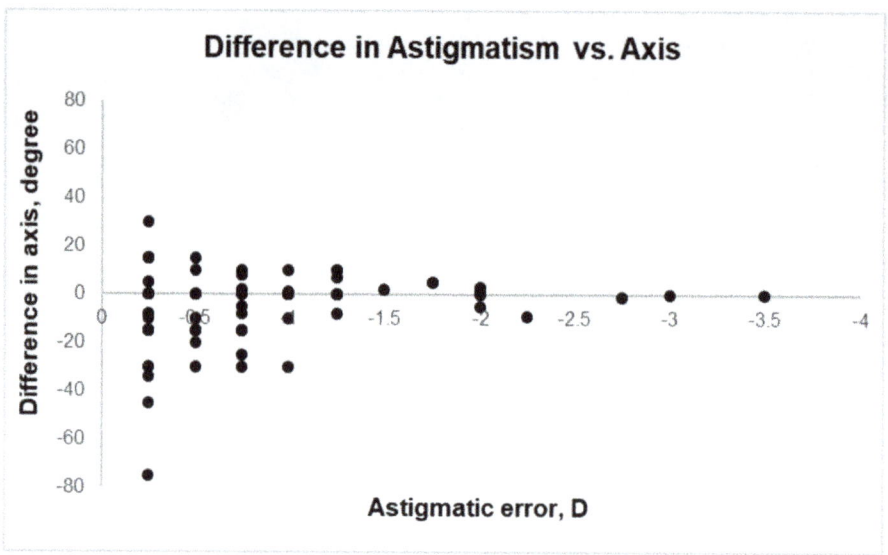

Figure 2. Difference of the cylinder-axis (deg) between Standard Refraction and Autorefraction as a function of the power of astigmatic error (D).

From Figure 2 it can be concluded that astigmatic errors of ≤ -1.0 D were very frequent (79% of the 85 right eyes) and that the difference between the objective axis of the correcting cylinder and the subjective axis differed especially at very small amounts of astigmatism. Vice versa, the difference between the axis decreased with increasing power of astigmatism, indicating that the quality of the objectively measured wavefront error for the cylinder axis increased with increasing power of astigmatism. To investigate, if a measured astigmatism needs to be corrected, the difference between the cylindrical error of the right eye when measured with the Standard Refraction and the objective measurement of the wavefront error was analyzed. The results gave evidence that the power of the astigmatic error based on the objective measurement of the wavefront error was more negative when compared to the Standard Refraction, however, 74% of the measurements had a difference within ± 0.25 D.

3.3. Visual Acuity from Different Correction Methods

The monocular visual acuity that was achieved with either one of the procedures was analyzed, as one can predict that a spherical refractive error of 0.25 D reduces the monocular visual acuity by 1 line (or 0.1 logMAR unit) [20,21], the achieved visual acuity (especially under monocular conditions) is a good indicator for (a) the quality of a method to detect a refractive error and (b) for the agreement between different methods. The analysis revealed that already 96% of the eyes had a visual acuity equivalent of 0.0 logMAR or better with correction data (sphere, cylinder, and axis) obtained from the aberrometer without further adjustments. This was slightly increased to 98%, when the refractive error was subjectively fine-tuned by an experienced optometrist (Wavefront Refraction, $n = 98$ eyes; Standard Refraction, $n = 98$ eyes). Table 2 summarizes the mean differences in visual acuity and the lower as well as upper limits for the single comparisons.

Table 2. Mean differences in visual acuity reached with each method and 95% limits of agreements.

	Mean Difference in VA, logMAR	95% Limit of Agreement, logMAR	p
Wavefront Refraction vs. Autorefraction	−0.02	±0.07	< 0.001
Standard Refraction vs. Autorefraction	−0.03	±0.10	< 0.001
Standard Refraction vs. Wavefront Refraction	−0.01	±0.09	= 0.02

3.4. Subjective Preferences in Correction

Figure 3 summarizes the findings of the subjective preference comparison, while the participants always had three possible decisions: whether they liked one of the corrections better than the other(s) or they were not able to see a difference.

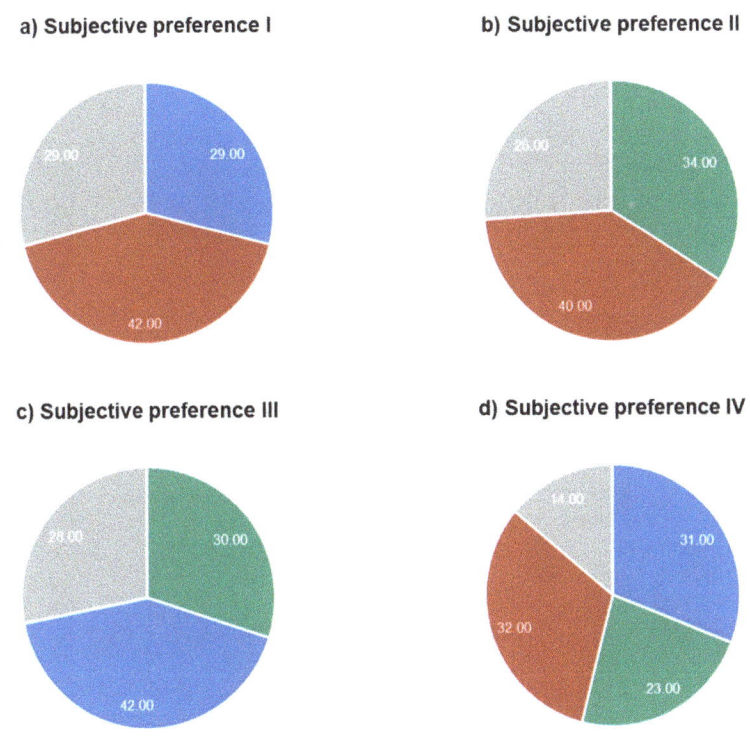

Figure 3. Subjective preferences for direct comparisons of methods (Figure 3a–c) and between methods. (**a**) Autorefraction (red) vs. Wavefront Refraction (blue), (**b**) Autorefraction (red) vs. Standard Refraction (green), (**c**) Standard Refraction (green) vs. Wavefront Refraction (blue), and (**d**) Standard Refraction (blue) vs. Wavefront Refraction (green) vs. Autorefraction (red). Gray area: no difference.

When comparing the individual as well as averaged preferences, it becomes clear that participants preferred the correction based on objective measurement of the wavefront error most (Figure 3a,b). In case the Standard Refraction was compared to the Wavefront Refraction, subjects preferred the Wavefront Refraction more (42%, Figure 3c). When the participants were asked to compare all three methods with each other, the Autorefraction and Wavefront Refraction were rated similar

(Autorefraction: 32% and Wavefront Refraction: 31%) and both ratings were higher compared to the Standard Refraction (23%).

3.5. Number of Decisions and Time for the Assessment of the Refraction

One main advantage of the Wavefront Refraction is that the number of decisions a patient has to make during the assessment of his or her refractive correction is reduced due to the fact that only the sphere under monocular as well as binocular conditions is rechecked by the eye care professional. Therefore, the number of decisions in each test was recorded and analyzed. During the process of the Wavefront Refraction, participants had to take 17 decisions on average, while the number of decisions increased to 25 in case of the Standard Refraction—an increase of roughly 50%. Since in the case of the Wavefront Refraction, the power as well as the axis of an existing astigmatism was not tested, one can assume that this procedure is much faster compared to the Standard Refraction. In case, the average time that was needed for the Wavefront Refraction was 353 ± 82 s (range 214–575 s), while this increased to 539 ± 119 s (range: 306–937 s) in case of the Standard Refraction (t-test: $p < 0.001$).

4. Discussion

Conventional autorefractors and subjective refraction following a standardized protocol are currently the gold standard in the assessment of refractive errors. Aberrometers have gained attention in optometric as well as ophthalmological settings since they are able to measure lower and higher order aberrations. The study has assessed the accuracy of Autorefraction while comparing the refractive correction as well as the visual acuity with two subjective refinement methods.

4.1. Agreement and Percentage of Agreement Between Subjective and Objective Refractions

Aberrometers have been shown to be reasonable, accurate, and repeatable [22–24]. Several investigations [25,26] have compared the spherical-equivalent refractive error of autorefraction to subjective refraction and the observed difference was less than or equal to ±0.50 D between 70% and 74% of the time. In case of the i.Profiler plus from ZEISS, the percentages of agreement for differences in the spherical refractive error of ±0.50 D were higher and calculated to be minimum 76%, when Standard Refraction was compared to the Autorefraction. One possible explanation is given by the internal fixation target, which is additionally blurred optically during the measurement, to avoid instrument myopia. Nevertheless, both subjective methods had fewer negative values in the final spherical equivalent refractive error compared to the objective method, resulting in a mean difference for the sphere of 0.36 D for Autorefraction vs. Wavefront Refraction and 0.35 D for Autorefraction vs. Standard Refraction. Lebow and Campbell (2014) investigated differences of the objective measure from the ZEISS i.Profiler plus to a conventional subjective measurement of the spherical equivalent refractive error in adults and reported a mean difference of 0.11 D (more negative readings with the i.Profiler plus) [25]. As the one-way ANOVA with post hoc Tukey HSD test showed that the device had no effect on the measured spherical equivalent error, one cannot assume that a systematic bias exists between the used methods and different explanations can account for the observed differences. First, subjects might have accommodated during the objective refraction, but there was only a small trend that younger participants showed higher differences than older participants ($R = -0.2$, $p = 0.06$). Second, and as already described by others, roughly 0.25 D of the observed difference could also be accounted to the fact that the location of infrared scatter layer is different than photoreceptor layer [27]. Third, chromatic aberration might play a role, but researchers have not found an improvement in accuracy between objective Autorefraction from wavefront errors and subjective refraction, in case polychromatic metrics were used to compute refractive correction or by taking into account the Stiles–Crawford effect [28].

4.2. Differences in Cylinder and Its Axis

When comparing the axis of the astigmatic error that was obtained with the aberrometer to the Standard Refraction, the gained results could lead to the interpretation that objective measurements are not very precise. From investigations of the interexaminer agreement of the axis of a correcting cylindrical lens, the same distribution of difference is known; therefore, it can be concluded that such differences can occur not only between an objective as well as a subjective method but also when different examiner measure the refractive errors of an individual. [18] For the difference between the power of a correcting lens, assessed objectively and subjectively, a mean difference of 0.12 D was observed, with 95% limits of agreement of ± 0.66 D. Lebow and Campbell, who also used the Autorefraction data from the ZEISS i.Profiler plus, compared these data to their Standard Refraction and the observed that mean differences are comparable to the current study (mean difference 0.02 D) [25]. In an investigation by Wosik et al. showed that the assessment of the astigmatic error is superior using aberrometer devices compared to standard autorefractors [29].

4.3. Impact of Higher Order Aberrations on Refraction Assessment

Additionally to the lower order aberrations, used to calculate the sphere, cylinder and axis, aberrometry provides information about higher order aberrations (HOAs) like coma, trefoil, or spherical aberration. Previous studies showed that the usage of HOAs can improve precision in interexaminer evaluation [13], especially in highly aberrated eyes, like keratoconic eyes [30,31]. However, image quality-based predictions in normal eyes range within the here reported limits of agreements towards the subjective refraction [32]. Since the current investigation enrolled only normally sighted participants, the amount of HOAs in the cohort is low and comparable to already reported values [33], as shown in Figure 4. Furthermore, the objective aberrometry measurements that were evaluated for a pupil diameter of 3 mm reduce the impact even further.

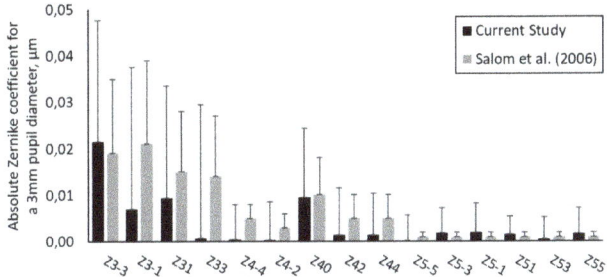

Figure 4. Comparison of the absolute Zernike coefficient (µm) for the higher order aberrations until fifth order from the current study to normal human subjects for a 3 mm pupil diameter (data from Salmon et al. [33]).

4.4. Visual Acuity with Each Correction

Visual acuity of 0.0 logMAR was achieved in 96% of the tested right eyes with the spherocylindrical prescriptions from the aberrometer. This portion increased to 98% after balancing the spherical error, in case of the Wavefront Refraction as well as in case of the Standard Refraction, where sphere, cylinder, and axis were balanced. This small increase in visual acuity can be explained by the fact that the spherical refractive error was around 0.3 D too negative with the objective method. The fact that visual acuity increased only slightly, when the refractive error was adjusted with both of the two subjective methods, is a good indicator for the fact that autorefraction measurement of spherocylindrical corrections are very reliable compared to two subjective methods that were evaluated.

4.5. Subjective Preferences in Correction

On average, participants preferred spherocylindrical correction from the autorefractor most, when compared to both subjective methods (Wavefront Refraction as well as Standard Refraction). This result can be explained by the fact that, especially, the measurements of the sphere were slightly more myopic with the autorefractor compared to both mentioned methods. This shift towards more negative power would result in a slightly higher contrast of the image on the retina that especially myopes prefer more compared to blur that would have been the result if spherical corrections were more positive. Nevertheless, since these comparisons were done with optotypes that had a size of 0.1 logMAR, one has to be careful with the interpretation of the results. In the future, it would be better to individually test this comparison at the threshold of the acuity that the single participant is able to read (in the case one wants to use optotypes) or to present more natural stimuli during the process of comparison, since optotypes are quite unnatural and the prescription is needed for the daily life.

4.6. Number of Decisions and Time for the Assessment of the Refraction

On average, 50% less decisions had to be made by each participant when refraction was measured using the Wavefront Refraction compared to the Standard Refraction. This small amount of decisions indicates that the prescriptions from the aberrometer are very close to the final value, when, e.g., compared to the refractive correction obtained with a Standard Refraction. Additionally, Wavefront Refraction was 50% faster than the Standard Refraction. Since the results from the wavefront-based subjective assessment of the refractive errors were shown to be comparable to the standard procedure in the measurement of refractive errors, one can conclude that the combination of the Autorefraction and Wavefront Refraction will result in acceptable prescription for patient in a fast manner.

5. Conclusions

Aberrometry may change the way refractive errors are measured clinically and provides a tremendous amount of data about the aberrations of the eye. Spherocylindrical prescriptions that were obtained by measuring wavefront errors, provided reliable information for the further correction of lower order aberrations with a subjective method. Autorefraction data was slightly more negative for spherical as well as astigmatic errors, but > 70% of the spherical equivalent error were within ±0.5 D compared to the conventional subjective refraction. The combination of the Autorefraction and Wavefront Refraction, while refining only the spherical refractive error, will result in acceptable prescription for the patient and can significantly save time in the assessment of the refraction.

Author Contributions: Conceptualization, A.O. and A.L.; methodology, A.O.; formal analysis, A.O. and A.L.; investigation, A.O. and A.L.; resources, S.W.; data curation, A.L.; writing—original draft preparation, A.O. and S.W.; writing—review and editing, A.L.; visualization, A.O.; supervision, S.W.; project administration, S.W.; and funding acquisition, S.W. All authors have read and agreed to the published version of the manuscript.

Funding: This work was done in an industry-on-campus-cooperation between the University of Tubingen and Carl Zeiss Vision International GmbH. A.O., A.L., and S.W. are employed by Carl Zeiss Vision International GmbH and are scientists at the University of Tubingen.

Conflicts of Interest: The authors declare no conflicts of interest. The funders had no role in the design of the study; in the collection, analyses, or interpretation of data; in the writing of the manuscript; or in the decision to publish the results.

References

1. Borish, I.M.; Benjamin, W.J. *Borish's Clinical Refraction*, 2nd ed.; Benjamin, W.J., Ed.; Elsevier: Amsterdam, The Netherlands, 1998.
2. Rosenfield, M.; Chiu, N.N. Repeatability of subjective and objective refraction. *Optom. Vis. Sci.* **1995**, *72*, 577–579. [CrossRef]
3. Bullimore, M.A.; Fusaro, R.E.; Adams, C.W. The repeatability of automated and clinician refraction. *Optom. Vis. Sci.* **1998**, *75*, 617–622. [CrossRef]
4. Goss, D.A.; Grosvenor, T. Reliability of refraction—A literature review. *J. Am. Optom. Assoc.* **1996**, *67*, 619–630.
5. Raasch, T.W.; Schechtman, K.B.; Davis, L.J.; Zadnik, K. Repeatability of subjective refraction in myopic and keratoconic subjects: Results of vector analysis. *Ophthalmic Physiol. Opt.* **2001**, *21*, 376–383. [CrossRef]

6. Zadnik, K.; Mutti, D.O.; Adams, A.J. The repeatability of measurement of the ocular components. *Investig. Ophthalmol. Vis. Sci.* **1992**, *33*, 2325–2333.
7. Pesudovs, K.; Weisinger, H.S. A comparison of autorefractor performance. *Optom. Vis. Sci.* **2004**, *81*, 554–558. [CrossRef] [PubMed]
8. Porter, J.; Guirao, A.; Cox, I.G.; Williams, D.R. Monochromatic aberrations of the human eye in a large population. *J. Opt. Soc. Am. A* **2001**, *18*, 1793. [CrossRef]
9. Philip, K.; Sankaridurg, P.; Holden, B.; Ho, A.; Mitchell, P. Influence of higher order aberrations and retinal image quality in myopisation of emmetropic eyes. *Vis. Res.* **2014**, *105*, 233–243. [CrossRef] [PubMed]
10. Salmon, T.O.; West, R.W.; Gasser, W.; Kenmore, T. Measurement of refractive errors in young myopes using the COAS Shack-Hartmann aberrometer. *Optom. Vis. Sci.* **2003**, *80*, 6–14. [CrossRef] [PubMed]
11. Nissman, S.A.; Tractenberg, R.E.; Saba, C.M.; Douglas, J.C.; Lustbader, J.M. Accuracy, repeatability, and clinical application of spherocylindrical automated refraction using time-based wavefront aberrometry measurements. *Ophthalmology* **2006**, *113*, 577.e1–2. [CrossRef]
12. Ommani, A.; Hutchings, N.; Thapa, D.; Lakshminarayanan, V. Pupil Scaling for the Estimation of Aberrations in Natural Pupils. *Optom. Vis. Sci.* **2014**, *91*, 1175–1182. [CrossRef]
13. Pesudovs, K.; Parker, K.E.; Cheng, H.; Applegate, R.A. The precision of wavefront refraction compared to subjective refraction and autorefraction. *Optom. Vis. Sci.* **2007**, *84*, 387–392. [CrossRef] [PubMed]
14. Navarro, R. Objective refraction from aberrometry: Theory. *J. Biomed. Opt.* **2009**, *14*, 024021. [CrossRef] [PubMed]
15. International Organization for Standardization. *ISO 8596:2018—Ophthalmic Optics—Visual Acuity Testing—Standard and Clinical Optotypes and Their Presentation*; International Organization for Standardization: Geneva, Switzerland, 2018.
16. Mon-Williams, M.; Tresilian, J.R.; Strang, N.C.; Kochhar, P.; Wann, J.P. Improving vision: Neural compensation for optical defocus. *Proc. Biol. Sci.* **1998**, *265*, 71–77. [CrossRef] [PubMed]
17. Thibos, L.N.; Wheeler, W.; Horner, D. Power vectors: An application of Fourier analysis to the description and statistical analysis of refractive error. *Optom. Vis. Sci.* **1997**, *74*, 367–375. [CrossRef] [PubMed]
18. Bland, J.M.; Altman, D. Statistical methods for assessing agreement between two methods of clinical measurement. *Lancet* **1986**, *327*, 307–310. [CrossRef]
19. Grein, H.-J.; Schmidt, O.; Ritsche, A. Reproducibility of subjective refraction measurement. *Ophthalmologe* **2014**, *111*, 1057–1064. [CrossRef] [PubMed]
20. Radhakrishnan, H.; Pardhan, S.; Calver, R.I.; O'Leary, D.J. Unequal reduction in visual acuity with positive and negative defocusing lenses in myopes. *Optom. Vis. Sci.* **2004**, *81*, 14–17. [CrossRef]
21. Leube, A.; Ohlendorf, A.; Wahl, S. The Influence of Induced Astigmatism on the Depth of Focus. *Optom. Vis. Sci.* **2016**, *93*, 1228–1234. [CrossRef] [PubMed]
22. Cleary, G.; Spalton, D.J.; Patel, P.M.; Lin, P.-F.; Marshall, J. Diagnostic accuracy and variability of autorefraction by the Tracey Visual Function Analyzer and the Shin-Nippon NVision-K 5001 in relation to subjective refraction. *Ophthalmic Physiol. Opt.* **2009**, *29*, 173–181. [CrossRef] [PubMed]
23. Allen, P.M.; Radhakrishnan, H.; O'Leary, D.J. Repeatability and validity of the PowerRefractor and the Nidek AR600-A in an adult population with healthy eyes. *Optom. Vis. Sci.* **2003**, *80*, 245–251. [CrossRef]
24. Salmon, T.O.; van de Pol, C. Evaluation of a clinical aberrometer for lower-order accuracy and repeatability, higher-order repeatability, and instrument myopia. *Optometry* **2005**, *76*, 461–472. [CrossRef] [PubMed]
25. Lebow, K.A.; Campbell, C.E. A comparison of a traditional and wavefront autorefraction. *Optom. Vis. Sci.* **2014**, *91*, 1191–1198. [CrossRef] [PubMed]
26. Teel, D.F.W.; Jacobs, R.J.; Copland, J.; Neal, D.R.; Thibos, L.N. Differences between Wavefront and Subjective Refraction for Infrared Light. *Optom. Vis. Sci.* **2014**, *91*, 1158–1166. [CrossRef] [PubMed]
27. Atchison, D.A.; Smith, G. Chromatic dispersions of the ocular media of human eyes. *J. Opt. Soc. Am. A* **2005**, *22*, 29. [CrossRef]
28. Guirao, A.; Williams, D.R. A method to predict refractive errors from wave aberration data. *Optom. Vis. Sci.* **2003**, *80*, 36–42. [CrossRef] [PubMed]
29. Wosik, J.; Patrzykont, M.; Pniewski, J. Comparison of refractive error measurements by three different models of autorefractors and subjective refraction in young adults. *J. Opt. Soc. Am. A* **2019**, *36*, 1–6. [CrossRef]

30. Jinabhai, A.; O'Donnell, C.; Radhakrishnan, H. A comparison between subjective refraction and aberrometry-derived refraction in keratoconus patients and control subjects. *Cur. Eye Res.* **2010**, *35*, 703–714. [CrossRef]
31. Sabesan, R.; Jeong, T.M.; Carvalho, L.; Cox, I.G.; Williams, D.R.; Yoon, G. Vision improvement by correcting higher-order aberrations with customized soft contact lenses in keratoconic eyes. *Opt. Lett.* **2007**, *32*, 1000–1002. [CrossRef]
32. Thibos, L.N.; Hong, X.; Bradley, A.; Applegate, R.A. Accuracy and precision of objective refraction from wavefront aberrations. *J. Vis.* **2004**, *4*, 9. [CrossRef]
33. Salmon, T.O.; van de Pol, C. Normal-eye Zernike coefficients and root-mean-square wavefront errors. *J. Cataract Refract. Surg.* **2006**, *32*, 2064–2074. [CrossRef] [PubMed]

© 2020 by the authors. Licensee MDPI, Basel, Switzerland. This article is an open access article distributed under the terms and conditions of the Creative Commons Attribution (CC BY) license (http://creativecommons.org/licenses/by/4.0/).

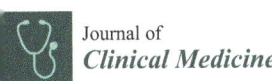

Review

Is 0.01% Atropine an Effective and Safe Treatment for Myopic Children? A Systemic Review and Meta-Analysis

Hou-Ren Tsai [1,2], Tai-Li Chen [1,2,3], Jen-Hung Wang [4], Huei-Kai Huang [2,5] and Cheng-Jen Chiu [6,7,*]

1. Department of Medical Education, Medical Administration Office, Hualien Tzu Chi Hospital, Buddhist Tzu Chi Medical Foundation, Hualien 970, Taiwan; melotsai0830@gmail.com (H.-R.T.); terrychen.a@gmail.com (T.-L.C.)
2. School of Medicine, Tzu Chi University, Hualien 970, Taiwan; drhkhuang@gmail.com
3. Department of Dermatology, Tzu Chi Skin Institute, Hualien Tzu Chi Hospital, Buddhist Tzu Chi Medical Foundation, Hualien 970, Taiwan
4. Department of Medical Research, Buddhist Tzu Chi General Hospital, Hualien 970, Taiwan; jenhungwang2011@gmail.com
5. Department of Family Medicine and Medical Research, Hualien Tzu Chi Hospital, Buddhist Tzu Chi Medical Foundation, Hualien 970, Taiwan
6. Department of Ophthalmology and Visual Science, Tzu Chi University, Hualien 970, Taiwan
7. Department of Ophthalmology, Hualien Tzu Chi Hospital, Buddhist Tzu Chi Medical Foundation, Hualien 970, Taiwan
* Correspondence: drcjchiu@gmail.com; Tel.: +886-03-856-1825 (ext. 10669)

Abstract: Several conflicting results regarding the efficacy of 0.01% atropine in slowing axial elongation remain in doubt. To solve this issue and evaluate the safety of 0.01% atropine, we conducted a systematic review and meta-analysis with the latest evidence. The review included a total of 1178 participants (myopic children). The efficacy outcomes were the mean annual progression in standardized equivalent refraction (SER) and axial length (AL). The safety outcomes included mean annual change in accommodative amplitude, photopic and mesopic pupil diameter. The results demonstrated that 0.01% atropine significantly retarded SER progression compared with the controls (weighted mean difference [WMD], 0.28 diopter (D) per year; 95% confidence interval (CI) = 0.17, 0.38; $p < 0.01$), and axial elongation (WMD, -0.06 mm; 95% CI = -0.09, -0.03; $p < 0.01$) during the 1-year period. Patients receiving 0.01% atropine showed no significant changes in accommodative amplitude (WMD, -0.45 D; 95% CI = -1.80, 0.90; $p = 0.51$) but showed dilated photopic pupil diameter (WMD, 0.35 mm; 95% CI = 0.02, 0.68; $p = 0.04$) and mesopic pupil diameter (WMD, 0.20 mm; 95% CI = 0.08, 0.32; $p < 0.01$). In the subgroup analysis of SER progression, myopic children with lower baseline refraction (>-3 D) and older age (>10-year-old) obtained better responses with 0.01% atropine treatment. Furthermore, the European and multi-ethnicity groups showed greater effect than the Asian groups. In conclusion, 0.01% atropine had favorable efficacy and adequate safety for childhood myopia over a 1-year period.

Keywords: 0.01% atropine; myopia control; axial length; standardized equivalent refraction

1. Introduction

Myopia is becoming a public health concern with a significant socioeconomic burden affecting 80% to 90% of young adults [1–7]. By 2050, Holden et al. has predicted that 9.8% of the world's population would be high myopia cases [8], leading to severe sight-threatening complications, such as glaucoma, myopic macular degeneration, and retinal detachment [9–12]. Thus, finding an effective and safe treatment to inhibit myopia progression is urgently needed [13].

The efficacy of atropine (a non-selective antagonist of muscarinic acetylcholine receptors) to prevent myopia progression in children has been studied widely. Different concentrations of atropine (0.01% to 1%) have been shown to inhibit myopic progression effectively [14–16]. However, high dose atropine has been subject to significant adverse effects such as blurred near vision, photophobia and rebound phenomenon after treatment cessation [16]. Chia et al. [17] have evaluated the change in standardized equivalent refraction (SER) and axial length (AL) after stopping the administration of atropine in a 5-year study and concluded that cessation of 0.1% and 0.5% atropine resulted in a greater degree of myopic rebound, but 0.01% atropine appears to result in less myopic rebound, which led to a more sustained effect of myopia retardation. They also proposed that a daily dose of atropine 0.01% is an effective first-line treatment in children aged 6 to 12 years with documented myopic progression of -0.5 D in the preceding year with few side effects.

Several studies have shown that low dose atropine, especially 0.01%, may slow SER progression with minimal side effects; nevertheless, the effect in inhibiting axial elongation is still inconsistent [18–20]. Fu et al. reported that 0.01% atropine significantly reduced myopia progression over a 12-month period as measured by AL when compared with a control group (average 0.14 mm, $p = 0.004$) (19). However, Khanal et al. [21] asserted that 0.01% atropine could not slow the abnormal eye enlargement, thus delaying implementing an effective dose. Li et al. [22] have pointed out that this phenomenon may be due to the sample size among previous studies powered primarily based on SER change and concluded that a larger sample size is needed to detect the difference in AL elongation between the 0.01% atropine and placebo groups. Although one meta-analysis [23] has enrolled seven RCTs to investigate the efficacy of 0.01% atropine in axial elongation, the control group differed among the enrolled studies, which may bias the actual effect of 0.01% atropine. Of note, excessive elongation of the eyeball may increase the risk of subsequent myopia complications [24,25], it is essential to determine whether 0.01% atropine can effectively inhibit axial elongation.

In addition, the most frequently reported side effects of topical atropine include blurred near vision, allergic reaction, and dilated pupil, which may increase the exposure of the lens and retina to ultraviolet light [26]. Although these were short-term and minimal in 0.01% atropine [14,19], it is also worthy of being investigated and compared with other concentrations of atropine in long-term use. Furthermore, the relevant evidence regarding the efficacy of 0.01% atropine compared to placebo continues to accumulate in recent years [19,20,27,28]. Thus, we conducted a rigorous quantitative and systematic summary of the evidence to increase the statistical power and elucidate the conflicting results of 0.01% atropine in childhood myopia. Furthermore, subgroup analysis according to known confounding factors such as different ethnicity, baseline age, and baseline myopia status was conducted to identify the ideal recipients for 0.01% atropine in myopia control.

2. Materials and Methods

2.1. Study Design

This meta-analysis aimed to survey the efficacy and safety of 0.01% atropine in myopia control. The study was performed per the recommendations made by the preferred reporting items for a systematic review and meta-analysis (PRISMA) statement (Table S1), and the methodology was pre-specified and registered on the INPLASY website (Registration No. INPLASY202140082).

2.2. Search Strategy

Studies describing the efficacy of 0.01% atropine in myopia control before June 2021 were identified from the PubMed, Embase, and Cochrane Library databases. No language restrictions were applied. The keywords "0.01% atropine," "myopia control," and their synonyms and derivatives were used. Details of the search strategies are described in Table S2. The "related articles" option in PubMed was used to broaden the search results, and all abstracts, studies, and citations retrieved were reviewed. Furthermore, we assessed the reference sections of the retrieved articles to identify other relevant studies. Lastly, relevant studies were retrieved from the ClinicalTrials.gov registry (https://clinicaltrials.

gov/, accessed on 27 June 2021) and the International Clinical Trials Registry Platform (ICTRP, https://www.who.int/ictrp/en/, accessed on 27 June 2021).

2.3. Inclusion and Exclusion Criteria

Studies were included in the systematic review if: (1) they were randomized control trials (RCTs), cohort studies, or case-control studies; (2) they compared a group treated with 0.01% atropine for myopia control with a control group; (3) the participants with a diagnosis of myopia were younger than 18 years; (4) at least one efficacy or safety outcome relevant to our review was reported in the studies, including the change in SER, AL, accommodative amplitude, and pupil size; and (5) the mean follow-up period was at least one year. We excluded review articles, case reports, case series, and animal or laboratory studies.

2.4. Data Extraction

Two authors (H.-R.T. and T.-L.C.) independently extracted the following items: first author, year of publication, study design, number of eyes, baseline SER, baseline AL, follow-up period, drop-out rate, and details of the treatment arm. The efficacy outcomes were the changes in SER and AL per year. The safety outcomes included changes in accommodative amplitude, photopic pupil size, and mesopic pupil size.

2.5. Quality Assessment

The methodological quality of the non-randomized studies was assessed using risk of bias in non-randomized studies-of interventions (ROBINS-I) [29], and that of the RCTs was evaluated using the Cochrane Collaboration's risk of bias assessment tool (RoB v.2.0) [30]. Decisions recorded individually by the reviewers (H.-R.T. and T.-L.C.) were compared, and disagreements were resolved by a third reviewer (C.-J.C.).

2.6. Data Synthesis and Statistical Analyses

The effect size of each study was presented as WMD with 95% CIs for continuous outcome measures (SER, AL, accommodative amplitude, mesopic pupil size, and photopic pupil size). When standard deviation data were not applicable, we calculated standard deviations with formulas described in the Cochrane Handbook for Systematic Reviews of Interventions [31]. The pooled estimates and their CIs were calculated using the DerSimonian and Laird random-effects model, considering the heterogeneity of the study populations [31]. The modified HKSJ adjustment was employed to adjust for type I errors and avoid inaccurate CIs as a sensitivity analysis if the included study number of each outcome was less than 10 and the pooled effect was statistically significant [32,33].

The statistical heterogeneity among studies was tested using I^2 statistics [34]. The statistical heterogeneity was considered significant when the I^2 statistic was $\geq$50%. We performed a leave-one-out sensitivity analysis to evaluate each study's influence on the overall effect by removing studies sequentially. Further, we conducted a subgroup analysis according to the study design, study population, mean age, and mean baseline refraction to explore the potential heterogeneity. The pooled effect sizes were deemed significant when the 95% CI of the mean difference (MD) did not cross zero. All statistical tests were two-sided, and p-values <0.05 were considered statistically significant. Outcome data were analyzed using Stata v17 (StataCorp, College Station, TX, USA).

3. Results

3.1. Search Results

Figure S1 presents a flowchart outlining the screening and selection of the included studies. A total of 1085 references were obtained from the three databases, trial registry websites, and a manual examination of bibliographies. Among these, we excluded 261 duplicate studies and 766 studies with obviously irrelevant titles and abstracts. The remaining 58 studies underwent full-text screening, and five randomized controlled trials

(RCTs) from 2019 to 2021 and three retrospective studies from 2015 to 2019 were included in the final meta-analysis.

3.2. Study Characteristics

The basic characteristics of the included studies are outlined in Table 1. A total of 1178 participants (0.01% atropine group, 600; control group, 578) were included. All RCTs [14,19,20,27,28] were conducted in Asian countries (Hong Kong, India, Japan, and China), while the retrospective studies [35–37] enrolled European or multi-ethnic participants and were performed in Italy [36] or the United States [35,37]. Among the included studies, one RCT [28] and one retrospective study [35] had follow-up data for 2 years, while the others provided 1-year follow-up data. In the case of multi-arm studies [14,19], we only extracted data from the 0.01% atropine and control groups. Of note, Fu et al. [19] did not report the results of pupil diameter as photopic or mesopic, and the lighting level in that study was kept in the range of 300 to 310 lux. Thus, we pooled the outcome data as the change in photopic pupil diameter.

3.3. Risk of Bias Assessment

Most domain-level judgments in the enrolled RCTs indicated a low risk of bias. The detailed risk of bias for the enrolled RCTs is reported in Table S3. The assessment revealed a moderate overall risk of bias in three non-RCTs (see details in Table S4).

3.4. Pooled Effects of the Efficacy Outcome

3.4.1. Spherical Equivalent Refractive Error

Eight studies analyzed the change in SER at the 1-year follow-up (Figure 1). A total of 600 children received 0.01% atropine as treatment, and 578 children served as placebo group controls. The children who received 0.01% atropine showed significantly less progression in refraction than controls (weighted mean difference [WMD], 0.28 D per year; 95% confidence interval [CI] = 0.17 to 0.38; $p < 0.01$). Heterogeneity was significant ($I^2 = 71.37\%$). After removing the papers sequentially for sensitivity analysis, the WMD results were stable (Figure S2a). The pre-specified subgroups, according to study design, study population, mean baseline refraction, and mean baseline age demonstrated similar results, showing that 0.01% atropine significantly inhibited SER progression (Table 2). In subgroup of study population, the European (WMD, 0.55 D per year; 95% CI = 0.31, 0.79; $p < 0.01$) and multi-ethnicity groups (WMD, 0.43 D per year; 95% CI = 0.28, 0.58; $p < 0.01$) showed greater effect than the Asian groups (WMD, 0.18 D per year; 95% CI = 0.11, 0.26; $p < 0.01$). After stratifying age at 10 or mean baseline refraction at −3.00 D, patients at age >10 group or mean baseline refraction >−3.00 D group seemingly demonstrated greater effect.

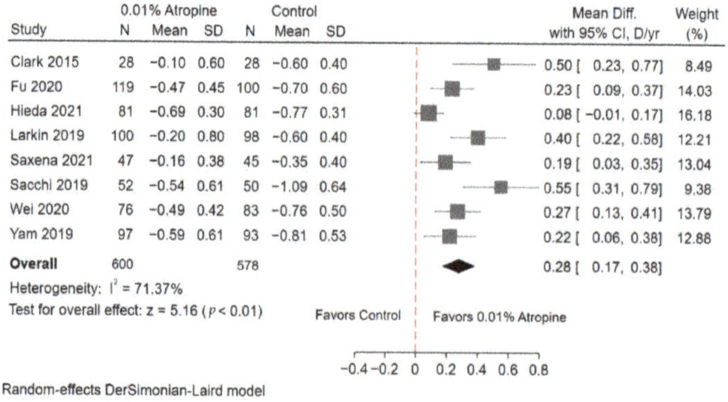

Study	0.01% Atropine			Control			Mean Diff. with 95% CI, D/yr	Weight (%)
	N	Mean	SD	N	Mean	SD		
Clark 2015	28	−0.10	0.60	28	−0.60	0.40	0.50 [0.23, 0.77]	8.49
Fu 2020	119	−0.47	0.45	100	−0.70	0.60	0.23 [0.09, 0.37]	14.03
Hieda 2021	81	−0.69	0.30	81	−0.77	0.31	0.08 [−0.01, 0.17]	16.18
Larkin 2019	100	−0.20	0.80	98	−0.60	0.40	0.40 [0.22, 0.58]	12.21
Saxena 2021	47	−0.16	0.38	45	−0.35	0.40	0.19 [0.03, 0.35]	13.04
Sacchi 2019	52	−0.54	0.61	50	−1.09	0.64	0.55 [0.31, 0.79]	9.38
Wei 2020	76	−0.49	0.42	83	−0.76	0.50	0.27 [0.13, 0.41]	13.79
Yam 2019	97	−0.59	0.61	93	−0.81	0.53	0.22 [0.06, 0.38]	12.88
Overall	600			578			0.28 [0.17, 0.38]	
Heterogeneity: $I^2 = 71.37\%$								
Test for overall effect: z = 5.16 ($p < 0.01$)								

Random-effects DerSimonian-Laird model

Figure 1. Forest plot of standardized equivalent refraction between the 0.01% atropine and control groups. SD, standard deviation; CI, confidence interval; D, diopter; yr, year.

Table 1. Characteristics of studies included in the meta-analysis.

Study (Author, Year)	Country	Study Design	Study Population	Follow-Up, yr	Intervention	Number of Eyes	Mean Age (SD), yr	Mean Baseline Refraction (SD), D	Mean Baseline Axial Length (SD), mm	Drop-Out Rate
Clark 2015	United states	Retrospective Case-control	Multi-ethnicity	1.1 (0.3)	Placebo 0.01% atropine	28 28	10.2 (2.2) 10.2 (2.2)	−2.0 (1.5) −2.0 (1.6)	NA NA	NA NA
Fu 2020	China	RCT	Asian	1	Placebo 0.01% atropine	100 119	9.5 (1.4) 9.3 (1.9)	−2.68 (1.42) −2.70 (1.64)	24.55 (0.71) 24.58 (0.74)	20/120 23/142
Heida 2021	Japan	RCT	Asian	2	Placebo 0.01% atropine	80 * 78 *	8.98 (1.50) 8.99 (1.44)	R/L: −2.96 (1.24)/ −2.97 (1.22) R//L: −2.92 (1.43)/ −2.90 (1.38)	R/L: 24.50 (0.69)/ 24.48 (0.70) R/L 24.41 (0.86)/ 24.40 (0.87)	6/86 * 7/85 *
Larkin 2019	United states	Retrospective Case-control	Multi-ethnicity	2	Placebo 0.01% atropine	98 100	9.2 (2.11) 9.3 (2.10)	−2.8 (1.6) −3.1 (1.9)	NA NA	NA NA
Saxena 2021	India	RCT	Asian	1	Placebo 0.01% atropine	45 47	10.8 (2.2) 10.6 (2.2)	−3.71 (1.37) −3.38 (1.32)	24.70 (0.80) 24.60 (1.02)	5/50 3/50
Sacchi 2019	Italy	Retrospective Cohort	European	1	Placebo 0.01% atropine	50 52	12.1 (2.9) 9.7 (2.3)	−2.63 (2.68) −3.00 (2.23)	NA NA	NA NA
Wei 2020	China	RCT	Asian	1	Placebo 0.01% atropine	83 76	9.84 (1.53) 9.44 (1.80)	−2.64 (1.46) −2.52 (1.33)	24.69 (0.97) 24.50 (0.76)	27/110 34/110
Yam 2019	Hong Kong	RCT	Asian	1	Placebo 0.01% atropine	93 97	8.42 (1.72) 8.23 (1.83)	−3.85 (1.95) −3.77 (1.85)	24.82 (0.97) 24.70 (0.99)	18/111 13/110

Abbreviations: yr, year; SD: standardized deviation; D, diopter; RCT: randomized controlled trial; NA: not applicable; R: right eye; L: left eye. * Two-year follow-up data presented.

Table 2. Subgroup analyses of efficacy outcomes in standardized equivalent refraction.

Subgroups	No. of Studies	Standardized Equivalent Refraction (SER)		
		Pooled MD (95% CI)	p-Value	I^2 (%)
Overall	8	0.28 (0.17 to 0.38)	<0.01 **	71.4
Study design				
RCTs	5	0.18 (0.11 to 0.26)	<0.01 **	38.5
Non-RCTs	3	0.46 (0.34 to 0.59)	<0.01 **	0.0
Study population				
Asian only	5	0.18 (0.11 to 0.26)	<0.01 **	38.5
European only	1	0.55 (0.31 to 0.79)	<0.01 **	-
Multi-ethnicity	2	0.43 (0.28 to 0.58)	<0.01 **	0.0
Mean age, year				
Age < 10	5	0.23 (0.12 to 0.34)	<0.01 **	67.5
Age > 10	3	0.40 (0.15 to 0.65)	<0.01 **	73.9
Mean baseline refraction, Diopter				
>−3.00	6	0.31 (0.17 to 0.46)	<0.01 **	79.4
<−3.00	2	0.20 (0.09 to 0.32)	<0.01 **	0.0

Abbreviations: MD, mean difference; CI, confidence interval; RCT: randomized controlled trial. ** $p < 0.01$.

3.4.2. Axial Length

Five RCTs reported the value of AL elongation at the 1-year follow-up (Figure 2). A total of 420 children received 0.01% atropine as treatment, and 402 children served as placebo group controls. The AL elongation of the 0.01% atropine group was significantly slower than that of the controls (WMD, −0.06 mm; 95% CI = −0.09, −0.03; $p < 0.01$). The overall heterogeneity I^2 was 0%. After omitting the papers individually in sensitivity analysis, the WMDs were similar to the above findings (Figure S2b).

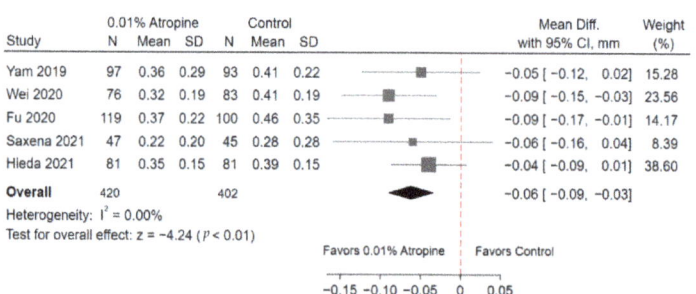

Figure 2. Forest plot of axial length between the 0.01% atropine and control groups. SD, standard deviation; CI, confidence interval.

3.5. Pooled Effects of the Safety Outcome
3.5.1. Accommodative Amplitude

Three RCTs (including 501 patients) were included (Figure 3a). Children with myopia treated with 0.01% atropine did not show significantly lower accommodative amplitudes than the controls (WMD, −0.45 mm; 95% CI = −1.80, 0.90; $p = 0.51$). Significant heterogeneity was noted ($I^2 = 92.60\%$). Of note, after omitting Fu et al. [17], the heterogeneity was significantly reduced ($I^2 = 0\%$), but the result still showed no statistical significance (WMD, 0.17 mm; 95% CI = −0.41, 0.75; $p = 0.56$) (Figure S2c).

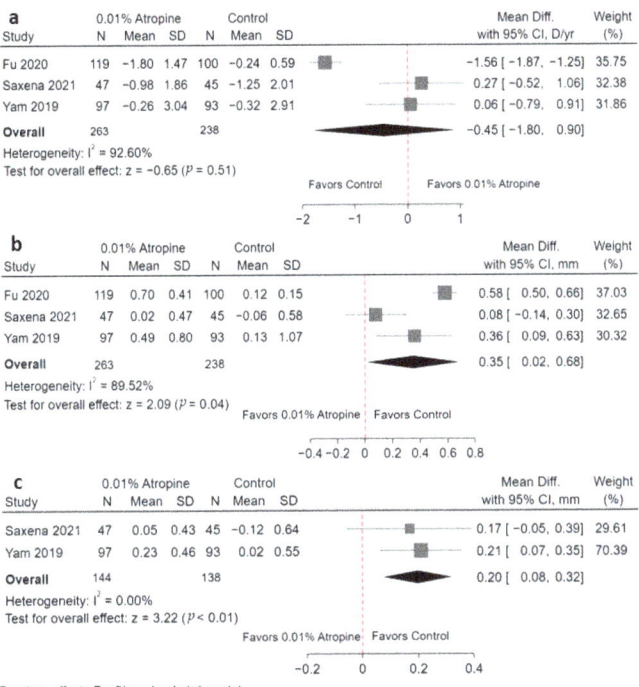

Figure 3. Forest plot of safety profiles between the 0.01% atropine and control groups; (**a**) change in accommodative amplitude, (**b**) change in photopic pupil diameter, (**c**) change in mesopic pupil diameter. Diff, difference; SD, standard deviation; CI, confidence interval; D, diopter; yr, year.

3.5.2. Photopic Pupil Diameter

Three RCTs (including 501 patients) were analyzed (Figure 3b). Children with myopia who received 0.01% atropine showed significantly increased in photopic pupil diameter (WMD, 0.35 mm; 95% CI = 0.02, 0.68; p = 0.04). High heterogeneity was detected (I^2 = 89.52%; p < 0.01). After removing Saxena et al. [18], the heterogeneity decreased significantly (I^2 = 58%), the photopic pupil diameter was still increased (WMD, 0.51 mm; 95% CI = 0.31, 0.71; p < 0.01) (Figure S2d).

3.5.3. Mesopic Pupil Diameter

Only two RCTs provided complete data of mesopic pupil diameter (Figure 3c). A total of 282 children (144 in the 0.01% atropine group and 138 in the control group) were included. Significant increased mesopic pupil diameter was noted in the 0.01% atropine group (WMD, 0.20 mm; 95% CI = 0.08, 0.32; p < 0.01). No significant heterogeneity was detected (I^2 = 0%).

3.6. Modified Hartung–Knapp–Sidik–Jonkman (HKSJ) Sensitivity Analysis

The overall effects on each outcome before and after modified HKSJ adjustment are presented in Table S5. Overall, the adjusted results in efficacy outcomes were similar to those from our previous meta-analyses, which indicates that our pooled effects were robust. However, the pooled results of the safety profiles showed a non-significant increase in photopic and mesopic pupil diameter after the modified HKSJ adjustment.

4. Discussion

Our meta-analysis collected up to date information and demonstrated that 0.01% atropine is effective in retarding childhood myopia progression, as measure by SER and AL over a period of 1 year. Regarding safety outcomes, there was no significant change in accommodative amplitude between 0.01% atropine and controls at the 1-year follow-up. Although both photopic and mesopic pupil diameter showed a significant increase in the 0.01% atropine group compared with controls, the clinical impacts of this phenomenon may be subtle (with an upper confidence interval of photopic and mesopic pupil diameter of 0.68 mm and 0.32 mm, respectively). In our subgroup analysis of SER, myopic children with lower baseline refraction (>−3 D) and older age (>10-year-old) obtained better responses with 0.01% atropine treatment. European and multi-ethnicity groups showed greater effect than Asian groups.

In 2016, a network meta-analysis [38] revealed that 0.01% atropine has a moderate efficacy in suppressing SER and AL progression (SER = 0.53 D/year, CI = 0.21 to 0.85; AL = −0.25 mm/year, CI = −0.25 to −0.05). However, no RCTs directly compared the 0.01% atropine and controls, and the findings were completely derived from indirect evidence. In 2017, Gong et al. [39] evaluated different doses of atropine (0.01% to 1%) to treat childhood myopia in a meta-analysis. Although they found 0.01% atropine was effective in slowing rates of SER progression (WMD, 0.50; CI = 0.24 to 0.76), only one retrospective study regarding 0.01% atropine was enrolled, and no information about AL changes was reported. Recently, one retrospective analysis of 13 myopic Australian children reported 0.01% atropine did not inhibit axial growth in 'fast' progressors compared to the age-matched untreated myope model (0.265 vs. 0.245 mm/year, $p = 0.754$, Power = 0.8) [40]. Our present meta-analysis used the latest evidence, including eight studies (five RCTs and three retrospective studies), and found a significant effect of 0.01% atropine in inhibiting myopic progression (SER = 0.28 D/year, CI = 0.17 to 0.38; AL = −0.06 mm/year, CI = −0.09 to −0.03). Our subgroup analysis identified a larger effect of 0.01% atropine in users with a mean age >10 years compared with users <10 years. This finding was consistent with the Low-Concentration Atropine for Myopia Progression (LAMP) Study [22]. The elongation of AL slowed and stabilized in older children might be part of the reason. Furthermore, patients with lower base line refraction (>−3 D) obtained better responses than those with higher ones (<−3 D). Although the mechanism of this phenomenon was unclear, this information provides a useful guide for clinicians to find the ideal candidate for the use of 0.01% atropine in myopic control.

The issue regarding the optimal dose of atropine has recently been up for debate. Two studies [38,39] recommended 0.01% atropine for myopic control due to its high acceptability. Of note, the long-term efficacy and safety profiles of 0.01% atropine have been proved in well-established ATOM2 trials [17]; a double-blind design and a large cohort of subjects (400 in each study) demonstrated that 0.01% atropine for periods up to 5 years is a clinically viable treatment of myopia with the best-sustained effect on myopia retardation. Compared to placebo, 0.01% atropine also demonstrated significant effect over a 2-year period [28,35]. However, several studies investigating the efficacy of 0.01% atropine for myopia control have produced inconsistent findings in AL change [14,19,20,27,28]. For example, Saxena et al. [20] and Yam et al. [14] found a non-significant efficacy of 0.01% atropine for retarding axial elongation at 1-year follow-up. In contrast, the efficacy of 0.01% in AL inhibition was identified in an RCT involving a large sample size (280 children) [19]. The present meta-analysis pooled axial elongation results from five high-quality RCTs, including 420 participants in the 0.01% atropine group and 402 in the control group, showing a significant efficacy of 0.01% atropine for childhood myopia. In addition, ATOM2 trial [17] demonstrated the significantly lower rebound of axial length for 0.01% atropine (0.19 ± 0.13 mm) compared to 0.5% and 0.1% atropine (0.35 ± 0.20 mm and 0.33 ± 0.18 mm, respectively, $p < 0.001$). This finding may instill confidence in practitioners and patients using 0.01% atropine.

An evaluation of the benefit versus risks will help better characterize the value of atropine in clinical practice to slow myopia. In the present meta-analysis, we evaluated the safety profiles of 0.01% atropine eye drops by quantifying the changes in accommodative amplitude, photopic, and mesopic pupil diameter. Although an increase in photopic and mesopic pupil diameter was noted in the 0.01% atropine group, the overall estimates were within the tolerable range [41,42]. The pooled estimates of change in accommodative amplitude were statistically insignificant and highly heterogeneous. This phenomenon may arise from different baseline accommodative amplitude and age as well as different measuring methods. Of note, we reviewed other common adverse events such as poor near visual acuity and allergic conjunctivitis in our included studies, and no significant influences were noted. Moreover, the drop-out rates in the enrolled studies were generally below 20%, and no treatment-related severe adverse events were noted, which indicates the high applicability of 0.01% atropine in clinical practice.

Phase 2 of the LAMP study [43] reported that the 0.05% atropine has a better effect in myopic control compared with 0.025% and 0.01% atropine. However, 31.2% of 0.05% atropine user developed photophobia at two weeks, which is significantly greater than 0.01% atropine users (5.5%), and its long-term safety profile (>2 years) and rebound phenomenon were unclear. By using a <3 mm increase in photopic pupil size as the cutoff beyond which there will be significant discomfort for some users [41], the reported data from Sankaridurg et al. [42] showed that some eyes would reach this cutoff in 0.025% and 0.05% atropine users; with 0.01% atropine, the change in photopic pupil size was approximately 1 mm and appears in alignment with the efficacy data. In a 3 × 3 phase I clinical trial paradigm, Cooper et al. [41] also concluded that 0.02% atropine might be the highest concentration that does not produce significant clinical symptoms from accommodation paresis or pupillary dilation. In addition, some real-world data [35,36,40] revealed that 0.01% atropine slows the rate of myopia progression in non-Asian patients with favorable safety profiles. Joachimsen et al. [44] even reported that 0.05% atropine induced significantly more anisocoria (2.9 mm compared to 0.8 mm) and loss of accommodation amplitude (loss of 4.2 D compared to 0.05 D) in Caucasian children compared to 0.01% atropine. They supposed that high variation in iris color and the affinity of atropine for melanin might be speculated for the differences [45], and this phenomenon was observed by Myles et al. [40]; those with blue eyes were more susceptible to experiencing dilated pupils as a consequence of atropine treatment. Loughman et al. [46] also proved 0.01% atropine to be a viable therapeutic option among Caucasian eyes. In our subgroup analysis of the study population, the results also demonstrated that 0.01% atropine was a somewhat more effective treatment in non-Asians than in Asians for SER progression. This finding is particularly meaningful since a previous meta-analysis [47] revealed that atropine slows myopia progression more in Asian than non-Asian children. The current evidence for slowing myopia with concentrations of atropine greater than 0.01% is promising, but it is not sufficiently clear that the profile is favorable when it comes to side effects [41]. Taken together, we asserted that 0.01% atropine is useful for myopic control due to its evidence-based long-term effect and applicability in the general population. Further clinical trials are still needed to explore the applicability of this treatment in non-Asian populations.

The major strength of the present study was the inclusion of high-quality RCTs that provided valuable primary data. Further, the overall heterogeneity of the pooling data in AL was low, and the significant results were robust after the leave-one-out and the modified HKSJ adjustment sensitivity analyses. This finding can resolve the inconsistency found in previous studies. Furthermore, we systematically summarized evidence regarding 0.01% atropine regardless of Asian or non-Asian population, providing helpful information for clinicians.

There are several limitations to this study. First, most of our included studies had short-term follow-up periods (1 year in six studies and 2 years in two studies). The long-term efficacy and safety profiles of 0.01% atropine eye drops cannot be obtained from this study. Second, we cannot directly compare the benefit–risk ratio between 0.01% atropine and other low dose atropine (such as 0.05% and 0.025%) in this study. However, currently, there was only one trial that compared those doses of atropine directly [14]. We look forward to collecting more relevant evidence and providing helpful information. Lastly, we did not conduct a meta-regression to assess the association between baseline characteristics and myopia progression after 0.01% atropine treatment since the power may be insufficient to identify the potential effect.

5. Conclusions

In conclusion, our meta-analysis demonstrated that 0.01% atropine had a favorable efficacy and adequate safety for managing childhood myopia over a 1-year period. The children who received 0.01% atropine showed significantly less progression in axial length and refraction than controls. 0.01% atropine also has a better treatment effect in children with lower refractive error and older age and seems more effective in non-Asian patients. Myopic children who have photophobia and blurry near vision after administration of higher-dose atropine may benefit with 0.01% atropine treatment. Further studies are warranted to elucidate the long-term efficacy and safety of 0.01% atropine eye drops and their applicability in different ethnic groups.

Supplementary Materials: The following are available online at https://www.mdpi.com/article/10.3390/jcm10173766/s1, Figure S1: Preferred reporting items for systematic reviews and meta-analyses (PRISMA) flow diagram of the literature search process, Table S1: PRISMA checklist, Figure S2: Leave-one-out sensitivity analysis of efficacy and safety outcome, Table S2: Search strategy modified in PubMed (a), Embase (b), Cochrane CENTRAL (c), Table S3: Summary of ROB 2.0 assessment in RCTs, Table S4: Summary of ROBINS-I assessment in non—RCTs, Table S5: Sensitivity analysis of overall effects of each outcome before and after modified Hartung–Knapp–Sidik–Jonkman (HKSJ) adjustment.

Author Contributions: H.-R.T., T.-L.C. and C.-J.C. had full access to all the data in the study and take responsibility for the integrity of the data and the accuracy of the data analyses. Study concept and design: H.-R.T.; acquisition, analysis, or interpretation of data, H.-R.T., T.-L.C., H.-K.H. and J.-H.W.; drafting of the manuscript, H.-R.T., C.-J.C. and J.-H.W.; critical revision of the manuscript for important intellectual content, H.-K.H., C.-J.C. and J.-H.W. All authors have read and agreed to the published version of the manuscript.

Funding: This research received no external funding.

Institutional Review Board Statement: Not applicable.

Informed Consent Statement: Not applicable.

Data Availability Statement: Data supporting the findings of this study are available within the included articles or published studies.

Acknowledgments: We thank Yu Ru Kou for the comments that considerably improved the manuscript.

Conflicts of Interest: The authors declare no conflict of interest.

References

1. Jung, S.K.; Lee, J.H.; Kakizaki, H.; Jee, D. Prevalence of myopia and its association with body stature and educational level in 19-year-old male conscripts in seoul, South Korea. *Investig. Ophthalmol. Vis. Sci.* **2012**, *53*, 5579–5583. [CrossRef] [PubMed]
2. Matsumura, H.; Hirai, H. Prevalence of myopia and refractive changes in students from 3 to 17 years of age. *Surv. Ophthalmol.* **1999**, *44* (Suppl. 1), S109–S115. [CrossRef]
3. Wu, H.-M.; Seet, B.; Yap, E.P.-H.; Saw, S.-M.; Lim, T.-H.; Chia, A.K.-S. Does education explain ethnic differences in myopia prevalence? A population-based study of young adult males in Singapore. *Optom. Vis. Sci.* **2001**, *78*, 234–239. [CrossRef]
4. Wu, J.F.; Bi, H.S.; Wang, S.M.; Hu, Y.Y.; Wu, H.; Sun, W.; Lu, T.L.; Wang, X.R.; Jonas, J.B. Refractive error, visual acuity and causes of vision loss in children in Shandong, China. The Shandong Children Eye Study. *PLoS ONE* **2013**, *8*, e82763. [CrossRef] [PubMed]
5. Wu, L.J.; You, Q.S.; Duan, J.L.; Luo, Y.X.; Liu, L.J.; Li, X.; Gao, Q.; Zhu, H.P.; He, Y.; Xu, L.; et al. Prevalence and associated factors of myopia in high-school students in Beijing. *PLoS ONE* **2015**, *10*, e0120764. [CrossRef]
6. Dolgin, E. The myopia boom. *Nature* **2015**, *519*, 276–278. [CrossRef]

1. Fricke, T.; Holden, B.A.; Wilson, D.A.; Schlenther, G.; Naidoo, K.; Resnikoff, S.; Frick, K.D. Global cost of correcting vision impairment from uncorrected refractive error. *Bull. World Health Organ.* **2012**, *90*, 728–738. [CrossRef]
2. Holden, B.A.; Fricke, T.R.; Wilson, D.A.; Jong, M.; Naidoo, K.S.; Sankaridurg, P.; Wong, T.Y.; Naduvilath, T.; Resnikoff, S. Global Prevalence of Myopia and High Myopia and Temporal Trends from 2000 through 2050. *Ophthalmology* **2016**, *123*, 1036–1042. [CrossRef]
3. Rada, J.A.S.; Shelton, S.; Norton, T.T. The sclera and myopia. *Exp. Eye Res.* **2006**, *82*, 185–200. [CrossRef]
4. Saw, S.M. How blinding is pathological myopia? *Br. J. Ophthalmol.* **2006**, *90*, 525–526. [CrossRef]
5. Saw, S.-M.; Gazzard, G.; Shih-Yen, E.C.; Chua, W.-H. Myopia and associated pathological complications. *Ophthalmic Physiol. Opt.* **2005**, *25*, 381–391. [CrossRef] [PubMed]
6. Tano, Y. Pathologic myopia: Where are we now? *Am. J. Ophthalmol.* **2002**, *134*, 645–660. [CrossRef]
7. Ang, M.; Flanagan, J.; Wong, C.W.; Müller, A.; Davis, A.; Keys, D.; Resnikoff, S.; Jong, M.; Wong, T.Y.; Sankaridurg, P. Review: Myopia control strategies recommendations from the 2018 WHO/IAPB/BHVI Meeting on Myopia. *Br. J. Ophthalmol.* **2020**, *104*, 1482–1487. [CrossRef] [PubMed]
8. Yam, J.C.; Jiang, Y.; Tang, S.M.; Law, A.K.; Chan, J.J.; Wong, E.; Ko, S.T.; Young, A.L.; Tham, C.C.; Chen, L.J.; et al. Low-Concentration Atropine for Myopia Progression (LAMP) Study: A Randomized, Double-Blinded, Placebo-Controlled Trial of 0.05%, 0.025%, and 0.01% Atropine Eye Drops in Myopia Control. *Ophthalmology* **2019**, *126*, 113–124. [CrossRef]
9. Zhao, C.; Cai, C.; Ding, Q.; Dai, H. Efficacy and safety of atropine to control myopia progression: A systematic review and meta-analysis. *BMC Ophthalmol.* **2020**, *20*, 478. [CrossRef]
10. Chua, W.-H.; Balakrishnan, V.; Chan, Y.-H.; Tong, L.; Ling, Y.; Quah, B.-L.; Tan, D. Atropine for the treatment of childhood myopia. *Ophthalmology* **2006**, *113*, 2285–2291. [CrossRef] [PubMed]
11. Chia, A.; Lu, Q.S.; Tan, D. Five-Year Clinical Trial on Atropine for the Treatment of Myopia 2: Myopia Control with Atropine 0.01% Eyedrops. *Ophthalmology* **2016**, *123*, 391–399. [CrossRef]
12. Chia, A.; Chua, W.-H.; Cheung, Y.-B.; Wong, W.-L.; Lingham, A.; Fong, A.; Tan, D. Atropine for the treatment of childhood myopia: Safety and efficacy of 0.5%, 0.1%, and 0.01% doses (Atropine for the Treatment of Myopia 2). *Ophthalmology* **2012**, *119*, 347–354. [CrossRef] [PubMed]
13. Fu, A.; Stapleton, F.; Wei, L.; Wang, W.; Zhao, B.; Watt, K.; Ji, N.; Lyu, Y. Effect of low-dose atropine on myopia progression, pupil diameter and accommodative amplitude: Low-dose atropine and myopia progression. *Br. J. Ophthalmol.* **2020**, *104*, 1535–1541. [CrossRef] [PubMed]
14. Saxena, R.; Dhiman, R.; Gupta, V.; Kumar, P.; Matalia, J.; Roy, L.; Swaminathan, M.; Phuljhele, S.; Velpandian, T.; Sharma, N. Atropine for treatment of childhood myopia in India (I-ATOM): Multicentric randomized trial. *Ophthalmology* **2021**, *161*, 00079-8.
15. Khanal, S.; Phillips, J.R. Which low-dose atropine for myopia control? *Clin. Exp. Optom.* **2020**, *103*, 230–232. [CrossRef] [PubMed]
16. Li, F.F.; Kam, K.W.; Zhang, Y.; Tang, S.M.; Young, A.L.; Chen, L.J.; Tham, C.C.; Pang, C.P.; Yam, J.C. Differential Effects on Ocular Biometrics by 0.05%, 0.025%, and 0.01% Atropine: Low-Concentration Atropine for Myopia Progression Study. *Ophthalmology* **2020**, *127*, 1603–1611. [CrossRef] [PubMed]
17. Zhao, Y.; Feng, K.; Liu, R.B.; Pan, J.H.; Zhang, L.L.; Xu, Z.P.; Lu, X.J. Atropine 0.01% eye drops slow myopia progression: A systematic review and Meta-analysis. *Int. J. Ophthalmol.* **2019**, *12*, 1337–1343. [CrossRef]
18. Tideman, J.W.L.; Snabel, M.C.C.; Tedja, M.S.; Van Rijn, G.A.; Wong, K.T.; Kuijpers, R.W.A.M.; Vingerling, J.R.; Hofman, A.; Buitendijk, G.H.S.; Keunen, J.E.E.; et al. Association of Axial Length with Risk of Uncorrectable Visual Impairment for Europeans With Myopia. *JAMA Ophthalmol.* **2016**, *134*, 1355–1363. [CrossRef] [PubMed]
19. Moriyama, M.; Ohno-Matsui, K.; Hayashi, K.; Shimada, N.; Yoshida, T.; Tokoro, T.; Morita, I. Topographic analyses of shape of eyes with pathologic myopia by high-resolution three-dimensional magnetic resonance imaging. *Ophthalmology* **2011**, *118*, 1626–1637. [CrossRef] [PubMed]
20. Yi, S.; Huang, Y.; Yu, S.Z.; Chen, X.J.; Yi, H.; Zeng, X.L. Therapeutic effect of atropine 1% in children with low myopia. *J. Am. Assoc. Pediatri. Ophthalmol. Strabismus* **2015**, *19*, 426–429. [CrossRef]
21. Wei, S.; Li, S.M.; An, W.; Du, J.; Liang, X.; Sun, Y.; Zhang, D.; Tian, J.; Wang, N. Safety and Efficacy of Low-Dose Atropine Eyedrops for the Treatment of Myopia Progression in Chinese Children: A Randomized Clinical Trial. *JAMA Ophthalmol.* **2020**, *138*, 1178–1184. [CrossRef] [PubMed]
22. Hieda, O.; Hiraoka, T.; Fujikado, T.; Ishiko, S.; Hasebe, S.; Torii, H.; Takahashi, H.; Nakamura, Y.; Sotozono, C.; Oshika, T.; et al. Efficacy and safety of 0.01% atropine for prevention of childhood myopia in a 2-year randomized placebo-controlled study. *Jpn. J. Ophthalmol.* **2021**, *63*, 315–325. [CrossRef]
23. Sterne, J.A.; Hernán, M.A.; Reeves, B.C.; Savović, J.; Berkman, N.D.; Viswanathan, M.; Henry, D.; Altman, D.G.; Ansari, M.T.; Boutron, I.; et al. ROBINS-I: A tool for assessing risk of bias in non-randomised studies of interventions. *BMJ* **2016**, *355*, i4919. [CrossRef] [PubMed]
24. Sterne, J.A.C.; Savović, J.; Page, M.J.; Elbers, R.G.; Blencowe, N.S.; Boutron, I.; Cates, C.J.; Cheng, H.-Y.; Corbett, M.S.; Eldridge, S.M.; et al. RoB 2: A revised tool for assessing risk of bias in randomised trials. *BMJ* **2019**, *366*, l4898. [CrossRef] [PubMed]
25. Higgins, J.P.T.; Thomas, T.J.; Chandler, J.; Cumpston, M.; Li, T.; Page, M.J.; Welch, V.A. (Eds.) *Cochrane Handbook for Systematic Reviews of Interventions*, 2nd ed.; John Wiley & Sons: Chichester, UK, 2020.

32. Guolo, A.; Varin, C. Random-effects meta-analysis: The number of studies matters. *Stat. Methods Med. Res.* **2017**, *26*, 1500–1518 [CrossRef] [PubMed]
33. Veroniki, A.A.; Jackson, D.; Bender, R.; Kuss, O.; Langan, D.; Higgins, J.P.T.; Knapp, G.; Salanti, G. Methods to calculate uncertainty in the estimated overall effect size from a random-effects meta-analysis. *Res. Synth. Methods* **2019**, *10*, 23–43. [CrossRef] [PubMed]
34. Higgins, J.P.T.; Thompson, S.G.; Deeks, J.J.; Altman, D.G. Measuring inconsistency in meta-analyses. *BMJ* **2003**, *327*, 557–560 [CrossRef]
35. Larkin, G.L.; Tahir, A.; Epley, K.D.; Beauchamp, C.L.; Tong, J.T.; Clark, R.A. Atropine 0.01% Eye Drops for Myopia Control in American Children: A Multi-ethnic Sample Across Three US Sites. *Ophthalmol. Ther.* **2019**, *8*, 589–598. [CrossRef]
36. Sacchi, M.; Serafino, M.; Villani, E.; Tagliabue, E.; Luccarelli, S.; Bonsignore, F.; Nucci, P. Efficacy of atropine 0.01% for the treatment of childhood myopia in European patients. *Acta Ophthalmol.* **2019**, *97*, e1136–e1140. [CrossRef] [PubMed]
37. Clark, T.Y.; Clark, R.A. Atropine 0.01% Eyedrops Significantly Reduce the Progression of Childhood Myopia. *J. Ocul. Pharmacol. Ther.* **2015**, *31*, 541–545. [CrossRef] [PubMed]
38. Huang, J.; Wen, D.; Wang, Q.; McAlinden, C.; Flitcroft, I.; Chen, H.; Saw, S.M.; Chen, H.; Bao, F.; Zhao, Y.; et al. Efficacy Comparison of 16 Interventions for Myopia Control in Children: A Network Meta-Analysis. *Ophthalmology* **2016**, *123*, 697–708. [CrossRef]
39. Gong, Q.; Janowski, M.; Luo, M.; Wei, H.; Chen, B.; Yang, G.; Liu, L. Efficacy and Adverse Effects of Atropine in Childhood Myopia: A Meta-analysis. *JAMA Ophthalmol.* **2017**, *135*, 624–630. [CrossRef] [PubMed]
40. Myles, W.; Dunlop, C.; McFadden, S.A. The Effect of Long-Term Low-Dose Atropine on Refractive Progression in Myopic Australian School Children. *J. Clin. Med.* **2021**, *10*, 1444. [CrossRef] [PubMed]
41. Cooper, J.; Eisenberg, N.; Schulman, E.; Wang, F.M. Maximum atropine dose without clinical signs or symptoms. *Optom. Vis. Sci.* **2013**, *90*, 1467–1472. [CrossRef]
42. Sankaridurg, P.; Tran, H.D. The Lowdown on Low-Concentration Atropine for Myopia Progression. *Ophthalmology* **2019**, *126*, 125–126. [CrossRef]
43. Yam, J.C.; Li, F.F.; Zhang, X.; Tang, S.M.; Yip, B.H.; Kam, K.W.; Ko, S.T.; Young, A.L.; Tham, C.C.; Chen, L.J.; et al. Two-Year Clinical Trial of the Low-Concentration Atropine for Myopia Progression (LAMP) Study: Phase 2 Report. *Ophthalmology* **2020**, *127*, 910–919. [CrossRef] [PubMed]
44. Joachimsen, L.; Farassat, N.; Bleul, T.; Böhringer, D.; Lagrèze, W.A.; Reich, M. Side effects of topical atropine 0.05% compared to 0.01% for myopia control in German school children: A pilot study. *Int. Ophthalmol.* **2021**, *41*, 2001–2008. [CrossRef] [PubMed]
45. Polling, J.R.; Kok, R.G.; Tideman, J.W.; Meskat, B.; Klaver, C.C. Effectiveness study of atropine for progressive myopia in Europeans. *Eye* **2016**, *30*, 998–1004. [CrossRef] [PubMed]
46. Loughman, J.; Flitcroft, D.I. The acceptability and visual impact of 0.01% atropine in a Caucasian population. *Br. J. Ophthalmol.* **2016**, *100*, 1525–1529. [CrossRef]
47. Li, S.M.; Wu, S.S.; Kang, M.T.; Liu, Y.; Jia, S.M.; Li, S.Y.; Zhan, S.Y.; Liu, L.R.; Li, H.; Chen, W.; et al. Atropine slows myopia progression more in Asian than white children by meta-analysis. *Optom. Vis. Sci.* **2014**, *91*, 342–350. [CrossRef]

MDPI
St. Alban-Anlage 66
4052 Basel
Switzerland
Tel. +41 61 683 77 34
Fax +41 61 302 89 18
www.mdpi.com

Journal of Clinical Medicine Editorial Office
E-mail: jcm@mdpi.com
www.mdpi.com/journal/jcm

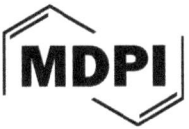

www.ingramcontent.com/pod-product-compliance
Lightning Source LLC
LaVergne TN
LVHW070715100526
838202LV00013B/1099